BUR N

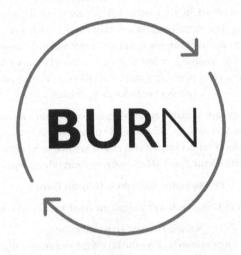

BURN

NEW RESEARCH BLOWS THE LID OFF
HOW WE REALLY BURN CALORIES,
STAY HEALTHY, AND LOSE WEIGHT

HERMAN PONTZER, PhD

Avery
an imprint of Penguin Random House
New York

AVERY

an imprint of Penguin Random House LLC
penguinrandomhouse.com

First trade paperback edition 2022
Copyright © 2021 by Herman Pontzer

Most Avery books are available at special quantity discounts for bulk purchase
for sales promotions, premiums, fund-raising, and educational needs.
Special books or book excerpts also can be created to fit specific needs.
For details, write SpecialMarkets@penguinrandomhouse.com.

Photographs copyright © Herman Pontzer

The Library of Congress has cataloged the hardcover edition as follows:

Names: Pontzer, Herman, author.
Title: Burn : new research blows the lid off how we really burn calories,
lose weight, and stay healthy / by Herman Pontzer, PhD.
Description: New York : Avery, an imprint of
Penguin Random House, [2021] | Includes index.
Identifiers: LCCN 2020020103 (print) | LCCN 2020020104 (ebook) |
ISBN 9780525541523 (hardcover) | ISBN 9780525541530 (ebook)
Subjects: LCSH: Metabolism. | Weight loss. | Human evolution.
Classification: LCC QP171 .P66 2021 (print) |
LCC QP171 (ebook) | DDC 612.3/9—dc23
LC record available at https://lccn.loc.gov/2020020103
LC ebook record available at https://lccn.loc.gov/2020020104

ISBN (paperback) 9780593421048

Printed in the United States of America

Book design by Lorie Pagnozzi

For Janice, Alex, and Clara

CONTENTS

BURN

CHAPTER 1

The Invisible Hand

The lions woke me up around two in the morning. The sound wasn't loud so much as *big*—like the moaning hydraulics of a garbage truck interrupted by the coughs and grunts of an idling Harley-Davidson. My first hazy, sleepy reaction was a kind of grateful joy. Ah, the sounds of wild Africa! I stared up through the gossamer mesh roof of my tent at the stars overhead, felt the night breeze pushing through the dry grass and thorny acacia trees and up against the tent's thin nylon walls, carrying the lions' chorus. I felt fortunate to be there, camped in my little tent in the middle of the vast East African savanna, a place so remote and untrammeled that there were *lions* just a few hundred yards off. How lucky was I?

Then a pang of adrenaline and fear. This wasn't a zoo or some tourist safari. Those lions weren't pretty pictures in a *National Geographic* magazine or a PBS nature show. This was real life. A gang of heavily muscled 300-pound feline killing machines was a short stroll away, and they sounded . . . anxious. Maybe even . . . *hungry*? Of course they could smell me. After days of camping I could smell myself. What was my plan when they came for my soft American carcass, the warm triple crème brie of human flesh? I wondered how close they'd get before I heard them in the tall grass, or if the end would come unannounced, an explosion of claws and hot angry teeth crashing through walls of the tent.

I kept thinking it through, trying to be rational. Judging by where the sound was coming from, the lions would have to walk past Dave's and Brian's tents first. I was Door Number 3 in this particular game of chance. That meant 1 in 3 odds of being eaten by lions tonight, or, if one was a glass-two-thirds-full kind of person, a 67 percent chance of *not* being eaten. That was a comforting thought. Plus, we were with the Hadza, on the outskirts of their camp, and nobody messes with the Hadza. Sure, hyenas and leopards would occasionally slink past their grass huts at night looking for scraps or unattended babies, but the lions seemed to keep their distance.

The fear began to dissipate. Drowsiness seeped back in. I'd probably be fine. Besides, if one had to be eaten by lions, it seemed preferable to be asleep at the time, at least until the last possible moment. I fluffed up the pile of dirty clothes I was using for a pillow, adjusted my sleeping pad, and went back to sleep.

It was my first summer working with the Hadza, a generous, resourceful, and badass people who live in small camps scattered about the rugged, semiarid savanna around Lake Eyasi in northern Tanzania. Anthropologists and human biologists like me like to work with the Hadza because of how they make their living. The Hadza are hunter-gatherers: they have no agriculture, no domesticated animals, no machines or guns or electricity. Each day they wrest their food from the wild landscape around them, using nothing but their own hard work and guile. Women gather berries or dig wild tubers from the rocky soil with stout pointed sticks, often with a child on their back in a sling. Men hunt zebra, giraffe, antelope, and other animals, with powerful bows and arrows they fashion themselves from branches and sinew, or chop open trees with small axes to extract wild honey from beehives built in the hollows of limbs and trunks. Kids run and play around the grass huts of camp or head out in groups to get firewood and water. Elders either head out foraging with the other adults (they are remarkably spry even into their seventies) or stay back at camp to keep an eye on things.

This way of life was the norm worldwide for over two million years, from the evolutionary dawn of our genus, *Homo*, through the invention of farming just twelve thousand years ago. As farming spread and brought towns, urbanization, and eventually industrialization in its wake, most cultures traded in their bows and digging sticks for crops and brick houses. Some, like the Hadza, held on proudly to their traditions even as the world around them changed and began to encroach. Today, these few populations are the last living windows into humanity's shared hunter-gatherer past.

Along with my good friends and fellow researchers Dave Raichlen and Brian Wood and our research assistant, Fides, I was in Hadzaland (as we casually refer to their homeland) in northern Tanzania to learn how the Hadza lifestyle is reflected in their metabolism—the way their bodies burn energy. It's a simple but incredibly important question. Everything our bodies do—growing, moving, healing, reproducing—requires energy, and so understanding how our energy is spent is the first foundational step in understanding how our bodies work. We wanted to know how the human body functions in a hunting and gathering society like the Hadza, where people were still an integral part of a functioning ecosystem, with a lifestyle still similar in important ways to that of our deep past. No one had ever measured daily energy expenditure, the total number of calories burned per day, in a hunter-gatherer population. We were eager to be the first.

In the modernized world, far removed from the daily work of acquiring our food with our bare hands, we pay little attention to energy expenditure. If we think about it at all, we think of the latest diet, our workout plan, whether we've earned that donut we crave. Calories are a hobby, a nugget of data on our smartwatches. The Hadza know better. They understand intuitively that food and the energy it holds are the fundamental stuff of life. Each day they confront an ancient and unforgiving arithmetic: acquire more energy than you burn or go hungry.

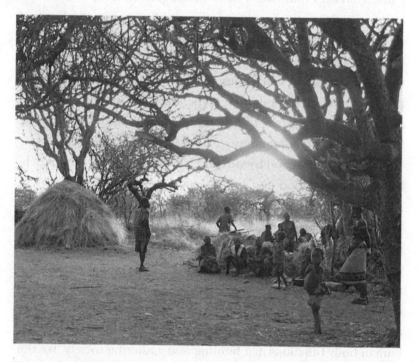

Figure 1.1. Early evening in a Hadza camp. Acacia trees provide a shady oasis on the savanna. Men, women, and children relax and discuss the day's events. Note the grass house at left.

We woke up with the sun still orange and weak on the eastern horizon, the colors of the trees and grass washed out in the diluted morning light. Brian started a cooking fire in our small, Hadza-style three-stone hearth and set a pot of water on to boil. Dave and

I milled around bleary-eyed, needing caffeine. Soon enough we were all drinking hot mugs of Africafe instant coffee and spooning up plastic bowlfuls of instant oatmeal and jelly. We discussed research plans for the day. We had all heard the lions during the night and joked nervously about how close they sounded.

Then, sauntering through the tall dry grass, came four Hadza men. They weren't coming from camp, but from the opposite direction, from the bush. They were each carrying large, misshapen loads over their shoulders, and it took me a moment to recognize what it was: legs, haunches, and other blood-matted parts of a big, freshly killed antelope. The men knew we liked to keep track of the foods they brought back to camp, and they wanted to give us a chance to record this kill before splitting it up among the families in camp.

Brian snaps to it, clears off the weigh scale, and locates the *Foraging Returns* notebook, striking up a conversation in Swahili, our common language with the Hadza.

"Thanks for bringing these by," says Brian, "but where the hell did you get a huge antelope at six in the morning?"

"It's a kudu," say the Hadza guys, grinning, "and we took it."

"Took it?" asks Brian.

"You guys heard the lions last night, right?" say the Hadza guys. "Well, we figured they were up to something, so we went and checked it out. Turns out they had just killed this kudu . . . so we took it."

And that was it. Another day in Hadzaland—a banner day in fact, starting off with the rare prize of big game in all of its fatty and proteinaceous glory. In camp later that morning, gnawing on roasted strips of kudu, hearing the story of how Dad and his buddies chased off a pride of hungry lions in the dark to bring home food, the Hadza kids would understand an important and timeless lesson. Energy is everything, and it's worth risking everything to get it.

Even if you have to steal breakfast from the lions' jaws.

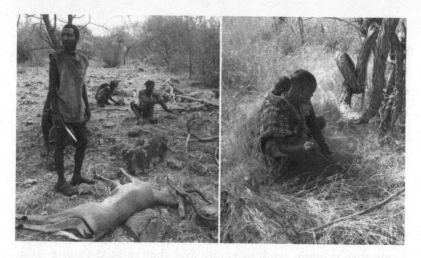

Figure 1.2. The Hadza workday. Men hunt game with bow and arrow or collect honey from wild beehives. At left, a man prepares to butcher an impala he shot with his bow an hour before. His friends, who helped track the animal, look on. Women gather wild berries and other plant foods. The woman at right is digging wild tubers from the rocky ground with a wooden digging stick while her child naps in a wrap on her back.

A Small Matter of Life and Death

Energy is the currency of life; without it, you're dead. Your body is made up of roughly 37 trillion cells, each humming along like microscopic factories, every second of every day. Together, they burn enough energy every twenty-four hours to bring eight gallons (about thirty liters) of ice water to a raging boil. Our cells outshine the stars: each ounce of living human tissue burns ten thousand times more energy each day than an ounce of the Sun. A small portion of this activity is under our conscious control—namely the muscle activity we use to move. Some of it we're dimly aware of, like our heartbeat and breathing. But most of this teeming activity goes on completely beneath the surface, in a vast and unseen ocean of cellular processes that keep us alive. We notice only when things go wrong, which, increasingly, they do. Obesity, type 2 diabetes, heart disease, cancer, and nearly all of the other diseases that plague us in the modernized world are, at their core, rooted in the ways our bodies take in and expend energy.

And yet, despite its importance for life and health, metabolism (the way our bodies burn energy) is badly and almost universally misunderstood. How much energy does an average adult burn each day? Every nutrition label in the supermarket will tell you that the standard American diet is 2,000 calories a day—and every label is wrong. Nine-year-olds burn 2,000 calories; for adults, it's closer to 3,000, depending on how much you weigh and how much fat you carry (and for the record, the correct term when we're talking about our daily energy needs is *kilocalories*, not calories). How many miles do you have to run to burn the energy stored in a single donut? At least three, but again, it depends on how much you weigh. For that matter, where does the fat go when we "burn it off" with exercise? Think it turns into heat? sweat? muscle? Wrong, wrong, wrong. You *breathe* most of it out as carbon dioxide, and turn a small fraction of it into water (but not necessarily sweat). If you didn't know that already, you're in good company; most doctors don't, either.

No doubt much of our ignorance on the subject of energetics stems from gaps in our education system and the Teflon-like quality with which the human brain repels unused details. When three out of four Americans can't name the three branches of U.S. federal government—an important bit of information drilled into us annually over twelve years of schooling—there may be little hope of people recalling the finer points of the Krebs cycle from high school biology. But our poor understanding is aided and abetted by a host of charlatans and Internet hucksters promoting wrong-headed ideas, usually for personal gain. With a reliably uninformed audience eager to stay healthy, you can sell almost anything no matter how preposterous. *Boost your metabolism!* they promise. *Burn fat with these simple tricks! Avoid these foods to stay thin!* scream the glossy magazines, usually without a shred of real evidence or scientific backing.

But the bigger, structural reason energetics is misunderstood is that we have gotten the science of energy expenditure fundamentally wrong. Since the beginning of modern metabolic research around the turn of the twentieth century, we've been taught to think of our bodies as simple engines: we take in "fuel" in the form of food, and burn it off by revving our engine with exercise. Any extra unburned fuel builds up as fat. People who run their engines hotter, burning more fuel each day, are less likely to get fat from accumulating unburned fuel. If you've already accumulated some unwanted fat, just exercise more to burn it off.

It's an appealing and simple model, a sort of armchair engineer's view of metabolism. And it gets a couple things right: our bodies need food for fuel, and unburned fuel gets stored as fat. But it gets the rest badly wrong. Our bodies don't work like simple fuel-burning machines because they aren't products of engineering, they're products of evolution.

As science is only beginning to fully appreciate, five hundred million years of evolution have made our metabolic engines incredibly dynamic and adaptable. Our bodies have gotten very crafty, able to respond to changes in exercise and diet in ways that make evolutionary sense even if they frustrate our attempts to stay trim and healthy. Consequently, more exercise doesn't necessarily mean more energy burned per day, and burning more energy doesn't protect against getting fat. And yet public health strategies stubbornly cling to the simplistic armchair engineer's view of metabolism, hurting efforts to combat obesity, diabetes, heart disease, cancer, and the other diseases that are most likely to kill us. Without a better understanding of how our bodies burn energy, we grow understandably frustrated when we see our weight-loss plans failing, the bathroom scale refusing to budge despite our earnest efforts at the gym, the latest overhyped metabolic magic letting us down.

This book explores the new, emerging science of human metabolism. As a human biologist interested in our species' evolutionary past as well as our prospects for the future, I've been working on the front lines of metabolic research in humans and other primates for over a decade. Exciting and surprising revelations over the past few years are changing the way we understand the links between energy expenditure, exercise, diet, and disease. In the following pages, we'll examine these new discoveries and their implications for living long and healthy lives.

Much of this new science has come from work with the Hadza and populations like them: small-scale nonindustrial societies still integrated into their local ecology. These cultures have a lot to teach us in the developed world, but it's not the caricatured version of hunter-gatherer life popularized in much of today's Paleo movement. Here, too, my colleagues and I have learned a great deal in the past few years about how diet and daily physical activity keep these populations free of the "diseases of civilization" that bedevil us in modernized, urbanized, industrialized countries. We will visit these groups to see what daily life (and field research) is like in these communities, and what lessons we can bring home. We'll also travel to zoos, rain forests, and archaeological excavations around the world to see how studies of living apes and fossil humans are contributing to our understanding of metabolic health.

But first, we need to get a sense of the immense reach and scale of metabolism in our lives. To truly appreciate the importance of energy expenditure, we have to look beyond the quotidian concerns of health and disease. Like the Earth's tectonic plates, metabolism is the unseen foundation underlying everything, slowly shifting and shaping our lives. The familiar geography of human existence, from our first nine months in the womb to the eighty or so years we might have on this planet, is formed by the metabolic engines burning away inside us. Our big, clever brains and chubby babies are built and powered by metabolic machinery far different from that of our ape kin. As we've come to understand only recently, our evolved metabolism made us the bizarre and wonderful species we are today.

Dog Years

"Una miaka ngapi?"

I was talking with a Hadza man, somewhere in his twenties I reckoned, asking him questions as part of the annual research effort to collect basic health information in the camps we visit. I was doing my best in passable if unbeautiful Swahili: *How old are you?*

He looked confused. Maybe I hadn't gotten it right? I tried again.

"Una miaka ngapi?"

He broke into a smile. *"Unasema." You tell me.*

My Swahili was fine. It was my question that was dumb.

For me, a typical overscheduled American, one of the most jarring culture shocks in living with the Hadza is their disinterest in time. It's not that they have no concept of time. They live with the daily rhythms of light and dark, hot and cool; the lunar cycle; the seasonal cycles of rainy and dry. They're fully aware of growth and aging and the cultural and physiological milestones that delineate our lives. After decades of visits from researchers and other outsiders, they even have a feel for Western measures of time, of minutes and hours, weeks and years. They get it, they just don't seem to care. They have no interest in keeping track. There are no clocks in Hadzaland, no calendars or schedules, no birthdays, holidays, or Mondays. Satchel Paige's "How old would you be if you didn't know how old you are?" isn't deep introspective reflection for the Hadza. It's daily life. For researchers, figuring out everyone's age in a Hadza camp is like getting your teeth cleaned: a necessary, annoying, and somewhat painful chore on the annual schedule.

The Hadza indifference toward time would be scandalous in the United States, where every parent knows the expected developmental trajectory of their offspring to the day, and our rights and responsibilities are governed precisely by our age. Walking at one, talking at two, kindergarten at five, puberty at thirteen, legal adulthood at eighteen, and you can celebrate the early landmarks of your life with a legal drink at twenty-one. Then it's marriage, kids, menopause, retirement, senility, and death—all on schedule, otherwise there's cause for personal alarm and public opinion. But whether we fret anxiously about each developmental milestone like a Manhattan millennial or let the years pass with the Zen-like indifference of a Hadza grandmother, the pace of human life is one of the great universals, a comforting rhythm that we all share in common.

And yet the human pace of life is *anything* but common. We are off-the-charts freaks among the animal kingdom when it comes to our life history, the rate at which we grow up, procreate, grow old, and die. We live life in slow motion. If humans lived like a typical mammal our size, we'd hit puberty before age two and be dead by twenty-five. Women would give birth every year, to five-pound babies. The average six-year-old would already be a grandparent. Daily life would be unrecognizable.

We have an intuitive cultural sense of how strange we are, but in our typically anthropocentric way we get it flipped around. Our pets, abiding by the normal mammalian schedule, live their lives at what feels to us like an accelerated rate. We talk about dogs living in "dog years," with each year of their life equivalent to seven of ours, as though it's the other animals that are different. But it's humans who are weird. Try calculating it the other way, putting your age in dog years, and you'll see how remarkable you are. I'm nearly three hundred (dog) years old and I'm feeling pretty good, considering.

Biologists studying life history have long known that the pace of life isn't some arbitrary and fixed schedule handed down from the heavens. Growth rates, birth rates, and the speed with which species age can and do change over evolutionary timescales. We've also known for decades that humans and other primates (our evolutionary family that includes lemurs, monkeys, and apes) have exceptionally slow life histories compared to other mammals. We've even had a fairly good idea *why* primates evolved slow life histories. Conditions in which species are less likely to be killed early by a predator or other malefactor favor a slower pace of life.

So we knew that primates, including us, had slow life histories, likely as a result of lowered mortality rates somewhere deep in our evolutionary past (perhaps moving to the trees made early primates harder for predators to catch). What no one could figure out was *how?* How did humans and other primates manage to slow everything down, decelerating our growth rates and extending our lives? Perhaps it had something to do with metabolism, since growth and reproduction require energy, as we'll discuss in Chapter 3. But what was the link? It wasn't clear. Finding the answer would take us to zoos and primate sanctuaries around the globe, uncovering the evolutionary changes in metabolism that made "normal" life so extraordinary.

Planet of the Apes

Monkeys and apes are smart, cute, and incredibly dangerous. Estimates vary, but it's safe to say nonhuman primates are about two times stronger, pound for pound, than humans. Most species have long, spear-like canines that they use to great effect in threatening and occasionally mauling one another. Kept in captivity, they are all too happy to use their talents to destroy humans, particularly when they're in a bad mood. And who among us wouldn't be bored, annoyed, maybe even just a bit resentful, living out our lives in a medical lab, a shitty zoo, or some dumbass's garage? We see ape actors on TV (less often now, thankfully) and are fooled into thinking they're adorable. But those are the children, the ones small and naïve enough that their humans can handle them, by force if needed. By ten years old, apes are unpredictably vicious, especially in captivity, relaxing peacefully one minute and tearing your face and testicles off the next. The tendency for cute child actors to turn into impulsive, destructive miscreants is just one more thing humans and apes have in common.

Knowing all this, I was in total disbelief at what I was watching. It was late summer of 2008, and I was at the Great Ape Trust in Iowa, in their spacious and modern orangutan facility, staring through a small window in the door to the ape access area. There, Rob Shumaker was calmly pouring isotope-laced sugar-free iced tea into the wide-open mouth of Azy, a 250-pound adult male orangutan with a face like a catcher's mitt and the strength to tear Rob's arms cleanly from his torso. Rob is not an idiot—there was a heavy-gauge steel fence between the two of them. But still, Azy seemed to be enjoying the treat, with something like friendliness in his eyes. I had been assured by many ape researchers time and time again that what I was watching was impossible: no captive apes would want to play along for a research study, even one as innocuous as this, and no head of an ape facility would be cocky or foolish enough to bother trying. Yet there was Rob, administering a thousand-dollar dose of doubly labeled water (isotope-enriched water used to track daily energy expenditure; see chapter 3) as easily as you'd water a houseplant.

My shock was amplified by the excitement of doing something truly new. This would be the first-ever measurement of daily energy expenditure (the total number of kilocalories burned per day) in an ape. It's rare to have the chance to do something really novel in science, to be the first to measure something important. This felt momentous. For the first time, we were going to get a comprehensive look at the metabolic engine of an ape. Were they like us? Like other mammals? Or was there something new and exciting to uncover below the orange, hairy surface?

I tried to temper my expectations with the understanding that we might not find anything interesting. For over a century, researchers had been studying animals' basal metabolic rates, or BMR, the calories burned per minute when the subject is completely at rest (see Chapter 3). In the 1980s and 1990s, several studies tested the idea that primates' slow life history was linked to a low metabolic rate, and therefore low BMR. There were vocal proponents of this hypothesis, like Brian McNab, who argued that nearly all aspects of life history and dietary variation across mammals were interrelated and directly tied to BMR. It was an appealing idea, since growth and reproduction require energy, and a faster pace of life presumably requires a faster metabolic engine. But more statistically rigorous analyses killed McNab's beautiful idea, showing that primates had normal, unremarkable, mammalian BMRs—nothing that could explain their weird life history. Other studies built upon these results, and a consensus developed that humans, apes, other primates, and even other mammals were all basically the same on the inside, at least when it came to metabolism. Species were just shaped differently, like different car bodies set on the same engines.

I had learned the consensus view in college at Penn State in the 1990s and grad school at Harvard in the 2000s, dutifully applying the received wisdom in some of my dissertation work. But like most

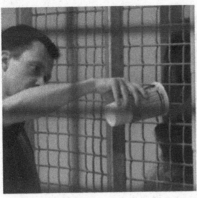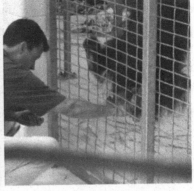

Figure 1.3. The first daily energy expenditure measurement in an ape. Through the heavy fencing, Rob Shumaker pours the doubly labeled water dose, mixed with sugar-free iced tea, into Azy's mouth (Azy's fuzzy profile is just visible on the right). Later, he collects a urine sample as the orangutan clings to the fencing with grasping feet.

scientists, I'm instinctively skeptical, and I began having heretical thoughts. The consensus view, that energy expenditure was basically the same across mammals, was based on measures of BMR, and that seemed to me to be a glaring issue. BMR is measured with the subject at rest (nearly asleep), so it doesn't represent *all* the calories the organism burns each day, just a fraction. Also, BMR can be tricky to measure. If the subject is agitated or cold or sick or young and growing, the measurement can be elevated—and unsurprisingly, much of the primate data came from very young, tractable monkeys and apes.

A handful of researchers were doing exciting work measuring *total* daily energy expenditures (the total number of calories burned per day, not just BMR) in a range of species, using a sophisticated isotope-based technique called the doubly labeled water method (see Chapter 3). Their research suggested that energy expenditure varied a lot among mammals, and seemed to reflect their evolution and ecology. I began to wonder. What if humans and other apes *don't* have the same metabolic machinery? What if daily energy expenditures *are* different? What might that tell us about the evolutionary histories of humans, apes, and all the other primates? Unfortunately, working with apes and other primates is such an immense challenge that it seemed unlikely we'd ever get the measurements needed to explore these critical questions.

My first trip to the Great Ape Trust was a revelation. They had two huge, state-of-the-art facilities, one for Rob's orangutans, one for bonobos, both with expansive indoor and outdoor areas, full-time staff, and integrated research facilities. The apes' well-being and quality of life were the first priority. Research projects were designed to be engaging and fun for the apes, or at least part of the daily routine, not an imposition. Invasive, painful, or otherwise harmful projects were out of the question.

At some point during the visit I began babbling on about doubly labeled water methods, metabolism and evolution in humans and other primates, and how it would be *so cool* to measure daily energy expenditures in apes, that no one had ever done it. I explained to Rob how the methods were totally safe and were used all the time in human nutrition studies. *We might even learn something practical about managing the diets and calorie intake of apes in captivity!* The apes would just need to drink some water, and then we'd need to collect urine samples every couple of days for a week or so. *Any chance we'd be able to do that here, with the orangutans?*

"Sure," says Rob, "we collect urine samples pretty regularly from most of the orangutans for health checks."

"Wow. Really? How?" I ask. This sounded too good to be true.

"We just ask them," says Rob. We had been chatting next to the fence of one of the outdoor areas. Rob looks over at Rocky, a four-year-old male orangutan who was half playing, half resting, half watching us. "Rocky, come here," says Rob, not like he's calling a dog, but like he's talking to his nephew. Rocky walks over to the fence near us. "Let me see your mouth," says Rob, and Rocky opens wide. "How about your ear?" and Rocky puts his ear to the fence. "The other one," and Rocky turns his head and puts his other ear toward us. "Thanks!" says Rob, and Rocky scampers off to play.

"We can ask them to pee in a cup, too," says Rob, as I stand there agog at the ape-human conversation I just watched. "Just one thing, though . . ."

"Yeah?" *Oh boy, here it is, I thought. Reality check. Here's where this whole thing falls apart . . .*

"Is it OK if some of the urine sample is spilled?"

"No problem at all," I said, "as long as we get a few milliliters to analyze."

"OK, good," said Rob. "Because Knobi, one of our adult females, always insists on holding the cup herself, with her feet."

I felt like Dorothy waking up in Oz. I wasn't in Kansas anymore. Somehow I was in Iowa, talking to the Wizard, and the Munchkins were orange, hairy, and quadrumanous.

A Sloth in the Family Tree

Later that fall, after the doses were administered and all the urine samples collected, I shipped a boxful of orangutan urine on dry ice off to Bill Wong, a professor at the Children's Nutrition Research Center at the Baylor College of Medicine. Bill is an expert in energetics and doubly labeled water methods and had generously helped me set up the orangutan project, determining the amount of dose needed and the schedule for urine sample collection. After decades of fruitful and interesting work in human nutrition and metabolism, Bill seemed to enjoy the prospect of switching gears a bit to analyze ape samples.

His e-mail with the first set of results was my initial indication that we'd found something interesting. The data looked great, said Bill, but the analyses indicated that orangutans had low daily energy expenditures. *Really* low. Bill asked me to send all of the samples I had (we had collected more than we needed for the analysis) so he could run them all again, free of charge. He wanted to be sure the numbers were right.

Another round of analysis, the same result. Orangutans burned fewer calories each day than humans. The difference was huge. Azy, the 250-pound male, burned 2,050 kilocalories per day—the same as a 65-pound, nine-year-old human boy. The adult female orangutans, at 120 pounds, burned even less energy: 1,600 kilocalories per day, about 30 percent lower than expected for a human that size. Not surprisingly, orangutan BMRs were low, too, well below human values. We had carefully monitored the orangutans' daily activity throughout the doubly labeled water measurement, and they walked and climbed about as much as orangutans do in the wild. (Which is to say *not that much*. Orangutans are impressively lethargic.) The low daily energy expenditures weren't an artifact of living in captivity; they were telling us something fundamental about orangutans' evolved physiology.

Any scientist lives for this moment. We had dipped our cup into unknown waters and come up with something unexpected. The received wisdom in primate energetics was wrong, at least in part. There were big, meaningful differences in metabolic rates among humans and at least one of our ape cousins. Humans and orangutans are descendants of a single apelike ancestral species that lived about eighteen million years ago. In the intervening millennia, evolution had pushed the metabolic rates of our two lineages apart. Humans and apes weren't just different in shape and proportion. We were different on the inside as well.

But the real surprise came when I compared orangutan energy

expenditures to a wide range of other species—rodents, carnivores, ungulates . . . every placental mammal species I could find with a published measurement of daily energy expenditure (which is to say, ignoring marsupials like koalas and kangaroos, which have strange physiologies). Shockingly, orangutans were burning just one-third of the energy expected for a placental mammal their size. Their daily energy expenditures fell within the lowest 1 percent of placental mammals. The only species with lower expenditures for their body size are three-toed sloths and pandas.

Everything we knew about orangutan ecology and biology seemed to click into place. Orangutans have extraordinarily slow life histories, even by primate standards. In the wild, males don't reach maturity, and females don't have their first baby, until they're about fifteen years old. Females reproduce incredibly slowly, with seven to nine years between pregnancies, the longest birth spacing of any mammal. They also cope with desperate and unpredictable food shortages in their native Indonesian rain forests. Orangutans depend on fruit, but there can be months with so little fruit available that they're reduced to tearing the bark from trees and scraping the soft inner layer off with their teeth for sustenance. These food shortages seem to affect their social behavior, as they're the only ape that lives alone; there's not always enough food to feed a group.

Orangutans' slow metabolism tied these observations together, and to their evolved physiology. It also held important implications for the survival of the species. Life in an unpredictable rain forest, where starvation was a perennial threat, had led to adaptations to minimize daily energy needs. Their metabolic engines had evolved to run slowly, conserving fuel to fend off depletion and death. But the consequences were stark: growth and reproduction require energy, and a lower metabolic rate inevitably meant a slower life history. This in turn meant orangutan populations were slow to rebound from natural or man-made disasters. Their low metabolic rate, an elegant evolutionary solution to a challenging environment, made orangutans more vulnerable to extinction in the face of habitat destruction and other human interference.

The first measurements of daily energy expenditure in an ape had revealed a new world of metabolic evolution, with big implications for ecology, health, and survival. What else was out there, waiting to be discovered? And how did humans fit into all of this? With daily energy expenditures measured for only a handful of primate species, we had no idea. We needed more data, from more species, across the full spectrum of the primate family tree.

Primate Power

The primate energetics project took several years and involved more than a dozen collaborators, and it came together in pieces. Brian Hare, an expert in ape cognition and an old friend of mine from grad school, was working at two ape sanctuaries in Africa, the Tchimpounga Chimpanzee Rehabilitation Centre in the Republic of Congo, and Lola Ya Bonobo in the Democratic Republic of Congo. (Note to travelers: Keep your Congos straight. One is often quite dangerous; the other is often extremely dangerous.) Like the Great Ape Trust, they were ape-first facilities that engaged in research only if it was safe and useful for the chimpanzees and bonobos. Around that same time, Mitch Irwin, a primatologist and conservationist working in Madagascar, agreed to incorporate energy measurements into an annual health assessment of wild diademed sifakas.

But the dam really broke when I met Steve Ross, the director of the Lincoln Park Zoo's Fisher Center for the Study and Conservation of Apes in Chicago. Steve is an incredibly friendly, positive, and helpful guy, which makes sense because he's Canadian. In addition to his conservation work and his research with gorillas and chimpanzees at the Lincoln Park Zoo, Steve has devoted himself to getting chimpanzees who are unhappily housed in labs, roadside zoos, garages, and other islands of misery moved into good zoos and sanctuaries. He worked tirelessly and successfully to get chimpanzees in the United States the same federal protections that gorillas, bonobos, and orangutans enjoy. Steve's a goddamn hero.

Collaborating with Steve, we were able to add gorillas, Allen's swamp monkeys, gibbons, and chimpanzees at Lincoln Park Zoo to the project. Doubly labeled water doses went out across the globe, to Chicago, Congo, the other Congo, and Madagascar, and slowly the urine samples trickled back in for analysis. With the handful of published measurements from other labs, we were able to assess the diversity of energy expenditure across the whole primate family, from tiny 2-ounce mouse lemurs to massive 480-pound silverback gorillas. We even had a range of settings represented, including labs, zoos, sanctuaries, and the wild. By 2014, we had the data together—were primates' metabolic engines different from other mammals'?

The results were startling. Primates burn only *half* as many calories as other placental mammals. To put that in human terms, consider that the normal daily energy expenditure for human adults is between 2,500 and 3,000 kilocalories per day, as we'll discuss in Chapter 3. Our analyses showed that a *typical* placental mammal our size burns well over *5,000* kilocalories per day. That's the daily energy expenditure of Olympic athletes at the peak of training! But it's not like those other mammals are incredibly active; they walk a couple of miles per day at most and spend much of their time eating and resting. Their bodies simply burn energy faster, *much* faster, than our diminished primate metabolism can sustain.

Finally we had an answer for *how* humans and other primates ended up with such slow life histories. Some sixty million years ago, early in primate evolution, there was a massive reduction in energy expenditure. Primate metabolic engines slowed way down, to half the speed of other placental mammals. Whether this metabolic change was driven by evolutionary pressure for a slower life history, or whether some change in diet or environment led to slower metabolism that had knock-on effects on growth, reproduction, and aging, remains unclear. What *is* clear is that the magnitude of evolutionary change in primate metabolism corresponds precisely to the change in life history. Primates' slow rates of growth, reproduction, and aging are exactly what we'd expect given their low daily energy expenditures. Today, humans and other primates, the inheritors of this metabolic legacy, enjoy longer, slower lives than other mammals.

Strangely, like researchers before us, we found that primate BMRs were similar to those of other mammals, even though daily energy expenditures differed drastically. We think the discrepancy between BMR and total daily expenditure reflects the large size of primate brains (brains use a lot of energy). And, it should be noted, the relationship between energetics and life history remains an active and controversial area of research. We'll delve into these topics and others in Chapter 3 and elsewhere. For now, let's turn our attention to a final puzzle in the evolution of primate energetics, one that will reverberate throughout this book: the evolved metabolic strategy of our own species.

This Is Us

Even as we analyzed the results for the primate energetics project, we schemed about a bigger and more elusive prize. The orangutan and other primate data had shown how malleable metabolic rates were over evolutionary time, and how intricately tied to ecology and life history. The obvious question, then, was: What could energy expenditure tell us about our own evolution? The consensus view, as I mentioned above, was that daily energy expenditure was similar across apes and humans, and hadn't changed much at all in our lineage.

The landmark study articulating this idea is a 1995 paper by Leslie Aiello and Peter Wheeler. They pulled together measurements of organ sizes for humans and other apes from earlier studies, noting that humans have larger brains but smaller livers and guts (the stomach and intestines) than other apes. Organs are not all equal in how they expend energy. Brains, guts, and livers are all energetically expensive organs—each ounce of tissue burns a ton of calories because the cells in those organs are incredibly active, something we'll discuss more in Chapter 3. Aiello and Wheeler did the calculations and found that, in humans, the energy saved by having a smaller gut and liver perfectly offset the energy cost of our larger brain. Based on that important observation, and the observation that human and ape BMRs were broadly similar to other mammals, Aiello and Wheeler argued that the critical metabolic changes in human evolution were changes in allocation, increasing the calories channeled toward the brain while decreasing energy to the guts. In this scenario, daily expenditure stays the same. Humans didn't spend more energy than apes, they just spent their energy differently.

Evolutionary trade-offs, like the brains-for-guts scheme Aiello and Wheeler uncovered, are a cornerstone of modern biology. As Charles Darwin himself observed, drawing on the writings of Thomas Malthus, there is always a struggle for resources among the denizens of the natural world. There's never enough to go around. Consequently, all species evolve under conditions of scarcity. You can't eat your cake and have it, too. If evolution favors the expansion of some traits—say, powerful hindlimbs and a big head full of nasty teeth—others have got to give, like the forelimbs . . . and voilà, you've got *Tyrannosaurus rex*. Or, as Darwin put it in *On the Origin of Species* (quoting Goethe), "to spend on one side, nature is forced to economise on the other side."

The idea that brains and guts trade off against each other was suggested as far back as the 1890s, by Arthur Keith in a study of primates in Southeast Asia. He even tried to show that this line of reasoning could explain the differences in human and orangutan brain sizes, but he was ahead of his time and out of his depth mathematically: with only a rudimentary understanding of how organ sizes change with overall body size across mammals, he failed to show the expected trade-off of brains and guts. This idea comes up again and again throughout the 1900s. Take Katharine Milton, for example, an anthropologist with deep expertise in nutrition, who has worked with people and other primates in Central and South America for decades (and did the first doubly labeled water study in a wild primate—howler monkeys—back in 1978). She showed that leaf-eating primates, with large guts to digest their fibrous diet, had smaller brains than fruit-eating species in the same forests. Carel van Schaik and Karen Isler at the University of Zurich produced a great set of studies in the 2000s and 2010s arguing that the cost of bigger brains could even help explain evolved life history differences among primates.

But as important as trade-offs are, there were reasons to think they weren't enough to explain the full set of energetically expensive traits that make humans unique. As we'll discuss in Chapter 4, humans grow more slowly and live longer than any of the other apes, yet somehow find the energy to reproduce faster than any of them. We also have huge, energy-hungry brains and physically active lifestyles (at least, in populations that aren't coddled by modern technology). Humans also invest more in bodily maintenance and live longer than other apes. Somehow, in violation of the natural order that insists on trade-offs, humans evolved to have it all.

We thought the suite of energetically costly human adaptations could be fueled by an accelerated metabolic engine, evolved to burn more calories each day. There was plenty of human data at our disposal, but we needed measurements from a lot of apes to do the comparisons properly. Steve Ross and I mapped out a plan to engage zoos all across the United States. Within months we were working with zoos all around the country, arranging schedules to gather data. We hired Mary Brown, an intern at Lincoln Park Zoo, nearly as cheerful and unstoppable as Steve, to travel zoo to zoo, fourteen in all, coordinating everything and collecting behavioral data on the apes we measured. Soon the urine was flowing in . . . liquid gold.

The results were even more exciting than we had hoped. We discovered that all four great ape genera (chimpanzees and bonobos, gorillas, orangutans, and humans) had evolved distinct daily energy expenditures. Humans were highest, burning about 20 percent more than chimpanzees and bonobos, about 40 percent more than gorillas, and about 60 percent more than orangutans after accounting for differences in body size. BMR differed, too, by the same proportions. Just as shocking were the differences in body fat. Humans in our sample carried twice as much fat (about 23 to 41 percent body fat) as the other apes (about 9 to 23 percent). Orangutans were on the high end of fattiness, chimpanzees and bonobos were particularly lean. As we will discuss in Chapter 4, it's likely that our increased body fat evolved hand in hand with our faster metabolic rate, providing a larger fuel reserve to guard against starvation.

These differences in metabolism and body fat were not due to lifestyle: we had carefully selected sedentary humans to compare with the zoo-living apes in our study. The differences were deeper, at the core of each species. Over the course of evolutionary history in each genus, metabolic rate had been tuned up or down like the burner on a stove, dictated by changes in food availability, or predation, or . . . what? For orangutans, we are reasonably certain that their low metabolic rates and capacity to store fat are an evolved response to food shortages, keeping daily energy demands low and maintaining a substantial fuel reserve in the form of fat. Metabolic variation among the African apes—chimpanzees, bonobos, and gorillas—is a story we're still working to unravel.

In the human lineage, our cells evolved to work harder, to do more, and to burn more energy. These metabolic adaptations brought on other major changes in the way our bodies work and how we behave, topics that we'll return to in later chapters. Energy expenditure evolved hand in hand with massive changes in diet, and in the ways we acquire, prepare, and share our food. A faster metabolism favored an increased capacity to store fat. Today, our evolved metabolism sets the limits on everything from sports and exploration to pregnancy and growth. And, of course, these fundamental changes in how our bodies burn energy were crucial in the evolution of our big brain and unique life history. Yes, trade-offs were important, but it was our evolved metabolism that made us human.

Darwin and the Dietician

It was the excitement of these discoveries and the promise of scientific adventure that had drawn me inexorably into a Hadza camp, tucked away in the remote Tli'ika Hills of northern Tanzania, listening to lion choruses and measuring energy expenditures. Our work with apes and other primates had overturned decades of scientific consensus, showing just how dramatically evolution had changed the metabolic strategies of humans and other apes. What would we discover if we turned our focus on our own species and investigated how people across different cultures, with vastly different lifestyles, burn energy? What might we learn by working with populations like the Hadza, who maintain a lifestyle similar in many ways to our shared hunter-gatherer past? We didn't know it at the time, living in our tents and doing science on the savanna, but our work with the Hadza would provide perhaps the biggest surprises of all, changing how we think about the relationships between energy expenditure and lifestyle.

In the chapters that follow, we'll examine energy expenditure, exercise, and diet from an evolutionary perspective, putting the modern concerns of health and metabolic disease in a different light than we typically encounter on the covers of wellness magazines or lifestyle books. Our metabolic engines were not crafted by millions of years of evolution to guarantee a beach-ready bikini body, to keep us fit, or even necessarily to keep us healthy. Instead, our metabolism has been shaped by the Darwinian directive to survive and reproduce. Rather than keeping us trim (as the armchair engineer's model of metabolism predicts), our faster metabolism has led to an evolved tendency to pack on more fat than any other ape. But that's not the only counterintuitive and counterproductive evolutionary inheritance at work deep within us. As we will discuss, our metabolism also responds to changes in exercise and diet in ways that thwart our attempts to lose weight. And our drive for food is ferocious, as we can see with the Hadza. If our evolved appetites can push us into a pride of hungry lions for breakfast, how can we keep ourselves out of the fridge?

An evolutionary perspective is absolutely critical if we're to turn the tide against obesity and metabolic disease. We in the developed world have built ourselves luxurious food-topias, Gardens of Eating where irresistible foods are hyper-abundant and we don't need to lift a finger to get them. Bodies that evolved to move all day sit slack and limp on comfy chairs and sofas, absorbing the world through bright screens like French fries under a heat lamp. All the while the casualties mount: obesity, diabetes, heart disease, cancer, cognitive decline—all on the rise, and each intimately related to the way we consume and burn energy. Reversing course, saving ourselves from these maladies, will require a better understanding of how our bodies work, and how energy expenditure, exercise, and diet are interrelated. The sooner we move beyond the simplistic armchair engineer's view of metabolism and embrace a Darwinian perspective, the better chance we'll have.

So let's dive in, deep into the gears of our evolved metabolic engines, to understand how all the moving parts fit together. If we are going to manage our evolved metabolism effectively, we'll need to understand how it works.

CHAPTER 2

What Is Metabolism Anyway?

How does music get inside the radio?"

It wasn't a question I was expecting. Brian Wood and I, along with his wife, Carla, and our field assistant Herieth, had just finished setting up our tents under low acacia trees near a Hadza camp in the rambling, arid flat that separates Lake Eyasi from the rocky Tli'ika Hills. Brian and I were relaxing on the dusty ground in camping chairs, chatting about work in the gray, late afternoon light. Two Hadza men, Bagayo and Giga, were sitting on the ground nearby, having what sounded like a heated discussion in Hadza. They had a small battery-powered radio, a prized possession in Hadzaland, where the entertainment options are limited. At some point they decided to bring us into the conversation, switching to Swahili to ask their question. But Brian and I must have both looked bewildered, because Bagayo asked again.

"How does music get inside the radio?"

Shit, we should know this . . .

Exposure to new ideas and knowledge is one of the best things about travel, and with the Hadza it's always a two-way street. Their deep understanding of the natural world is mind-blowing. A typical Hadza kid can tell you about the physical characteristics and behavioral tendencies of dozens of animal species, and tell you about the uses—food, fire, housing, tools—of every shrub, grass, and tree on the landscape. Watching a Hadza man track a wounded impala for miles without any obvious signs, or a Hadza woman determine the size and ripeness of a wild tuber three feet below the surface by tapping the ground with a rock, feels like nothing short of magic.

For our part, we share what we know about the outside world. We share our books and gadgets, and occasionally hold movie nights, playing nature documentaries or action movies on our laptops (the *Jurassic Park* films are perennial favorites). The innate curiosity that we're all born with, the lifeblood of any scientist, seems to be well-nurtured in Hadza culture. They want to know.

Conversations usually start off innocently enough, but can develop into far-reaching discourses on geography, cosmology, or biology. "How long would it take to walk to your house?" is a simple enough question, but a real answer requires a discussion about the Earth being both round and unimaginably big, with huge continents separated by massive oceans (they were familiar with those concepts but remained noncommittal). "Are walruses real?" [And if so, what the hell are they?] is another fair question, particularly if you've just watched a documentary on Arctic wildlife and are unfamiliar with ice, oceans, or marine mammals. I tried to explain that walruses were, in fact, real (though admittedly absurd) creatures, like hippopotamuses with tusks of an elephant and feet like a fish. I'm not sure anyone believed me.

There's a great quote of uncertain provenance, often attributed to Einstein, that "if you can't explain something simply, you don't really understand it." Discussions with the Hadza brought this to life. Between the limits of my Swahili and their lack of formal schooling, it was always a fun challenge explaining how different research equipment worked, how the dinosaurs in *Jurassic Park* were created by computer, or what a blood pressure cuff measures. It often exposed gaps in my own understanding of which I hadn't been aware. They'd been hidden, papered over in my mind with empty jargon that sounded smart but didn't hold any real meaning for me.

Come to think of it, how *did* music get inside the radio?

Tentatively, I started in. In Arusha, the nearest big town (which all Hadza knew about, even though few had ever ventured that far), there was a building. Inside, a person played music from a tape or a record. (So far, so good. They'd seen tape players.) Now, the building had a machine that listened to the music and sent it through the air, from an antenna—a big metal pole. The radio, with its own antenna, captured the music out of the air and played it through the speaker.

"OK. But what is sent through the air from the building in Arusha, all the way out here?"

"Uh, radio waves," I answered, knowing immediately that I was in trouble.

"OK . . . What are radio waves?"

Good question. "Well, they travel through the air invisibly, and you can't hear them, but they carry the music . . ." I trailed off. I had no idea how to describe radio waves, because I didn't really understand them myself. In my mind they weren't much more than the little arcs emanating from an antenna in some cartoon. I knew they were a type of "electromagnetic energy," but that was just another piece of empty jargon. It was like light, right? But how would I explain invisible light emanating from a metal pole, carrying music? Was that even an accurate way to describe it?

"Ah!" says Bagayo, picking up his hunting bow. "It's like *this*," and he plucks the string of the bow. The sound travels invisibly through the air, from the bowstring to our ears. Great analogy! *Yes,* that's exactly the sort of thing we're talking about here! I knew sound waves and radio waves were different things, but I also knew I couldn't do better than Bagayo at explaining them.

Giga and Bagayo are satisfied. Brian and I are off the hook.

The next time we're in town to resupply, I google "radio waves."

Demystifying Metabolism

If we're going to discuss the cutting-edge science in human metabolism we'll need to have a real understanding of what metabolism is and how it works—certainly a better understanding than the typical biologist has of radio waves. No placeholders, not too much jargon, and zero bullshit. Let's start at the beginning.

Metabolism is a broad term that covers all of the work your cells do. The vast majority of this work involves pumping molecules in or out of cell membranes (their walls) and converting one kind of molecule into another. Your body is a walking, sloshing bucket of thousands of molecules interacting—enzymes, hormones, neurotransmitters, DNA, and more—and hardly any of it comes in its usable form directly from your diet. Instead, cells are constantly bringing nutrients and other useful molecules circulating in the bloodstream in through their walls for use as fuel or building blocks, converting those molecules to something else, and then pushing the stuff they've built out of their walls to be used elsewhere in the body. Cells in the ovaries pull cholesterol molecules inside, build estrogen out of them, and then push the estrogen—a hormone with effects all over the body—out into the bloodstream. Nerves and neurons are constantly pumping ions (positively or negatively charged molecules) in and out to maintain a negative internal charge. Pancreas cells, guided by DNA, assemble insulin and a long list of digestive enzymes from amino acids. The list goes on and on. The amount of metabolic work happening *right now* in your body is staggering.

All of this work requires energy. In fact, work *is* energy. We measure work and energy using the same units and can talk about them interchangeably. Throw a baseball, and its kinetic energy as it leaves your hand is, by definition, exactly equal to the amount of work you did to accelerate it. Heat is another common form of energy. Microwave a cup of milk to warm it for your kid, and the increase in temperature tells you how much electromagnetic energy was captured by the milk. The energy released from burning gasoline is equal to the work done to move the car along the road plus the heat generated by the engine. Energy consumed is always equal to the combination of work done and heat gained, whether we're talking about your body, your car, or your smartphone. We all play by the same laws of physics.

Energy can also be stored in things that have the *potential* to do work or create heat, like the gasoline in a fuel tank. A stretched rubber band or the spring of a mousetrap set to go off has strain energy. A bowling ball set precariously on a high shelf, one that could crash to the floor, has potential energy. The bonds that hold molecules together can store chemical energy, which gets released when the molecules break apart. When the molecules in a pound of nitroglycerin (chemical formula: $4C_3H_5N_3O_9$) are broken into nitrogen (N_2), water (H_2O), carbon monoxide (CO), and oxygen (O_2) during detonation, it violently releases enough energy (730 kilocalories) to launch a 165-pound man two and a half miles straight up into the sky (which would be work) or vaporize him (which would be heat), or some combination of the two. This brings us to our last point about energy: it can be converted among its many forms—kinetic energy, heat, work, chemical energy, and so on—but it can never be lost.

Calories and joules are the two standard units used to measure energy, whether it's the chemical energy stored in food, the heat from a fire, or the work done by a machine. Calories are most common in the United States when discussing food, but we've managed to muck up the standard usage. One calorie is defined as the energy needed to raise the temperature of one milliliter of water (one-fifth of a teaspoon) by one degree Celsius (1.8 degrees Fahrenheit). It's a tiny amount of energy—too small to be a useful unit of measure when we talk about food (like road signs giving driving distances in inches). Instead, when we talk about "calories" in food, we're actually talking about *kilocalories,* or 1,000 calories. A cup of dry Cheerios has 100 calories according to the nutrition label on the box, but they actually mean 100 kilocalories, or 100,000 calories.

So why don't we just say "kilocalories" or "kcal" instead of abusing the term "calorie"? Bizarrely, in the late 1800s, when scientists were deciding to adopt "calories" as the preferred unit of measure for food energy, the influential and pioneering American nutritionist Wilbur Atwater decided to stick with an early, arcane convention and simply capitalize "Calories" when referring to kilocalories. That's about as sensible as capitalizing "Yards" to refer to miles. We've been stuck with the confusing use of calories (or Calories) on our food labels ever since. Of course, this is just one more entry in the long, embarrassing history of measurement in the United States. A country that insists on using teaspoons, inches, and Fahrenheit obviously has deep psychological issues about discussing their units. (By the way, if you're traveling in the civilized world and want to convert joules on their food labels to calories, divide joules by four.)

Since work and energy are two sides of the same coin, we can think about all the work that our cells do and all the energy they consume as two ways of measuring the same thing. We can use "metabolism" and "energy expenditure" interchangeably. That's why evolutionary biologists like me, as well as doctors and people in public health, are so fixated on energy expenditure, which is how we measure metabolism: it is the fundamental measure of the body's activity. The speed with which a cell does its work determines metabolic rate, the energy used per minute. Add up the work of all the cells in your body and you've got your body's metabolic rate, the energy you expend each minute. Your metabolic rate is the full force of your cellular orchestra, 37 trillion microscopic musicians, blending together in an intricate symphony.

The sophisticated metabolic system that sustains us, and that we all take for granted, is a marvel of evolution. It took nearly a billion years—untold trillions of generations, quadrillions of false starts and dead ends—for the basic framework of today's simplest single-cell metabolic systems to evolve on this planet, an eternity of trial and (mostly) error. It took another two billion years for the simplest multicelled organisms, with their integrated metabolic systems and divisions of labor, to evolve. Along the way, life had to confront some major challenges in basic chemistry. Oils had to mix with water. Oxygen, a chemical that burns and kills, had to be harnessed for life. Fats and sugars, holding more energy per gram than nitroglycerin, had to be burned carefully for fuel without blowing organisms up or boiling them alive.

That's not even the strangest part. All the work our bodies do is powered by microscopic alien life-forms called mitochondria, living within your cells. Mitochondria have their own DNA and their own two-billion-year evolutionary history, including saving all life on Earth from certain doom. And much of the work done to digest your food into usable bits is done by a vast ecosystem that lives in your gut. This microbiome is made of trillions of bacteria that make their home all along your digestive tract, the long and serpentine passageway that connects your mouth to your butt.

We are all walking chimeras, part human and part other, performing the ordinary miracle of turning dead food into living people every day without a moment's thought. It's a story you've probably heard before, but likely with the magic boiled out of it and served cold from a textbook. It's well worth another listen. If nothing else, it's the essential foundation you'll need to understand how diet affects your health and how your body burns energy—how life actually works.

Soylent Green Really Is People (or It Could Be)

Going at least as far back as the ancient Greeks and as recently as the 1600s, people—including very smart people like Aristotle—thought that flies, mice, and other organisms could grow spontaneously from inanimate objects like dirt and rotten meat. It made sense: one day there was a pile of old rags and some hay in the corner of the barn, the next day there were mice. Maggots seemed to explode out of old carcasses without anyone or anything putting them in there. Without a good grasp of the microscopic world or rigorous experimentation, people found it a hard idea to disprove. It didn't fully die until Louis Pasteur's breakthrough experiment in 1859, boiling broth and showing that nothing would grow in it if you kept out dust and bugs (we've been pasteurizing our food ever since). Today, the idea of "spontaneous generation" is taught to schoolkids as a classic example of how benighted people used to be and how far science has come.

It's absurd, of course, to suggest that flies could appear spontaneously from a dead corpse. But as we've come to understand over the past century of scientific research on metabolism, the truth is even stranger. Animals, plants, and all other living things are essentially "spontaneous generation machines," assembling their bodies and those of their offspring from food, water, and air. What is a fly, after all, except a little machine that builds baby flies out of rotten meat?

In the classic and campy *Soylent Green*, a 1973 sci-fi movie set in a dystopian future New York City, Charlton Heston's character is appalled to discover that the green mush that everyone eats is actually made from humans. He's carried off in the final dramatic scene, shouting to anyone who will listen, "Soylent Green is *people!*" Fast-forward to 2018, and in an example of life capitalizing on art, you can buy Soylent brand food mixes, gloopy tubes of nutrients that are meant to replace normal food for people on the go or without lunch friends. I have no idea how they taste, but there is a Soylent Green variety. Now, I'm pretty sure that the Soylent Green you buy online these days isn't people. But here's the thing: it *could* be. All you have to do is eat it.

Every molecule in your body, every pound of bone and muscle, every ounce of brain and kidney, every fingernail and eyelash, all six quarts of blood squirting around your vessels, *all* of it is made of reassembled bits of food you've eaten. The energy that keeps you moving and keeps you alive comes from your diet as well. *You are what you eat* isn't just a well-worn cliché, it's how life actually works. One shudders to think about the sizable proportion of Americans who are literally walking, talking, reformulated Big Macs. My kids are built and powered almost entirely from chicken nuggets, pasta, yogurt, and carrots. I myself am fueled largely by pretzels and beer. How does it all work?

Follow the Pizza

Let's start with lunch. You're sitting down to a hot, glistening slice of pepperoni pizza (vegans may substitute meat and cheese alternatives into this thought experiment). You take a bite and begin to chew, a luxurious mélange of bread, sauce, meat, and cheese dancing across your taste buds, the crust fighting against your teeth, the smell wafting up the back of your palate and filling your nose. It is transcendent.

The alchemy has begun. Chewing and mixing the food with saliva is the first step in digesting your meal and its main constituent parts, the macronutrients. There are three macronutrient categories: carbohydrates, fats, and proteins. Carbohydrates are starches, sugars, and fiber. They come mostly from the plant-based portions of your food—the crust and tomato sauce in the pizza you're eating. Fats (which include oils) come from both plant and animal sources, like the cheese and pepperoni in your slice. Proteins come mostly from animal tissue and the leaves, stems, and seeds of plants (including beans, nuts, and grains). The pepperoni and cheese are full of protein, as are the basil leaves scattered atop your slice. There's protein in the crust as well, including the much maligned gluten that makes it chewy.

There's also water trapped in the slice, as well as trace amounts of other stuff like minerals, vitamins, and other elements that your body needs. But the macronutrients—carbohydrates, fats, and proteins—are the main attraction. They are what build and power your body. They are the raw materials of metabolism.

The flow chart in Figure 2.1 shows where the carbohydrates, fats, and proteins from your food go in your body and what they do. Think of it as a subway map for macronutrients—a challenge to read at first, but easy enough once you follow each line from origin to destination. Each macronutrient has its own line, and each line makes three stops: Digest, Build, and Burn. Like any good transit system, there are side branches that can take you from one line to another. Off we go!

Carbohydrates

If you eat a typical American diet, carbohydrates account for about half of the calories you consume each day. In fact, despite the recent popularity of low-carb diets, humans across cultures and around the globe, including hunter-gatherers like the Hadza, typically get more calories from carbohydrates than from fats or proteins (Chapter 6). We're primates, after all, and primates eat plants—especially ripe, sweet fruits. Carbohydrates are our main source of fuel, and we have a 65-million-year history of relying on them.

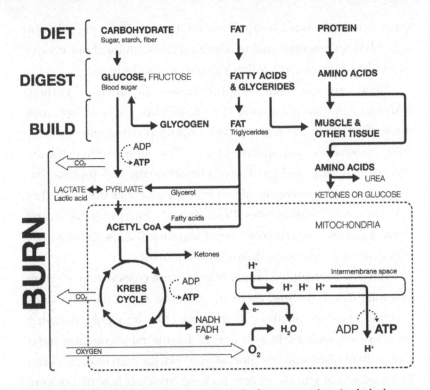

Figure 2.1. Subway Map for Macronutrients. Each macronutrient (carbohydrate, fat, protein) has its own pathway in the body, and each makes three major stops: Digest, Build, and Burn. Single-headed arrows indicate one-way paths. Paths with double-headed arrows run both directions. Some pathways are omitted for clarity. Fiber digestion by the microbiome produces fatty acids that would join the Fat pathway. Sugars are used to build some structures in the body, such as DNA. The many pathways by which amino acids can be converted to glucose or ketones aren't shown. Galactose, the least common product of carbohydrate digestion, is also omitted. e-: electrons. H+: hydrogen ions.

Carbohydrates come in three basic forms: sugars, starches, and fiber. Sugars and starches are *digested* and either used to *build* glycogen stores or *burned* for energy (see above). They can also be converted into fat, as we'll see below. Fiber is a different beast, with an important role in the gut regulating the digestion and absorption of sugars and starches, and feeding the trillions of bacteria and other critters in our intestinal microbiome. In fact, the microbiome plays an essential role in digesting fiber, and without it we're in trouble. But first, let's follow the starches and sugars.

Sugars are just small carbohydrates—little chains of carbon, hydrogen, and oxygen atoms. The smallest are just one sugar molecule big (hence the *mono* in their technical name, monosaccharides; saccharide just means sugar). The monosaccharides are glucose, fructose, and galactose. The other sugars—sucrose, lactose, and maltose—consist of two monosaccharides stuck together and are called disaccharides ("two sugars"). Sucrose (table sugar) is just a glucose and fructose bound together. Lactose (milk sugar) is glucose and galactose. Maltose is two glucoses.

Starches are simply a bunch of sugar molecules strung together in a long chain. Because there are so many sugar molecules stuck together, starches are also called polysaccharides ("poly" meaning many) or complex carbohydrates. By far the most common sugar molecule in plant starch is glucose, and plant starch molecules can be hundreds of glucose molecules long. Starch is how plants store energy, which is why it's in huge supply in energy storage organs of plants like potatoes and yams. Nearly all plant starch (the starch in our food) is a mix of just two polysaccharides, called amylose and amylopectin.

No matter what foods they come from, starches and sugars all get digested into one of the three monosaccharides. Starch digestion starts in your mouth, with an enzyme in your saliva called amylase, which begins the process of breaking long amylose and amylopectin molecules down into smaller and smaller pieces. Enzymes are proteins that break apart molecules or promote chemical reactions (their names usually end in -*ase*). Digestive enzymes like amylase chop food molecules into smaller and smaller bits. Starches have been so important in human evolution that we've evolved to make more amylase than any of the other apes, something we'll discuss in Chapter 6.

• • •

After you swallow, the mushy bolus of food ends up in your stomach, where the acid kills bacteria and other nasties that have hitched a ride in your food. After that, the food is pushed out of your stomach and into the small intestine, where most of the digestive work takes place. In the small intestine, the starches and sugars are hit with enzymes produced by the intestine and pancreas to break them down further. The pancreas, an organ about five inches long and the shape of a skinny chili pepper, sits just beneath the stomach and is attached to the small intestine with a short duct. It's most famous for its production of insulin, but the pancreas also produces most of the several dozen enzymes used in digestion (along with bicarbonate, which neutralizes the stomach acid as it enters the intestine). The assembly of these enzymes (their specific shape and makeup) and the levels of production (whether to make a lot or a little of a particular enzyme) are controlled by your genes. For example, if you're lactose intolerant and can't digest milk, that means your genes have shut down the assembly and production of the enzyme lactase, which is needed to break the disaccharide lactose into glucose and galactose. No other enzyme can do that job, so the lactose heads intact to the large intestine, sending the bacteria there into a feeding frenzy that produces a lot of gas and all the other lovely side effects of milk intolerance.

Starch and sugar digestion continues until all the polysaccharides and disaccharides are broken down into monosaccharides. Since much of the carbohydrate in your diet comes from starch, and starch is made entirely from glucose, about 80 percent of the starches and sugars that you eat end up as glucose. The rest is broken down to fructose (about 15 percent) or galactose (about 5 percent). Of course, if you eat a diet high in processed foods full of sugar (i.e., sucrose, which is glucose plus fructose) or high-fructose corn syrup (which is about 50 percent fructose and 50 percent glucose mixed with water), the percentage of fructose might be a bit higher for you, and the percentage of glucose a bit lower.

These sugars are absorbed through the intestinal wall and into the bloodstream. The walls of our intestines are chock-full of blood vessels, and blood flow to our guts more than doubles after a meal to carry away nutrients. The result is the familiar rise in blood sugar (almost all glucose) after a meal, particularly one high in carbs. If the food you eat is processed, low in fiber, and easily digested, the carbs are digested quickly and the sugars rush into the bloodstream, creating a huge, steep spike in blood sugar. Those foods are said to have a high glycemic index, which is the rise in blood glucose measured two hours after ingesting a particular food, relative to the rise you'd experience from eating pure glucose. Foods that are harder to digest (more complex carbohydrates, fewer sugars, more fiber) take longer to digest and absorb, resulting in a long, low rise in blood sugar—and a low glycemic index. We'll discuss diets in Chapter 6, but there's some evidence that low glycemic index foods might be better for you.

The unsung heroes in all this digestive work are dietary fiber and your microbiome. Fiber is a class of carbohydrate (there are many varieties of fiber) that our bodies can't digest—at least, not on their own. These tough, stringy molecules are what give plant parts their strength and structure. Fiber from our food covers the intestinal walls like a wet knit blanket, forming a lattice-like filter that slows the absorption of sugars and other nutrients into the bloodstream. That's why the glycemic index—the rush of sugar into the blood—is about 25 percent higher for orange *juice*, which doesn't have much fiber, compared to a piece of orange, which does.

Fiber also feeds our microbiome, the steamy ecosystem of organisms that live in our guts and help us digest food. Most of the microbiome lives in the large intestine, or colon, where it plays a critical role dealing with fiber and all the other stuff we can't digest in the small intestine. We are only beginning to appreciate the importance of the microbiome, but the scale is stunning. With trillions of bacteria, each with their own thousands of genes, the microbiome is like a four-pound superorganism living inside of you. These bacteria digest much of the fiber we eat, using enzymes our own cells can't make and producing short-chain fatty acids that our cells absorb and use for energy. Our microbiome also digests other stuff that escapes the small intestine, aids in immune system activity, helps produce vitamins and other essential nutrients, and keeps the digestive tract running properly. The effects on our health, from obesity to autoimmune diseases, are wide-ranging, and new discoveries are happening every day. What we know for sure at this point is, if your microbiome isn't happy, you aren't happy.

The main reason we eat and crave carbohydrates, their reason for existence as far as our cells are concerned, is to power our bodies. Carbs are energy. Once the sugars are absorbed in your bloodstream, there are only two places for them to go—they can be burned now or stored for later (Figure 2.1). This is where the hormone insulin, produced by the pancreas, comes in. Some cells use insulin to get glucose molecules inside of them, through their membranes.

Burning carbohydrates for energy is a two-stage process that we'll discuss in detail below. Blood sugar that isn't burned immediately is packed away into glycogen stores in your muscles and liver. Glycogen is a complex carbohydrate similar to plant starch. It's easy to tap into when energy is needed, but relatively heavy because it holds an equal proportion of carbon and water (hence the term "carbohydrate"). It's like canned soup: quick to prepare, but heavy and bulky because it's stored with water.

Humans, like other animals, have evolved hard limits on the amount of glycogen our bodies can hold. Once those buckets are full, blood sugar has to go somewhere else. And the only place left to go is fat.

When your body's energy needs are met and your glycogen stores are full, the excess sugar in your blood is converted to fat, as we'll discuss below. Fat stores are a bit more difficult to use for fuel—there are more intermediate steps to convert them to a burnable form. But fat is a much more efficient way to store energy than glycogen, because it's energy dense and doesn't hold water. And as we know all too well, there's virtually no limit to how much fat the human body is able to store.

Fats

Fats have a fairly simple itinerary—they are *digested* down into fatty acids and glycerides and then *built* back up into fat in your body, which is eventually *burned* for energy. The challenge, though, is that fats are hard to digest. It comes down to basic, familiar chemistry: oil and water don't mix. Fats (including oils) are all hydrophobic molecules, which means they won't dissolve in water. But like all life on Earth, our body's systems are water-based. Breaking big globs of fat down into microscopic bits isn't possible with just water—it's like trying to clean a greasy pan without soap. The evolutionary solution? Bile.

Bile was long thought to play a role in our moods and temperament as one of the four humors, a fun example of clever people believing dumb things. Very smart people, from Hippocrates all the way through doctors and physiologists of the 1700s, thought that too much yellow bile made people aggressive. Doctors would bleed people with leeches if they were suspected of being out of humoral balance, which is one reason that doctors probably killed more people than they saved until the advent of modern medicine a century or so ago. Today we know that bile is the stuff that makes fat digestion work.

Bile is a green juice produced by your liver and stored in your gall bladder, which is a small, thumb-sized pouch that sits between the liver and small intestine, connected to both with short ducts. When fats enter the small intestine from the stomach, the gall bladder squirts a bit of bile into the mush of food. Bile acids (also called bile salts) act like detergents, breaking up the globs of fat and oil into tiny emulsion droplets. Once the fat is emulsified, enzymes called "lipases," produced by the pancreas, are added to the mix and break these emulsion droplets down to an even smaller size, to microscopic droplets called micelles, just a hundredth the diameter of human hair. These micelles form, break apart, and form again like the bubbles in a fizzy drink. Each time they break apart, they release the individual fatty acids and glycerides (which are fatty acids attached to a glycerol molecule) they were holding, the basic building blocks of fats and oils.

Fatty acids and glycerides are absorbed into the intestinal wall and re-formed into triglycerides (three fatty acids attached like streamers to a glycerol molecule), the standard form of fats in the body. Here the body confronts the next challenge of digesting fats: because they don't mix well with water, they tend to clump together in water-based solutions like blood. Lumpy blood would kill you, clogging up the small vessels in your brain, lungs, and other organs. The evolved solution is to pack triglycerides into spherical containers called chylomicrons. This keeps the fats from clumping together, but results in a package too big to be absorbed through capillary walls and into the bloodstream, where they need to go for distribution throughout the body.

Instead, the fat molecules, packed in chylomicrons, are dumped into the lymphatic vessels. Part surveillance system, part garbage collection, the lymphatic vessels have their own network throughout your body, picking up debris, bacteria, and other detritus and bringing it to the lymph nodes, spleen, and other immune system organs to be dealt with. It's well suited to pick up big particles like chylomicrons stuffed with fat. The lymphatic vessels also collect all the plasma that leaks out of your blood vessels (about three quarts a day) and returns it to your circulatory system, so it offers a port of entry into the bloodstream. Specialized lymph vessels called lacteals, embedded in the intestinal wall, pull chylomicrons into the lymph system and then dump them directly into the circulatory system, just upstream of your heart.

White, fat-filled chylomicrons are so big, and so plentiful after a fatty meal, that they can give the blood a creamy hue. Eventually, though, they are ripped apart and their contents pulled into waiting cells for storage or use. Lipoprotein lipase enzymes in the blood vessel walls first break the triglycerides into fatty acids and glycerol, which are pulled into waiting cells by aptly named fatty acid transporter molecules before being reassembled into triglycerides. Most fat is stored in fat cells (adipocytes) and muscles, forming a reserve fuel tank. These stored triglycerides are the fat that we feel in our belly and thighs, or see marbled into a nice cut of steak. Problems arise when our bodies start storing substantial amounts of fat in our liver and other organs, which can lead to liver failure and a range of other health issues. The causes of fatty liver aren't always clear, but obesity is a major risk factor.

A small proportion of the fats we eat are used to build structures like cell membranes, the myelin sheaths that coat our nerves, and parts of our brain. Some of the fatty acids needed to build these tissues can't be made by reformulating others, and so are considered essential fatty acids—you need to get them from the food you eat. That's why food producers often tout the omega-3 fatty acid (an essential fatty acid) content in their fish, milk, or eggs.

Like carbohydrates, the ultimate destination for fat—the reason you crave it and the reason your body goes to all the trouble to digest and store it—is to burn it as fuel. All animals are evolved to store energy as fat because it holds an incredible amount of energy in a small package, 255 kilocalories per ounce. That's on par with jet fuel, more than five times the energy density of nitroglycerin, and nearly a hundred times better than a typical alkaline battery. Happily, the process of breaking down fats for energy is a slower process than exploding dynamite. Some fats are burned immediately after digestion, fresh from your gut. But most of the time, between meals, your body draws on stored fats for fuel. The triglycerides that make up your stored fat are broken down into fatty acids and glycerol and used to make energy (Figure 2.1), something we'll see in more detail below.

Proteins

Proteins have an interesting itinerary. Unlike fats and carbohydrates, proteins aren't a primary source of energy (unless you're a carnivore). The main role of protein is to build and rebuild your muscles and other tissues as they break down each day. Your body does burn protein for energy, but it's a small contributor to your daily energy budget.

Protein digestion begins in the stomach with an enzyme called pepsin, which starts breaking proteins apart. The cells within your stomach wall make an enzyme precursor called pepsinogen, which is converted by the stomach acid into the enzyme pepsin, which then gets all Edward Scissorhands on any proteins it comes in contact with, chopping them up. This process continues in the small intestine as food leaves the stomach, with enzymes secreted by the pancreas.

All proteins get digested down to their basic building blocks: amino acids. Amino acids are a class of molecules shaped a bit like a kite—a head attached to a tail. They all have the same head: a nitrogen-containing amine group connected to a carboxyl acid. Amino acids are distinguished by their tails, which are always some configuration of carbon, hydrogen, and oxygen atoms. There are hundreds of amino acids on Earth, but only twenty-one are used to build proteins in living plants and animals. Nine of these are considered essential for humans, meaning our bodies can't make them on their own; we need to get them from our diet (don't worry—if you haven't died yet, you're getting them). The others your body can make by itself if needed, usually by breaking down and reformulating other amino acids. But we're getting ahead of ourselves.

The next stop for amino acids is to build the tissues and other stuff that make up the human machine (Figure 2.1). Once the proteins from our pizza slice are digested into amino acids, they are absorbed through the walls of the small intestine and into the bloodstream. From the blood, the amino acids are pulled into cells to construct proteins, which are chains of amino acids strung together. The construction of proteins from amino acids is one of the primary jobs of DNA. A gene is just a stretch of DNA that lines up a particular sequence of amino acids to make a protein (some genes are regulatory, meaning they don't assemble proteins themselves but instead activate or suppress protein-assembling genes). Variants in DNA sequence (the string of As, Ts, Cs, and Gs) can result in different amino acid lineups and thus slightly different proteins, contributing to biological differences among individuals. Amino acids are also used to make a variety of other molecules like epinephrine, the fight-or-flight hormone; and serotonin, one of the neurotransmitters our brain cells use to communicate.

These same tissues and molecules break down over time. They are eventually converted back into amino acids, and travel through the bloodstream to the liver. There, things get a little tricky. The amine group in the amino acid has a very similar structure, NH_2, to ammonia, NH$_3$ (notice the similarity in the names as well, *amine* and *ammonia*). In the same way that drinking ammonia-based household cleaner would surely kill you, accumulating ammonia from breaking down amino acids would be fatal. Happily, we have an evolved mechanism to convert that ammonia to urea, which then travels via the bloodstream to the kidneys to be excreted in the urine. It's the urea in our pee that lends it that zesty eye-watering smell, which makes sense because it's made from ammonia.

We pee out the equivalent of fifty grams (about two ounces) of protein each day. Exercise adds to that total by increasing muscle breakdown. We have to eat enough protein to replace what we lose each day, lest we find ourselves in protein deficit. If we eat more protein than we need, the extra amino acids are converted to urea and cleared out by the urine. This can make for some very expensive pee if you overdo it on the protein supplements.

The last stop on the protein train line is to burn the amino acids for fuel (Figure 2.1). After the nitrogen-containing head is chopped off, converted to urea, and sent on its way, the tails are used to make glucose (a process called gluconeogenesis, which literally means "making new sugar") or ketones, both of which can be used for energy, as we'll see below. Proteins are typically a minor part of the daily energy budget, providing around 15 percent of our calories each day. But they are a vitally important emergency energy supply if we're starving, a bit like setting the furniture on fire to heat your house. The skeletal figures of victims of famine are a haunting example of this process taken to the extreme, their bodies consuming themselves in a desperate effort to stay alive.

Burn, Baby, Burn

All roads on our metabolic train map lead, eventually, to one place: fuel. Carbs, fats, and proteins all hold stored chemical energy in the bonds that hold their molecules together. Breaking those bonds apart releases that energy, the energy we use to power our bodies.

In all biological systems, including our bodies, energy has one fundamental, common form: adenosine triphosphate, ATP. ATP molecules are like microscopic rechargeable batteries, which are "charged" by adding a phosphate molecule onto a molecule of adenosine diphosphate, ADP (note the "tri" versus the "di" in their names, indicating three phosphates on ATP versus two on ADP). A gram of ATP holds about fifteen calories of energy (that's calories, not kilocalories), and the human body only holds about fifty grams of ATP at any given time. That means each molecule cycles from ADP to ATP and back over three thousand times per day to power our body. Burning carbs, fat, and protein, then, is the process of transferring the chemical energy in the sugar, fat, and amino acid molecules to the chemical bond that holds the third phosphate onto molecules of ATP. When we use food to make energy, what we're making is ATP.

Let's start with one molecule of glucose, the predominant form of sugar that our bodies use for energy (the story is essentially the same for fructose and galactose). This glucose molecule might come directly from carbs we just ate, or might come from stored glycogen that's been reconverted to glucose. As we began to discuss at the end of the section on carbohydrates, burning sugars for energy is a two-stage process. First, glucose ($C_6H_{12}O_6$) is converted to a molecule called pyruvate ($C_3H_4O_3$) in a ten-step process that is powered by two ATP molecules but produces four ATP molecules, resulting in a net gain of two ATP. It's a relatively fast process, and it's what we use to power short bursts of activity like a 100-meter sprint or a powerlift at the gym.

This first stage of metabolism is called anaerobic because it doesn't require oxygen, which you can appreciate when you watch the Olympics on TV: elite sprinters hardly seem to breathe at all, and powerlifters hold their breath. If there's not enough oxygen present, either because we're not breathing effectively or (more likely) because our muscles are working too hard, too fast for oxygen supply to keep pace with all of the pyruvate being produced, the pyruvate gets converted to lactate. Lactate can be reconverted to pyruvate to be used for fuel, but if it builds up, it can also become the dreaded lactic acid, which makes our muscles burn when we're working hard and pushing our limits.

The second stage, aerobic metabolism, is where we need oxygen. If there's sufficient oxygen in the cell, the pyruvate produced at the end of the first stage is pulled into a chamber within the cell called the mitochondria. There are dozens of mitochondria in a typical cell, and they are known as the "powerhouse of the cell" because the bulk of ATP production happens within them. This is where the magic happens, the chemical choreography that keeps us alive.

In the mitochondria, pyruvate is converted to acetyl coenzyme A, or acetyl CoA, which would vie with ATP for the title of the most important chemical you've probably never heard of or have completely forgotten. Acetyl CoA is like a train car full of passengers—carbon, hydrogen, and oxygen atoms—without an engine to pull it. Along comes oxaloacetate, which is hitched to acetyl CoA and begins to pull it along a circular track called the Krebs cycle. The train will make eight stops, and at each, some carbon, hydrogen, and oxygen passengers get on or off. The coming and going of those atoms generates two ATP. By the final stop, only the oxaloacetate engine is left. It's hitched up to another acetyl CoA and the cycle repeats.

Importantly, some of the passengers are robbed as they get on and off the Krebs cycle train, their electrons stolen away by the molecules NADH and FADH. These NADH and FADH molecules scurry away to the back alleys of the mitochondria and unload their purloined electrons into a special receptor complex in the membrane—a door in the wall. Mitochondria are double-walled structures, like a thermos; there's a small space between the inner and outer membranes called the intermembrane space. When the stolen electrons are deposited into the inner membrane complex, positively charged hydrogen ions (which are in plentiful supply) chase the negatively charged electrons and end up trapped in the intermembrane space. The hydrogen ions are like fish caught by a weir: they flow through the inner membrane, pulled by the electrons, only to find themselves trapped and crowded in the intermembrane space.

With all the positively charged hydrogen ions packed together, there is an electrochemical force pushing them out to balance the charge on either side of the inner membrane. But there's only one way for the hydrogen ions to escape the inner membrane space: a special portal in the inner membrane that's built like a turnstile. The hydrogen ions stream through the turnstile, driven by the electrical charge. As the turnstile spins, it forces together ADP and phosphate molecules, making ATP. This is the real moneymaker, producing thirty-two ATP. The complex choreography of electrons and hydrogen ions dancing along the inner membrane, called oxidative phosphorylation, is the primary energy generator that powers your body.

And what becomes of the glucose molecule itself, the carbon, oxygen, and hydrogen atoms that we started with at the beginning? Remember that it's the energy in the bonds holding these atoms together that we use to charge our ATP, *not* the atoms themselves. Instead, the carbon and oxygen atoms, which make up 93 percent of the mass of a glucose molecule, are converted to carbon dioxide (CO_2) in the conversion of glucose to pyruvate and in the Krebs cycle. The hydrogens bind with oxygen at the end of oxidative phosphorylation, forming water, H_2O. We eat carbohydrates only to breathe them out, filling the air around us with the skeletons of potatoes past; a remaining fraction ends up as drops of water in the ocean of our body.

Burning Fat, Getting Fat, and Going Keto

We use the exact same steps of aerobic respiration to burn fat. Instead of starting with a glucose molecule, we start with a triglyceride molecule. It might be fresh from the pizza we just ate, packaged in a chylomicron, or newly released from our copious body fat stores. Regardless of their source, triglycerides are broken into fatty acids and glycerol and converted to acetyl CoA (glycerol is transformed to pyruvate first; Figure 2.1). And just like glucose, the atoms of carbon, oxygen, and hydrogen that make up those fatty acids and glycerols are exhaled as CO_2 or formed into water. Aside from the small proportion that's converted to water, the fat you burn leaves your body by air, excreted by your lungs. You exhale your food.

If we're burning a lot of fat, whether we're on an extremely low-carb diet or starving, some of the acetyl CoA generated will be converted to molecules called ketones. Most ketone production occurs in the liver. Ketones are sort of a traveling version of acetyl CoA, and can travel in the bloodstream to other cells, be reconverted to acetyl CoA, and used to generate ATP. Like a lot of metabolic conversion, most ketone production is done in the liver, but they are used throughout the body. This is the pathway that popular ketogenic diets engage, promoting a system of eating all fats and proteins and almost no carbohydrates. With the carbohydrate train line essentially shut down, all traffic shifts to the fat and protein pathways.

Because ketones travel in the blood, they show up in your pee.

The curious and bored can buy test strips over the counter at most pharmacies. The presence of ketones in urine signals that the body is in "ketogenesis," and depending heavily on fat for energy.

Once you're familiar with the fat and glucose pathways in Figure 2.1, it's fairly obvious why extremely low-carb, ketogenic diets like Atkins or the trendy Paleo diet (which as we'll see in Chapter 6 isn't Paleo at all) can lead to massive fat loss. If you consume no carbohydrates, the only way to generate acetyl CoA is by burning fat. Sure, you can also burn proteins by converting amino acids into ketones or glucose (some amino acids even form molecules that can jump into the middle of the Krebs cycle, like a kid jumping into a double-Dutch jump rope session). But protein is typically a minor player in terms of daily calories. Fat is the main fuel on a low-carb diet, and if you eat fewer calories than you burn, the deficit will be met by burning stored fat for energy. Some of this fat will be processed into ketones prior to burning. For example, the brain is a particularly picky eater and generally uses only glucose for metabolism, but if there's no glucose available, it will switch to burning ketones.

The dark side of converting fats to energy is that the tracks run both ways. As you see in Figure 2.1, a sugar molecule (glucose or fructose) can be converted to acetyl CoA and then jump on the fatty acid track instead of entering the Krebs cycle, and voilà! You convert the sugar into fat. It's the same process used to convert fat into acetyl CoA, just run in reverse.

In fact, like any good, flexible transit system, our metabolic pathways are evolved to respond to traffic conditions and send molecules to their most sensible destinations.* Got more sugars than

---

* I realize the analogy may be lost on readers living in developing countries like the United States that lack a functioning mass transit system, but trust me: this is how they're supposed to work.

you need? Send the extra glucose and fructose to glycogen. Glycogen stores full? Send the excess sugar to acetyl CoA. If the Krebs cycle train is overcrowded because energy demands are low, start sending acetyl CoA to fat. And there's always plenty of space available in fat. Glycogen stores fill up, and you can't store excess protein, but there's no limit to how much fat you can layer on.

And that's why we should be suspicious of any diets that target one specific nutrient as a hero or a villain for weight loss. Nothing is innocent if eaten in excess. Any calories that aren't burned, no matter if they come from starches, sugars, fats, or proteins, will wind up as extra tissue in your body. If you're pregnant or bulking up at the gym, that extra tissue might be useful things like organs or muscle. But if you're not, those extra calories, no matter their original dietary source, will end up as fat. That's the foundation we need to understand to begin talking about all the real-world complexities of diet and metabolic health. We'll talk a lot more about diets and the evidence for what works and what doesn't in Chapters 5 and 6.

Poisoned by Plants

Is it better to live in blissful, romantic ignorance? I can certainly see the argument for it. It's easier to face the day when you feel like Mother Nature just wants to give you a big warm hug—that the natural world and even your fellow humans are essentially good. Pain and death may be inevitable, but only because we're clumsy, fallible, and out of tune with the guiding harmonies of the universe. If only we let go and felt the karmic flow, were generous and kind, the world would surely reciprocate. If only we could return to a state of nature, like our hunter-gatherer ancestors.

Right?

Movie night on the savanna. The entire Hadza camp is gathered in the darkness around Brian's laptop. There's a nature documentary on, and everyone loves it. Every time a new animal protagonist walks into the frame, chatter wells up from the crowd. *Ooooohhh! Look at that wildebeest! Aw man, that's a huge giraffe!* Then it's a nighttime scene at the edge of watering hole. Elephants have come to drink, desperate for water at the height of the dry season. But lions are lurking nearby. They pounce on a baby elephant, gnawing at the back of its neck while it runs in fear. The little elephant raises its tiny trunk and bleats its pained baby elephant cry. The crowd is rapt, myself included. Adult elephants try to run the lions off, but it's no use. There are too many and they attack like ninjas, one after the other, drawing blood from deep wounds. Soon it's over. *A baby elephant!* Oh god, the horror. Surely Nature has erred. Something this repugnant wasn't supposed to happen.

The Hadza erupt with glee. *Ha! The lions got 'em!*

I'm stunned. *What psychopaths root for the lions?**

Then it begins to sink in. Feeling bad for the elephants is a luxury of life in the industrialized world, experiencing nature through a television screen. To grow up in it, to live in nature every day, is to understand that it doesn't want to snuggle. There's no majestic drama playing itself out for the benefit of your spiritual growth. Instead, you are part of a jumbled crowd of species, some malevolent, others indifferent, none of them your friends. Hadza hate elephants because elephants are massive and ornery and occasionally kill Hadza. They view elephants with about the same affection as they view snakes, and Hadza people *hate* snakes.

The Hadza don't weep for the animals they hunt and kill, any more than you cry over a cup of yogurt. They are not cynical or jaded, but they know the deal. Being part of the ecosystem means

---

* The same could be asked of Detroit football fans.

eating others, whether it's plants or animals. The wild hunting dogs that catch your scent on the breeze and turn to follow will feel no remorse as they tear your innards out. Nothing personal, it's just business. Understanding life in a real, functioning ecosystem requires us to abandon the romantic, Disneyesque mythologies that we're fed growing up in our sheltered suburbias.

Understanding the world through the lens of evolution is a similarly disorienting wake-up call. What Darwin saw clearly for the first time was that species are all competing for limited resources, struggling to find food without becoming dinner. There is neither "good" nor "bad" in nature—*we* place those cultural assessments on an otherwise amoral and indifferent cast of characters. Even things that seem clearly done for our benefit are driven by evolutionarily selfish ulterior motives. Fruits, those gifts from the tree, heavy with sweet flesh, are simply a clever way of dispersing seeds. Dogs have evolved to prey on our emotions and make us love them because humans are a great source of dog food. And the lush green plants that fill our planet with life? They've been quietly poisoning us for two and half billion years.

Life requires energy, and the first fuel system to evolve on our planet was photosynthesis. The earliest bacteria to harness the sun's energy relied on hydrogen and sulfur rather than water to make photosynthesis work. Then around bout 2.3 billion years ago, somewhere in the shallow ponds of a young, rocky Earth, a new recipe for photosynthesis evolved, converting water (H_2O) and carbon dioxide (CO_2) into glucose ($C_6H_{12}O_6$) and oxygen (O_2). Sunlight provided the energy needed for this conversion—energy that got stored in the molecular bonds of glucose.

This new type of photosynthesis, called *oxygenic* because it produces oxygen as a waste product, was a game changer. Oxygenic photosynthetic life colonized the planet, soaking up CO_2 and water and spewing out oxygen. We tend to think of oxygen as a good thing, the sustainer of life, but its true chemical nature is devastating. It steals electrons and binds to other molecules, altering them completely and often tearing them apart. Oxygen is Shiva the destroyer, obliterating everything it touches either slowly (rust) or violently (fire).

At first, the new oxygen produced by plants was absorbed by the iron in dirt and rocks, creating massive, oxidized "red beds" in the Earth's crust. Then the oceans absorbed as much oxygen as they could hold. After that, the atmosphere began to fill, climbing from 0 percent to over 20 percent oxygen as photosynthetic plants across the globe belched out the noxious stuff unabated and uncaring. As oxygen levels soared, it began to snuff out life, an event known as the Great Oxygen Catastrophe. Earth was on the brink of becoming a dead planet.

Aliens Within: Mitochondria and the O_2 Joy

In the incomprehensible fullness of evolutionary time, unlikely events become routine. Consider the chances of being struck by lightning, which are 1 in 700,000 per year for a person in the United States. If you live to be seventy, your lifetime chances are still reassuringly low, 1 in 10,000. But what if you lived for three billion years, watching the full history of life on Earth unfold? Over that timescale, you could expect to be struck by lightning over 4,200 times.

The numbers are even more difficult to grasp when we consider evolution among the teeming microscopic hordes of bacteria and other single-celled organisms. There are over a million bacteria in an ounce of "clean" drinking water, and about 330 million cubic miles of water on the planet. That puts the total number of waterborne bacteria on this planet (ignoring any on land) at around 40×10^{27}, or 40 with 27 zeros after it. Even if they only replicate only once a day, that's 14×10^{30} replications a year. What are the chances of a random mutation arising that changes a metabolic pathway, making some previously unusable chemical into a source of food? Even if the odds are one in a hundred trillion, we can expect more than 100,000 *trillion* such mutations every year. Over the millions of years available to evolution, such mutations are almost inevitable.

As the young Earth slowly filled with poisonous oxygen over eons, it presented an opportunity. Among the untold quadrillions of bacteria living, mutating, and reproducing over billions of years, some hit upon a seemingly impossible solution, a way to harness oxygen to make fuel: oxidative phosphorylation. Shuttling electrons in and out of an intermembrane space enabled these bacteria to reverse the process of photosynthesis, using oxygen to break apart the bonds of glucose, unleashing the stored solar energy trapped within. The waste products were CO_2 and water—the ingredients for photosynthesis.

It was a landmark event in the evolution of life. Aerobic metabolism opened a fresh, untrammeled frontier, a new way for life to work. Oxygen-using bacteria swept across the planet, diversifying into new species and families. Soon they were everywhere.

Then another improbable event. In the vicious cell-eat-cell world of early, simple life, the proliferating aerobic bacteria would have been a delicious new menu item. When a cell eats another cell (whether it's an amoeba in a backyard stream gobbling up a paramecium or an immune cell in your bloodstream killing an invading bacterium), it engulfs its prey, bringing the victim inside its membrane to dismantle and burn for fuel. But as uncountable zillions of aerobic bacteria were eaten over hundreds of millions of years, a small handful (maybe only one or two) escaped destruction. Instead, against the odds, they survived intact, living on within their new host. It was a microscopic Jonah in the belly of the whale.

And it worked brilliantly.

These chimeric cells held advantages over others in the oceans of middle earth. With a dedicated energy-producing bacterium on board, these hybrid cells outcompeted others in the battle for turning energy into offspring. Having an internal bacterial engine became the norm. Every animal on Earth today, from worms to octopi to elephants, is an inheritor of this great leap forward. Like all other animals, we carry the descendants of those planet-saving aerobic bacteria in our cells. They are our mitochondria.

The revolutionary idea that mitochondria evolved from symbiotic bacteria was championed by the visionary evolutionary biologist Lynn Margulis. Researchers as far back as the 1800s had recognized the visual similarity between mitochondria and bacteria as viewed through a microscope and floated the possibility of a bacterial origin of mitochondria, but it was Margulis who gave the idea life and heft. She wrote a landmark paper on the theory in the late 1960s. It was rejected by more than a dozen journals as too outrageous, but she persevered. During the decades that followed, it became clear that Margulis's outrageous idea was dead-on.

Mitochondria within our cells retain their own strange loop of DNA, a telltale vestige of their bacterial past. And we dutifully feed and tend to them like treasured pets, our heart and lungs dedicated to the task of supplying our mitochondria with oxygen and carting away their CO_2 waste. Without them and the magic of oxidative phosphorylation, we couldn't sustain the energetic extravagance we take for granted. Life would have never evolved into the grand menagerie we see today.

Oxygen is the essential ingredient in oxidative phosphorylation precisely because it's an electron thief—the characteristic that makes it so destructive. Oxygen is the final electron acceptor in what is known as the electron transport chain, the bucket brigade that passes electrons along the inner membrane of the mitochondria, pulling hydrogen ions into the intermembrane space. Without oxygen, the electron transport chain stops, the Krebs cycle backs up, and the mitochondria shut down. When electrons jump onto oxygen at the end of the electron transport chain, they attract hydrogen ions, forming water, H_2O. Your mitochondria form more than a cup of water (about three hundred milliliters) each day from the oxygen you breathe in.

Off to the Races

At the fundamental level of macronutrients and mitochondria, pathways and ATP production, all animals (humans included) are essentially the same. Figure 2.1 applies equally well to cockroaches, cows, and Californians. And yet, in the nearly two billion years since aerobic metabolism and mitochondria came on the scene, a staggering diversity of life has evolved, all using the same basic metabolic framework. Metabolisms have been sped up and slowed down, tweaked and shaped to fuel the myriad ways that animals move, grow, reproduce, and repair. As we saw in the last chapter, these metabolic changes have shaped our own species in essential ways.

Now that we understand the metabolic basics that all animals share, let's explore the ways that evolution has shaped them to be different. Let's see all the places that oxygen-eating engines can take us, and how they function day to day in the real world. How much energy do we really burn each day, and what is it all spent on? How much energy does it take to walk a mile, battle a cold, or build a baby? Can we really "boost" our metabolism with coffee, diet, or superfoods? How does our body manage to supply the right amount of fuel to meet our daily needs? And why do our metabolic engines wear out and fail? Is death the inescapable cost of burning energy, the devil's bargain for a chance to dance among the living?

Most important, how far do I have to run to escape the guilt of a good donut?

CHAPTER 3

What Is This Going to Cost Me?

Deep in the woods about a half hour outside of Boston, on the grounds of a decommissioned Cold War missile launch site, lies a hidden menagerie of strange creatures and earnest nerds toiling away to uncover life's mysteries. It's the Harvard field station, a mash-up of old New England farm and mad scientist laboratory. As the fall leaves dance with color, emus strut around their pastures like grumpy dinosaurs while wallabies bounce in the grass nearby. The goats and sheep up the hill seem to be your typical pastoral flock, but notice the little black boxes on their collars, logging every movement like the flight recorders on a 747. Inside the low cement-block buildings, you'll find guinea fowl running on miniature treadmills or frogs hopping off of tiny, instrumented platforms to measure their accelerations. Bats and birds fly down hallways as over-caffeinated grad students and high-speed infrared cameras watch them dart and maneuver.

It was the late summer of 2003, midway through my PhD at dear old Harvard, and I was learning the ins and outs of measuring energy expenditure for my dissertation. I still recall my first few weeks working at the field station, feeling like the new, unprepared intern in a James Bond–style secret laboratory—if the 007 program were preoccupied with animals instead of supervillains. *Goats are in the north paddock, treadmill is through that door, oxygen analyzers are on the cart. Good luck, try not to break anything, and don't forget to clean up the goat shit.* It was hard some days to tell the difference between immersion learning and drowning. I loved it.

I had spent the morning putting Oscar the dog on a treadmill, measuring the energy he burned to walk and trot. For my study, dogs had to wear a big, clear plastic mask—a makeshift astronaut helmet fashioned out of a 3-liter soda bottle—over their head to funnel their expired breath into the oxygen analyzer. Oscar was a shelter-rescue pit bull mix, the loyal companion of a fellow grad student, Monica, and he loved treadmills with an intensity that bordered on mania. It helped that I smeared hot dogs on the inside of the mask. Monica's office was just down the hall from the treadmill lab, and she had to make sure Oscar was inside with the door closed whenever another dog was on the treadmill, lest Oscar erupt in jealousy.

What started as an innocent project measuring the costs of walking and running in humans, dogs, and goats grew into a sort of professional obsession with measuring energy expenditures. Soon I was off to California on a project to measure expenditures in chimpanzees walking on two legs or four. Next it was humans running with their arms folded across their chests, trying to figure out the energy advantage of swinging your arms (it's tiny). Dave Raichlen, Brian Wood, and I spent the summers of 2010 and 2015 in Hadza camps with a portable metabolic lab, measuring the cost of every Hadza activity we could think of—walking, climbing trees, chopping into bee's nests, digging tubers. Just last year, I was working with Masahiro Horiuchi and collaborators in Japan to calculate the energy consumed with each breath and heartbeat.

You might think that such esoteric interests would make me an outlier, maybe even an outcast. But there are labs in universities all over the world dedicated to measuring energy expenditures. It's a vibrant, if eclectic, field of biology and medicine. There are yearly conferences. But to say I'm not alone in my obsession only makes it weirder. Why would *anyone* devote their career to measuring how much these things cost?

In the economics of life, calories are the currency. Resources are always limited, and energy spent on one task can't be spent on another. Evolution is a heartless accountant: the only thing that matters, at the end of a life, is how many surviving offspring an organism has produced. Organisms that spend their calories unwisely, in the eyes of natural selection, will reproduce less. The next generation will be full of offspring from the careful, strategic spenders—those who were best at acquiring energy, and who allocated those calories most effectively. Since physiology and behavioral tendencies are inherited, these offspring will tend to spend their calories like their parents did. This new generation plays the game again, but this round the competition is stiffer. The least effective competitors have been weeded out. Over eons, the organisms left standing are those with exquisitely tuned strategies for acquiring and spending their calories. Each species represents a particular metabolic strategy, calibrated to its environment—the latest move in this never-ending game of life.

Want to know how a species' physiology has been shaped by evolution? Want to understand how different tasks are prioritized or triaged when times are tough? Follow the calories.

On the Shoulders of Giants

Nothing could be more obvious than the need to eat and breathe, but the science of metabolism took a long time to develop. Every detail we covered in Chapter 2, every word and arrow in Figure 2.1, took someone—or more often, several people—years to figure out. It's a history that stretches back more than two centuries.

The early breakthroughs in metabolism science came in the middle and late 1700s, with researchers in Europe and America uncovering the roles of oxygen and food. Scientists of that era, like everyone else from time immemorial, knew that humans and other animals needed to eat and breathe to survive. People had even made a connection between fire and metabolism, recognizing that humans and other mammals generate body heat. But the details on both were fuzzy. No one knew *what*, exactly, we needed from the air, or precisely *how* our bodies used food. None of the science in Chapter 2 was known.

It didn't help that early metabolic research began with a view of the world that was completely backward. As the Enlightenment got rolling and modern Western science was born in the 1600s, the general consensus was that we didn't get *anything* important out of the air. Instead, scientists thought that body heat (as well as the heat from fire) represented a substance they called "phlogiston" leaving the body. Phlogiston was thought to be the essential stuff in combustible material that made it flammable and was released as it burned. Air absorbed phlogiston, but it could hold only so much. That's why a candle would go out when a jar was placed over it: once the air inside was saturated with phlogiston, no more could be released and the candle couldn't burn.

Oxygen wasn't discovered until 1774, by the chemist Joseph Priestley. He called it "dephlogisticated air," thinking oxygen was a purified form of air that was free of phlogiston. Priestley introduced the substance to fellow chemist Antoine Lavoisier during a visit to Paris. Both were fascinated by the science of combustion. Lavoisier, considered by many to be the father of modern chemistry, rejected the idea that Priestley's air was "dephlogisticated."

Instead, Lavoisier argued that the gas was a substance all its own and dubbed it "oxygen," or "acid maker," for its predilection for stealing electrons and forming acids (the same properties that make oxygen so critical in the electron transport chain). Lavoisier was the first to recognize that fire consumed oxygen. He had a hunch that living organisms did the same.

In 1782, Lavoisier and his buddy Pierre-Simon Laplace conducted an ingenious experiment that led to a fundamental breakthrough in metabolic science. They placed a guinea pig in a small metal container and set it (with the lid closed, but with breathing holes) in a larger bucket partly filed with ice. They then packed ice around the sides and top of the guinea pig container and opened a drain in the bottom of the bucket. By measuring the water that drained from the bucket, they were able to measure the heat given off by the guinea pig. Lavoisier and Laplace calculated the ratio of calories burned to the amount of CO_2 that the guinea pig produced and found it was the same ratio as burning wood or candle wax. Lavoisier concluded *la respiration est donc une combustion*: essentially, metabolism is combustion.

Imagine what else Lavoisier might have discovered if he hadn't been guillotined in the throes of the French Revolution just a few years later.

It took decades of painstaking experiments to show that the heat generated when food is burned in a fire is precisely the same as when it's burned in the body, and that the amounts of oxygen consumed and CO_2 produced are the same as well. With these fundamental rules established, scientists had two general approaches for measuring energy expenditure: they could measure the heat produced (called direct calorimetry) or measure oxygen consumption and CO_2 production (called indirect calorimetry).

As a practical matter, measuring gases is a lot easier than measuring heat. So by the late 1800s, pioneers in the emerging fields of nutrition and energetics were using oxygen consumption and CO_2 production as the main measure of calories burned by humans and animals.

Fast-forward another hundred years, and that's the same approach I was using to measure Oscar's energy expenditure while he walked and trotted on the treadmill. As you can see in Figure 2.1, burning carbs, fats, and proteins consumes oxygen and produces CO_2. Measuring oxygen consumption and CO_2 is the standard approach for measuring calories. Oxygen and CO_2 aren't energy themselves, but they are so tightly linked to ATP generation and energy expenditure that they are reliable and accurate measures of metabolism.

Now the fine print. Since oxygen and CO_2 are indirect measures of energy expenditure, there are some important details that need to be considered when using them to measure metabolism. First, it takes a few minutes of activity before the body reaches a steady state of oxygen consumption and CO_2 production. You know this already if you exercise regularly: your breathing and heart rate don't reach their mid-exercise rhythm until you've been at it for a while. Short bursts of activity, like sprinting or powerlifting, don't last long enough to reach steady state, and they rely on anaerobic metabolism that doesn't consume oxygen, making them difficult to measure. Also, the amount of energy burned for a given amount of oxygen consumed or CO_2 produced changes a bit depending on whether you're burning more carbs, proteins, or fats. Conveniently, the mix of fuels can be calculated from the ratio of oxygen consumption to CO_2 production (called the respiratory exchange ratio or respiratory quotient) to give an accurate measurement of energy expenditure.

Despite these challenges, researchers have investigated the energy costs of a staggering diversity of human activity. These measurements are the references used for every piece of fitness equipment and every online calculator that's ever told you how many calories you've burned. Crank away on your elliptical, shake your smartwatch, or churn like a madman at your spin class, and the calorie count that's spit out is based on measurements of oxygen consumption and CO_2 production in some test group, toiling away in a lab. At least, that's what the numbers are supposed to be based on. There are no metabolism police checking whether companies make stuff up.

Often, energy expenditures are reported in metabolic equivalents, or METs. One MET is defined as 1 kilocalorie per kilogram of body mass per hour, roughly the energy cost of resting. The Compendium of Physical Activity, compiled every few years since 1993 by Barbara Ainsworth and her team, is the definitive resource for anyone wondering about the caloric cost of a particular activity. It has MET values for over eight hundred activities, from the everyday ("typing: electric, manual, or computer," 1.3 METs), to the unexpected ("fishing with a spear, standing," 2.3 METs), and from the curiously vague ("sexual activity, general, moderate effort," 1.8 METs) to the disconcertingly specific ("walking, backwards, 3.5 mph, uphill, 5 percent grade," 6.0 METs). I've listed some common activities and their costs in Table 3.1.

Table 3.1. Energy Costs for Various Activities

1 MET = 1 kcal per kg body weight per hour

ACTIVITY	METS	NOTES
Resting	1.0	Sleeping is a bit lower, 0.95 METs
Sitting	1.3	Same for reading, watching TV, computer work
Standing	1.8	On two legs
Yoga	2.5	Hatha style
Walking	3.0	2.5 mph (4 km/hr) on a firm, level surface
Sports	6.0–8.0	Soccer, basketball, tennis, other aerobic sports
Housework	2.3–4.0	Cleaning, laundry, mopping, etc.
High Intensity	10–13	Navy SEAL training, boxing, vigorous rowing, etc.

Getting Around: The Costs of Walking, Running, Swimming, and Cycling

"Seven forty-five, walking."

Not even eight A.M. yet and it was already hot in the sun. What had started as yet another cool morning in Hadzaland was turning into yet another blistering day. I was hanging with a group of Hadza women on their daily outing for food. That day it was kongolobi berries: hard, pea-sized spheres that were nearly all seed, with just a thin rind of tangy sweet flesh.

We had left camp a bit before seven A.M., the women and I walking fast in a loose column for about half an hour along a faint track carved into the road by the occasional Land Rover or pickup truck. The track climbed up from the flats along the eastern edge of Lake Eyasi and over the rocky Tli'ika Hills, offering a shortcut to the village of Domanga for the rare traveler with a reason to go there and good suspension. A truck might pass this way once every few weeks, just enough traffic to keep the golden grass and hardy scrub from erasing it completely. As the track wove its way along the top of the Tli'ika Hills, a bend of it ran by the Sengeli camp, and the Hadza who lived there often used it as a thoroughfare to and from home.

"Seven fifty A.M., walking."

We walked through an endless golden ocean of dry grass, passing stands of acacia trees, towering baobabs, and thick groves of dry, woody bushes. Finally, we arrived at a grove of kongolobi bushes and the women left the Land Rover track and fanned out. They efficiently stripped handfuls of berries off the thin stems and stuffed them into their congas. The congas, colorful rectangles of thin cloth the size of beach towels, were tied like satchels over their shoulders, forming a deep pocket that hung at the hip. My charge that day was to follow Milé, a sixty-five-year-old woman, as she went about her morning foray for berries. Milé had agreed to let me tag along and take notes, with the unspoken understanding that I'd try not to get in the way or be too annoying.

These focal follows, as they're called, are the bread and butter of anthropology—the daily observations that, amassed over time, provide a detailed portrait of life in a particular community. The trick is to be unobtrusive so that the day unfolds without your disrupting it. Fumbling with notebooks or falling over from heat exhaustion are considered poor form. I'm in reasonable shape and had a bottle of water and a granola bar in my backpack; I wasn't too worried about exhaustion. And I was keeping notes as instructed by Brian Wood, who's done dozens of these follows and is a proper anthropologist: I kept a voice recorder in my right hand and, every five minutes on the dot, whispered what Milé was doing at that moment into the recorder.

"Seven fifty-five, walking."

My only problem was a growing self-consciousness. Not only was I lurking around silently, watching everyone like the chaperone at a Catholic school prom, I was talking into a voice recorder every five minutes like the world's worst spy. The quieter I tried to be, the more absurd it felt, whispering into a little black box in the vast emptiness of the African savanna. And it was almost always the same note: *walking.*

To be Hadza is to walk. And walk. And walk. Every day. A Hadza woman will walk about five miles a day on average; Hadza men will cover about eight and a half. A woman Milé's age will have walked well over a hundred thousand miles in her lifetime, enough to circle the globe four times. A Hadza man, if he reaches his seventies, might cover the 239,000 miles it would take to reach the moon.

"Eight A.M., walking."

When we finally returned to camp a few hours later, Brian asked me how my follow had gone. I told him it was *great.* All good.

No problems. I was too embarrassed to mention my annoyance at all the *walking* notes. Surely, it reflected poorly on me as both an adult and an anthropologist. Brian and I were friends from our grad school days at Harvard, and while we were both in the Anthropology department, we had received very different training. While I was out at the field station putting dogs and goats on treadmills and learning metabolic physiology, Brian was living with the Hadza and learning the ropes of real anthropological fieldwork—focal follows, interviews, foraging ecology. Now, years later, in the middle of a field season with the Hadza, I was desperate to avoid being the weak link. I didn't want to admit to feeling like an idiot using the voice recorder. Serious, dedicated anthropologists wouldn't let something akin to vanity impinge on their work.

Later on, though, at dinner, as Brian, Dave Raichlen, and I talked through the day's events and made plans for the next, I came clean. It felt a little . . . *odd*, I said, to keep repeating "walking" every five minutes into the recorder like a madman wandering Penn Station talking to a dead iPhone.

"Yeah . . . you don't have to do that," said Brian.

What!? Not recording the goings-on at precise five-minute intervals seemed like a serious violation of the Anthropologist's Code of Observation, if there was such a thing. Rule 1: Take Notes Every 5 Minutes. Rule 2: Don't Die (it messes up the notes). Rule 3: Don't Screw Up Rule 1.

Brian explained how he did it: any time a five-minute check-in was skipped in the notes, it could be assumed you were walking. Walking was a default activity, like breathing. It didn't hurt to note when someone was doing it, but it was much more important and useful to note when they stopped. To a seasoned field guy like Brian, the logic was obvious.

"When you're out with the Hadza, you're *always* walking."

Walking is such a central feature of Hadza life that it's the first activity we measured when Dave, Brian, and I started the Hadza energetics project in 2009. During our first season with them to measure total daily energy expenditures using doubly labeled water, we also brought a portable respirometry system with us. It was heavy and cost twice as much as my Honda Civic, but it fit in a briefcase and did a bang-up job measuring oxygen consumption and CO_2 production. Participants would wear a light plastic mask over their nose and mouth, similar to the oxygen masks commonly found in hospitals. The mask had a thin tube that ran to the sensor unit, about the size of a thick paperback novel, clipped into a chest harness. It was a tiny metabolic laboratory.

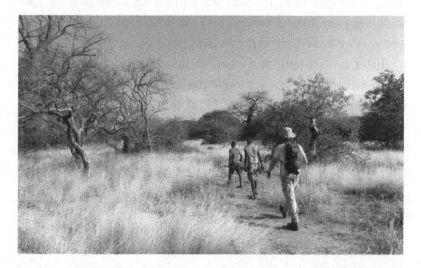

Figure 3.1. Walking. Working and living with the Hadza means a lot of miles on foot. Here, we followed two Hadza men tracking an impala shot two hours before. Despite their best efforts following faint hoofprints and flecks of dried blood, they never recovered it.

We cleared out a flat walking path around camp for the trials. Hadza men and women would walk for about five to seven minutes at a steady speed while the mask and sensor unit calculated their rate of energy expenditure (kilocalories per minute) from the measurements of oxygen consumption and CO_2 production. We found that the Hadza spend as much energy walking as every-body else:

$$\text{Walking Cost (kcal per mile)} = 0.36 \times \text{Weight (pounds)}$$

This equation comes from a large meta-analysis by Jonas Rubenson and colleagues, combining data from twenty different studies. Our Hadza data fell right in line with this much larger sample. Apparently, a lifetime of walking doesn't make a person more efficient at it.

Using the equation for walking cost, you'd find that an average 150-pound person burns 54 kilocalories to walk a mile ($0.36 \times 150 = 54$). A smaller person, at 100 pounds, would burn 36 kcal. (These are the costs above and beyond the costs of resting, which we'll discuss below.) If we want to factor in the effort to carry a backpack or a baby, we just add the weight of those items to the "Weight" term before multiplying by 0.36. So a 180-pound person carrying a 20-pound backpack has a total weight of 200 pounds and will burn 72 kcal to walk a mile.

Running is more costly than walking. The same study by Rubenson and colleagues surveyed data from twenty-three studies of running energy expenditure and found that the cost to run a mile increases with weight as:

$$\text{Running Cost (kcal per mile)} = 0.69 \times \text{Weight (pounds)}$$

So a 150-pound person running a mile can expect to burn 102 kcal ($0.69 \times 150 = 102$). Since 150 pounds is a typical weight for an adult, a good rule of thumb is that walking costs 50 kcal per mile, and running costs 100 kcal. Running is twice as costly as walking, but still nowhere near the cost of swimming. Studies of elite swimmers by Paola Zamparo, Carlo Capelli, and their colleagues put the cost of swimming at:

$$\text{Swimming Cost (kcal per mile)} = 1.98 \times \text{Weight (pounds)}$$

This is nearly three times the cost of running. By comparison, riding a bicycle is much cheaper:

$$\text{Bicycling Cost (kcal per mile)} = 0.11 \times \text{Weight (pounds)}$$

Just one-third the cost of walking. That's at 15 mph, though. Cycling costs increase exponentially with speed, and are also affected by factors like wind, road surface, and tire design and pressure (which affect rolling resistance). Regardless, the economy of a bicycle compares favorably to even the greenest gasoline-powered car. A Toyota Prius, at about 3,000 pounds, burns a gallon of gasoline (28,800 kcal) to travel 55 miles, meaning its cost per pound (0.175 kcal per mile) is about 60 percent greater than traveling by bike.

To finish out our tour of human-powered travel, let's look at the cost of climbing. Whether you're a Hadza man climbing a baobab tree to harvest honey from a beehive in the canopy, a rock climber at some alpine crag, or an accountant taking the stairs at work, the cost of ascent increases with body weight as:

$$\text{Climbing (kilocalories per foot)} = 0.0025 \times \text{Weight (pounds)}$$

At first blush, the cost of climbing may seem low. But note that unlike the costs of walking, running, swimming, and biking, the climbing equation gives the cost per *foot* increase in elevation; the others are shown as cost per *mile*. Climbing is actually about thirty-six times more costly per distance covered than walking, and is easily the most expensive type of human-powered travel. Of course, walking or running downhill is *less* costly than traveling on level ground, as long as the descent isn't so steep that you struggle to work your way down. Conveniently, for the hills we typically encounter on trails and sidewalks (grades less than 10 percent), the additional costs of going uphill are about the same as the energy saved going downhill. The costs of going up- and downhill can usually be ignored if you're estimating costs for an outing where the net elevation gained is negligible.

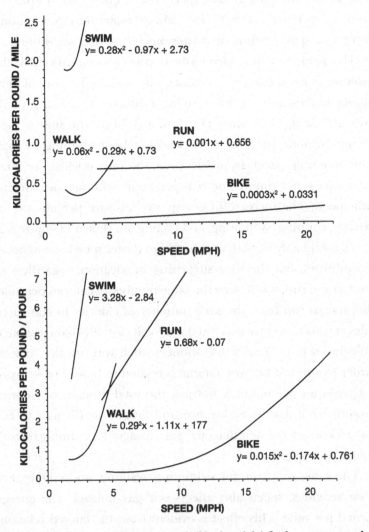

Figure 3.2. Energy costs (kcal per pound of body weight) for human-powered travel. Top panel gives the energy burned per mile traveled; the bottom panel gives the energy burned per hour.

Effects of Speed, Training, and Technique

You know from experience that the faster you walk, run, cycle, climb, or swim, the harder you breathe and the more energy you burn. It also seems like elite athletes float by with no effort while we mortals huff and puff. In fact, speed affects energy cost in two different ways, but the effects don't always match our perceptions. And training and technique matter much less than you'd think.

The main way that speed affects cost is straightforward: the faster we move, the faster our muscles have to do the work of moving our bodies, and the faster we burn calories. If running a mile costs 100 kcal, we'll burn 600 kcal per hour running 6 mph (10-minute mile pace) or 1,000 kcal per hour running 10 mph (6-minute mile pace). In other words, the rate at which we burn energy (kcal per minute, or kcal per hour) will increase directly with speed. The increase in energy expenditure per minute for walking, running, swimming, and cycling are shown in Figure 3.2.

That probably fits with your intuition (faster speed means faster expenditure), but there's a surprising implication: regardless of how fast you run, you'll burn the same number of calories per mile. That means you burn the same number of calories to run three miles at your fastest pace as you do to jog it casually—you just burn the calories faster (and finish sooner) when you run fast. It feels harder to run fast because fatigue is related to how hard we work (e.g., calories per minute), not just the total number of calories burned. We'll discuss endurance and fatigue in Chapter 8. For now, it's enough to know that our "gas mileage" for running doesn't change with speed.

The same isn't true for swimming, walking, and cycling. For those activities, speed also affects our gas mileage, the energy burned per mile. This effect is evident from the curved relationships between speed and energy per mile in Figure 3.2. Take walking, for example. Walking at our most economical pace, about 2.5 mph, burns roughly 50 kcal per mile for a 150-pound person. We can think of that as an energetically optimal speed, since it requires the least amount of energy per mile. Walking faster, at 4 mph, will burn roughly 40 percent more energy, about 70 kcal per mile. At around 5 mph, the cost of walking exceeds the cost of running; it's actually cheaper to *run* at that speed than it is to walk.

We've evolved to be very sensitive to these changes in walking cost. Put someone on a treadmill and slowly increase the speed, and they'll naturally switch from walking to running very near the metabolic transition speed where it becomes cheaper to run.* Ask study subjects to walk around a track at their normal pace, or observe people walking down the sidewalk, and you'll find they stick pretty close to the energetically optimal speed. Our habitual walking speeds also depend on our goals and environment. People in big, fast-paced cities and Hadza out foraging for food typically walk a bit faster than their energetically optimal speed. Apparently, under the right circumstances we are willing to spend a bit more energy per mile to save time and cover more ground. Like other animals, we've evolved to be very strategic about how we spend our energy.

Walking costs (kcal/mile) increase with speed because of the inherent mechanics of a walking gait. We rise and fall with each step, our center of gravity following a roller-coaster trajectory as we walk. That up-and-down movement gets harder to do as we move faster. When we switch to a run, our legs transform from rigid struts to springy pogo sticks, and we bounce from step to step. We still rise and fall with each step, but the springlike mechanics of

---

* The mechanical or physiological triggers for the walk-run transition are hotly debated, but no one disagrees that we tend to switch right near the energetically optimal transition speed.

running result in a flat cost versus speed relationship. Cycling and swimming costs per mile increase with speed, but for different reasons than for walking. When you swim or bike, you move your body through fluid (water or air), and you lose energy fighting drag. The faster you move, the more drag fights to slow you down. The effect is extremely strong in swimming: increasing your speed just from 2 mph to 3 mph will increase the energy burned per mile by about 40 percent. For cycling, the costs of fighting drag aren't too noticeable below about 10 mph (which is one reason that air drag isn't a factor in running). But above 10 mph, the effect of drag really grows. A 150-pound cyclist will spend 15 kcal more per mile to increase her speed from 10 to 20 mph; increasing from 20 to 30 mph will cost 25 kcal more per mile. And all of this assumes there's no wind, which will affect drag by increasing or decreasing the flow of air relative to the rider. Cycling at 20 mph into a 10 mph headwind will result in the same drag as going 30 mph in still air.

Surprisingly, training and technique have only modest effects on the costs of getting around. Studies of elite runners show a mix of results; some have found that trained athletes burn less energy per mile, but others report no difference. Other studies have taken a more controlled approach, training subjects over weeks or months and measuring energy expenditure along the way. Those studies don't always show a measurable effect on the cost per mile, and even in the studies that do find a difference, the effect is typically small, around 1 to 4 percent. An effect that size might be important at elite levels of competition where races are won or lost by fractions of a second, but it's unlikely to be noticeable to the average person.

Technique and equipment have similarly unimpressive effects. In Capelli and colleagues' study of swimming energetics, they report the same costs per mile for athletes swimming freestyle, backstroke, or butterfly (breaststroke was noticeably more costly). Apparently, you can swim in nearly any style and it has little effect on the cost per lap. The same goes for running. The Internet is full of nuanced and sober advice for how to hold your arms when you run, but it's mostly bullshit, at least in terms of energetics. You can walk or run with your arms folded across your chest, behind your back, or over your head and it increases the calories burned by only 3 to 13 percent. The newest rage in running tech is the Nike Vaporfly shoe, which for $250 holds the promise of lowering your running cost by about 4 percent. It's an impressive bit of engineering, but for a 150-pound athlete, a 4 percent savings is just 4 kcal per mile, equivalent to the energy in one M&M. That reduction is unlikely to mean much unless you're competing at an elite level. Since the cost per mile increases directly with weight, the average overweight American would see a much larger improvement in the costs of running (and everything else) by shedding a few pounds. Each percentage drop in body weight means a similar percentage decrease in the energy burned per mile.

Miles per Donut

We can use the equations for walking, running, and climbing cost to put the energy expended for different activities into perspective. For the most part, the costs of physical activity are disappointingly small. Consider a typical 150-pound adult. Even if they get their recommended daily allowance of 10,000 steps per day (about five miles), that's only about 250 kcal—just about the same number of calories as a 20-ounce bottle of soda (240 kcal) or half of a Big Mac (270 kcal). Climbing one flight of stairs (about 10 feet of ascent) burns about 3.5 kcal, less energy than they'll get from an M&M. You'd have to run about 3.5 miles to burn off the calories in a chocolate glazed donut (340 kcal) and more than eight miles to burn the equivalent of a large McDonald's milkshake (840 kcal).

The costs are, of course, bigger for more extreme events. For a 150-pound athlete, running a marathon will burn about 2,690 kcal. An Ironman triathlon (2.4-mile swim, 112-mile bike, 26.2-mile run) will burn about 8,000 kcal, assuming an average speed on the cycling leg of 25 mph and a fast swim. Running the 100-mile Western States ultramarathon will burn about 16,500 kcal, and that's ignoring the costs of elevation gain. Hiking the Appalachian Trail with a 30-pound pack will burn about 140,000 kcal.

And what about Milé and other Hadza women, walking each day to find and bring home food? Hadza men and women tend to be smaller in stature than adults in the industrialized world. Hadza women average about 95 pounds. Still, a typical Hadza woman, covering five miles each day, would burn about 63,000 kcal over the course of a year just by walking. That's a lot of energy.

But it's still less than the cost of building a baby.

A Body at Rest

All of the basic functions our cells do to keep our body alive and functioning don't stop when we start moving. Instead, these functions keep running in the background, burning energy—the inescapable costs of simply being alive. The energy expenditure estimates generated by the equations above for walking, cycling, swimming, and climbing are the costs *over and above* those background costs. Often we ignore these unseen costs when we talk about exercise and energy expenditure, but they are far greater than anything you're likely to do at the gym.

Background energy expenditure goes by several names: basal metabolic rate, basal energy expenditure, resting energy expenditure, resting metabolic rate, and standard metabolic rate, among others. These distinctions reflect subtle differences in the way these metabolic rates are measured. Researchers aren't always careful about which terms they use, adding to the potential for confusion.

Basal metabolic rate, or BMR, is the most well-defined measurement: it's the rate of energy expenditure measured in early morning with the subject lying down, awake but calm, with an empty stomach (no food for the previous six hours), in a comfortable temperature. If one or more of these criteria isn't met, the measurement is usually called resting energy expenditure or some variant, with an explanation of the conditions in which the measurement was taken.

Basal metabolic rate (as well as its many variants) is the energy your body burns when it isn't doing any physical work, digesting any food, or working to stay warm. The best way to think of it, then, is the summed up energy expenditure of your organs as they go about their various tasks. The bigger you are, the bigger your organs are and the more work they do each day. It's not surprising, then, that BMR (in kcal per day) increases with body weight (in pounds) as:

$$\text{Infants (0 to 3 years): BMR} = 27 \times \text{Weight} - 30$$
$$\text{Children (3 years until puberty): BMR} = 10 \times \text{Weight} + 511$$
$$\text{Women: BMR} = 5 \times \text{Weight} + 607$$
$$\text{Men: BMR} = 7 \times \text{Weight} + 551$$

We need different equations for infants, children, men, and women for two reasons. First, body size has a strange nonlinear effect on metabolic rate. Energy expended per pound is much steeper for small organisms (including small humans) than for large ones, as we'll discuss below. That's why the slope for infants in the equation above (27) is four or five times steeper than it is for men (7) and women (5). Second, our metabolism changes as we mature and our bodies shift their physiology from *growth* to *reproduction*. Body composition also changes at puberty, with women putting on more body fat than men. Fat doesn't expend as much energy as other tissues, and so, on average, the calories burned per pound is lower for women (5) than men (7).

The BMR equations above give a sense of your body's background energy needs per day, but they're just ballpark estimates. Your BMR could easily fall above or below the value predicted from the equations above by 200 kcal per day. Much of that variation has to do with your body composition. If most of your weight is fat, your BMR will probably fall below the predicted value. If most of your weight is lean tissue, you'll likely land above. That's one big reason people notice their metabolisms "slowing down" as they grow old: we tend to trade muscle for fat as we hit middle age and beyond.

Even within lean tissue there's a lot of variation in calories burned per day. Some of your organs are pretty metabolically quiet. Others burn enough energy each day to power a 3-mile run. Individual variation in the sizes of different organs, particularly the ratio of muscle to organ mass, can have a noticeable effect on BMR. Here's a behind-the-scenes look at the secret metabolic lives of your organs.

Muscle, Skin, Fat, and Bone

The largest organs are the quietest. For a typical U.S. adult, muscle accounts for 42 percent of body weight but only 16 percent of BMR, about 280 kcal per day (about 6 kcal/day per pound). Your skin weighs 11 pounds but burns only 30 kcal per day; your skeleton weighs a bit more but burns even less. Fat cells are more active than you might think. They make hormones and traffic in glucose and lipids to maintain energy supply to the body. Still, each pound of fat burns only about 2 kcal per day, for a total of about 85 kcal per day for a typical 150-pound adult with 30 percent body fat.

Heart and Lungs

Your heart is a pump made of muscle. It has its own electrical system, which is why Mayan rulers in ancient times could rip the hearts from the chests of sacrificial victims and the hearts would go on beating. With each beat, the heart pumps about 2.5 ounces (70 ml) of blood into the body via the aorta. That's about five quarts (or about five liters) per minute, nearly all the blood in your body. And that's just at rest! During exercise, you heart's output can easily triple. Amazingly, all this work is done for the low, low cost of about 2 calories per beat. Not *kilocalories,* just 2 calories (0.002 kcal). With a resting heart rate of 60 beats per minute, your heart burns about 8 kcal per hour, the energy equivalent of two M&M's. The heart accounts for about 12 percent of BMR. Lungs, for comparison, are more than twice as large but burn only about 80 kcal per day, or about 5 percent of BMR.

Kidneys

The kidneys are your body's housecleaning staff: tireless, essential, and underappreciated. In addition to maintaining precisely the right amount of water in your body, the kidneys handle the enormous task of clearing out waste and toxins, filtering 180 liters of blood a day. Millions of microscopic sieves (the nephrons) clean every drop of blood thirty times per day, pumping salts and other molecules in and out to eliminate the bad stuff and keep the good. And yet people will still spend untold money and time (mostly on the toilet) with fad "cleanses" promising to rid their body of toxins. Most of these products just give the kidneys more crap to clean up (seriously: stop it). The kidneys also perform an important metabolic task called gluconeogenesis, converting lactate, glycerol (from fat), and amino acids (from proteins) into glucose (Figure 2.1). All of this metabolic work takes a lot of energy. Together, your kidneys weigh only half a pound, but they burn about 140 kcal per day, accounting for 9 percent of BMR.

Liver

The liver is your body's unsung hero. This 3.5-pound metabolic factory is involved in nearly every life-sustaining process, including each of the major pathways in Figure 2.1. It is the main storage depot for glycogen, and does most of the work converting glucose to glycogen and glycogen back into glucose. It metabolizes fructose into fat for storage or into a burnable form of glucose. The liver breaks apart unused chylomicrons and stores the fat or repackages it into other lipoprotein containers (including the low-density lipoproteins, or LDLs, and the high-density lipoproteins, or HDLs, in your cholesterol report). The liver is the main site of gluconeogenesis, converting fats and amino acids to glucose when needed, and turning the nitrogen-bearing head of amino acids into urea to excrete in the urine. The liver is also the primary site of ketogenesis. Oh, and it breaks down a wide range of toxins, from alcohol to arsenic (but you should still *definitely* do that grapefruit and maple syrup cleanse . . .). All this ceaseless metabolic work burns about 300 kcal per day, 20 percent of BMR.

Gastrointestinal Tract

Like every other animal with a distinct mouth and butt, we are really just elaborate tubes. That tube is your gastrointestinal tract, which runs from your mouth to your stomach, then through your small and large intestines to your anus. It is the processing plant for digesting food and turning it into nutrients, as we discussed in Chapter 2. The human gastrointestinal tract weighs about 2.5 pounds and burns about 12 kcal per hour, and that's just at rest on an empty stomach. Digestion costs much more, about 10 percent of the daily calories consumed, or 250 to 300 kcal per day for the typical adult. It's unclear how much of the energy burned by the gut is attributable to the trillions of bacteria toiling away in our microbiome. A recent study in mice by Sarah Bahr, John Kirby, and colleagues suggests the calories burned by the microbiome might account for as much as 16 percent of BMR in humans, which would mean that the resting energy expenditure of the gastrointestinal tract (about 12 kcal per hour) is attributable almost entirely to gut bacteria. More research is needed to determine if that estimate is right, but it gives some sense of the daily energy expended by our bacterial friends.

Brain

The brain and liver share the title of "costliest organ." Your brain weighs a little less than 3 pounds but burns about 300 kcal per day, accounting for 20 percent of BMR. The high cost of brain tissue is the main reason large brains are so rare among animals. Only under rare circumstances does evolution favor channeling tons of energy into a large brain rather than directly into survival and reproduction. The brain is also a high-maintenance prima donna. It runs almost entirely on glucose (but can burn ketones in a pinch). Neurons, the gray-matter cells that do the work of cognition and control, sending and receiving signals, do little of their own housekeeping, Instead, the glial cells (white matter), which outnumber the neurons nearly 10 to 1, do much of the support work, providing nutrients and cleaning up waste.

Most of the work the brain does lies entirely outside of our conscious experience. The brain is ceaselessly busy sending and receiving signals to regulate and coordinate every aspect of life, from body temperature to reproduction. Thinking accounts for a tiny fraction of this work, and consequently the costs of cognition are small. Studies measuring energy expenditures before and during mental challenges have found only minuscule effects. Experienced chess players battling a superior opponent (a computer program) and subjects engaged in a challenging memory task increased their metabolic rates by only around 4 kcal per hour, the energy equivalent of a single M&M.

But while *thinking* is incredibly cheap, *learning* is quite energetically expensive. Learning is a physical process within the brain. Neurons, with their sinuous dendrites and axons stretching out like the branches of trees, form new connections (called *synapses*) with other neurons to make new neural circuits. Other synapses and circuits are broken, or "pruned." Our brains form, strengthen, and prune synapses throughout our lives (it's happening in your brain right now as you form new memories from reading this book) but by far the most active period is in childhood, when we're soaking up the world around us. Work by Christopher Kuzawa and colleagues has shown that in children three to seven years old, the brain accounts for over 60 percent of BMR, three times more than in adults. So much energy is channeled to the brain during these early critical years that it actually slows down growth in the rest of the body.

Beyond BMR

With all of your organs toiling away all day, it's little wonder that BMR accounts for most of the calories you burn each day, around 60 percent for most of us. Still, those are just the minimum costs, the energy expended while resting comfortably. Of course, life is rarely comfortable and calm. We aren't evolved to lie in bed all day. Our bodies are built to be out in the world, fighting off infection, battling the heat and cold, growing up, and having kids.

Thermoregulation

Mammals and birds have evolved to run hot. We burn a lot more energy each day than reptiles, fish, and other cold-blooded animals, and this ramped-up metabolic rate enables us to grow and reproduce more quickly (see below). But there's a catch: the complex metabolic stew of chemical reactions that keeps us alive needs to be kept within a narrow range of temperatures. If our body temperature rises or falls just a few degrees from normal (98.6°F, or 37°C), we can die.

All birds and mammals have a thermoneutral zone, a range of environmental temperatures where body temperature is maintained without any effort. For humans, the thermoneutral zone is roughly between 75°F and 93°F. If that seems like a high temperature range, that's because you probably don't walk around nude very often. With business attire (button-down shirt, pants, sport coat), the thermoneutral zone shifts colder, between 64°F and 75°F. That's probably the temperature you keep your house. Humans are masters of creating thermoneutral microenvironments next to our skin using clothing and our built environment. Our natural insulation, fat, can shift our thermoneutral zone as well. Adults who are obese have a thermoneutral range that's a couple of degrees colder than adults who aren't.

When we get cold, our bodies have two ways to generate more heat. First, we can burn a special type of fat called brown adipose tissue or brown fat, which makes up a tiny proportion of your body fat. Brown fat creates heat by modifying the electron transport system in its mitochondria: the protons sequestered in the intermembrane space are allowed to leak back through the membrane without producing any ATP. The energy that would be captured in the ATP is lost as heat. People living in the Arctic tend to have about 10 percent higher BMRs than those in warmer climates, which is probably due in part to brown fat activity. The second way we can generate heat is through shivering, which is simply involuntary muscle contraction. Mild cold exposures, like hanging out in shorts and T-shirt in a 65°F room, can raise your metabolic rate 25 percent above your BMR (that's an additional 16 kcal per hour for most of us). In extreme cold, shivering can cause our resting metabolic rate to climb above three times our BMR, a much larger effect than burning brown fat.

Getting too hot can also be fatal. Humans have evolved to deal with heat by becoming the sweatiest animals on the planet.

However, the energy costs of sweating haven't been carefully measured. They are likely very small. The main cost of dealing with heat seems to be the challenge of staying hydrated and avoiding heatstroke.

Immune Function

As the Covid-19 pandemic made clear to all of us, the world is full of nasty pathogens. But easy access to effective medical care—one of the triumphs of modernization—has led to a sort of cultural amnesia. We tend to forget how scary infectious disease is. Among the Hadza, acute infections kill four out of ten children before their fifteenth birthday. The numbers are equally grim in other hunter-gatherer and subsistence farming societies. Parents in developed countries with the gall to withhold medicine and vaccines from their kids should talk to some Hadza moms.

We are under constant assault from bacteria, viruses, and parasites that would like nothing more than to use our bodies as steamy brothels. In the mucky, organic world outside our walls, away from indoor plumbing and disinfectant, disease is unavoidable. I've got a buddy who works deep in the rain forests of Indonesia studying orangutans and gibbons. Inspired by bird watchers who keep a record of all the species they've seen over the years, he keeps a "Life List" of every tropical disease he's ever contracted. It's not a short list. Inevitably, coming home from a field season means a prescription for Flagyl to kill the beasts that have turned his guts into a frat house. You can't drink alcohol when you're on Flagyl, which he seems to regard as the worst part of the whole affair.

To respond to infection, immune system cells proliferate and manufacture a broad range of molecules. All of that metabolic work burns calories. A study of twenty-five U.S. college men who reported to a student health clinic found their BMRs were 8 percent higher, on average, than normal. Notably, the study excluded men who were running a fever. Ramping up body temperature to kill an infection with fever—an ancient mammalian defense—would increase BMR even more.

Michael Gurven and colleagues working with the Tsimane people of rural Bolivia have measured the daily cost of immune defense in populations without the antiseptic advantages of modernization. The Tsimane live in small, remote villages in the Amazonian rain forest. They have a mixed economy, hunting and gathering wild foods but also farming plantains, rice, manioc, or corn by hand. A small number, living in villages closer to towns, work manual labor jobs for cash. For everyone, daily life means being outdoors in the forest and on the river, interacting with the natural world and a host of bacteria, viruses, and parasites eager to find a host. Not surprisingly, the rates of infection are high. Around 70 percent of the population has a parasitic infection (usually worms) at any given time, and their white blood cell counts (the number of immune system cells the body has mustered to deal with infection) are ten times greater than we see among U.S. adults. All of this immune system activity burns energy. BMRs for Tsimane adults are 250 to 350 kcal per day higher than industrialized populations.

For kids, the costs of battling infection have serious consequences for growth. Sam Urlacher, a postdoc in my lab at Duke, has spent years working with children in the Shuar population of Ecuador. Daily life for the Shuar is very similar to that of the Tsimane, a mix of hunting and gathering and simple farming in the Amazonian rain forest. Like the Tsimane, the Shuar have high rates of infection. Sam found that Shuar kids five to twelve years old have BMRs that are about 200 kcal per day higher than kids in the United States and Europe, a 20 percent difference. The energy demand of fighting infection steals calories away from growth. When our immune system responds to an infection, it makes a number of molecules (immunoglobulins, antibodies, and other proteins) that circulate in the blood—telltale signs of the battles fought against bacteria, viruses, and parasites. Sam found that Shuar kids with more of these markers in their blood grew slower than those who had fewer. The cost of immune response, in terms of both calories and growth, is probably one big reason that indigenous populations like the Shuar, Tsimane, and Hadza tend to be short-statured.

Growth and Reproduction

It is a fundamental law of nature that mass and energy can never be created or destroyed, but only moved around and transformed from one form to another. Making a human is no different: whether it's mom building a fetus or kids building themselves, growth requires food and energy. More precisely, the energy content of the tissue added has to equal the energy content of the nutrients used to build it. So what's the cost of a pound of flesh?

Our bodies are built from a conglomerate of protein, fat, and carbohydrate—the same macronutrients we eat. The energy content of those building blocks is the same as it is in food: 4 kcal per gram of carbohydrate (like glycogen) or protein (like muscle), 9 kcal per gram of fat (see Chapter 2). Living tissue also holds a good deal of water (about 65 percent of its weight), which has no calories. As children grow, the energy content of new tissue, which is a mix of about 75 percent lean tissue and 25 percent fat, works out to about 1,500 kcal per pound. To that we have to add the energy burned to do the work of disassembling the nutrients from our diet and reassembling them into tissue, which comes to about 700 kcal per pound. The cost of growth, then, is about 2,200 kcal per pound.

The type of tissue added affects cost. Adding a higher proportion of fat costs more, whereas adding a higher proportion of lean tissue (like muscle) costs less, because the energy content of fat is more than twice that of protein. One way to see that difference is to look at the energy burned when we lose weight—the mirror image of growth. The energy we expend to lose weight has to be equal to the energy content of the tissue that's been lost. Since the tissue we lose during weight loss is mostly fat, the general rule is that it takes about 3,500 kcal to burn off one pound.

For mothers, the cost of growth is only a fraction of the cost of pregnancy and nursing. A newborn baby weighs, on average, between seven and eight pounds. The cost to grow that much baby is only about 17,000 kcal. But the mother also adds tissue of her own (typical weight gain during pregnancy is about twenty-five to thirty pounds) and has to pay the daily metabolic cost of keeping all that new tissue—the fetus plus herself—alive. The total cost of a healthy nine-month pregnancy is about 80,000 kcal. That's 27 percent more energy than the typical Hadza woman spends walking over the course of a year.

Nursing is even more costly. Milk production for mothers whose children are exclusively breastfeeding (no other foods) costs about 500 kcal per day, which comes out to about 180,000 kcal per year—more than hiking the Appalachian Trail. Some of that energy comes from fat stores built up during pregnancy (about 3,500 kcal per pound lost). And, just as in pregnancy, most of that energy fuels the baby's BMR and other expenditure. Only a small portion goes to the growth of new tissue.

The Game of Life

But to consider growth and reproduction solely as costs misses a fundamental point: those calories aren't simply spent, they're invested. As far as evolution is concerned, life is a game of turning energy into offspring. More energy for reproduction means more offspring, which is how the game is won: by flooding the next generation with more copies of your genes than anyone else's. More energy for growth and reproduction can also mean larger offspring, which have a better chance of surviving to reproduce themselves. Any other expenditures—immune defense, brains, digestion—are worthwhile only to the extent that they improve the ability, over the long term, to channel energy into reproduction.

It's unsurprising, then, that life history—the pace of growth, reproduction, and aging—is tightly bound to metabolic rate. The two great leaps in metabolic evolution, from cold-blooded reptiles to warm-blooded birds, and (independently) to warm-blooded mammals, were directly tied to changes in the way these animals grow and reproduce. Mammals and birds evolved turbocharged metabolisms, burning ten times more calories per day than their reptilian ancestors. In each case, this radical metabolic acceleration was favored by natural selection because it increased energy for growth and reproduction. Mammals grow five times faster than reptiles and channel about four times more energy into reproduction. Birds have similarly high rates of growth and reproductive output.

Nature plays chess, not checkers. There are as many winning strategies in the game of life as there are species on the planet. The best play depends on local conditions and on the strategies of those around you. High-energy strategies have obvious advantages, but low-energy risk-averse strategies can be winners as well. Reptiles, fish, insects, and other cold-blooded, slow-metabolism groups remain incredibly successful despite the advance of mammals and birds. The earliest members of our group, the primates, evolved a much slower metabolic rate and life history around sixty-five million years ago (see Chapter 1). It turned out to be a savvy move. Short-term growth and reproduction were reduced, but the slower metabolic rate also stretched out the life span, and lifetime reproductive success improved. Primates conceded the sprint but won the marathon, becoming one of the most successful and prolific mammalian groups.

Metabolic rate shapes life history within groups as well. For each of the major groups of vertebrates—placental mammals (primates and non-primates), marsupials, reptiles, birds, fish, amphibians—metabolic rate increases with body size in a distinct curve (Figure 3.2). Just as we saw with human BMR (above), calories per day rises steeply among small animals but grows shallower with larger species. This is Kleiber's law of metabolism, named for the pioneering Swiss nutritionist Max Kleiber, who, along with others, described the relationship between metabolic rate and body size in the 1930s. Using measurements of BMR for a range of species, Kleiber argued that metabolic rate increased with body mass to the ¾ power, or $mass^{0.75}$. Nearly a century later, we now know that the same is true for total daily energy expenditures, not just the portion spent on BMR. Groups differ in the height of the curve (e.g., reptiles have lower curves than mammals) but all have an exponent (the shape of the curve) around 0.75, as shown in Figure 3.3.

As we see in Figure 3.3, daily energy expenditure is a function of body size: larger animals burn more calories per day. But an exponent less than 1 means that small animals burn a lot more energy *per pound* of tissue than large animals. For reasons that still aren't well understood, the cells of small animals work harder and burn energy faster than the cells of large animals. Each cell in a mouse burns ten times more energy each day than a cell in a caribou.

Rates of growth and reproduction follow these same distinctive curves. Within birds, mammals (primates and others), and reptiles, rates of growth and reproduction increase with body mass with exponents in the neighborhood of Kleiber's 0.75, ranging from 0.45 to 0.82. That means that, for their body size, small animals grow faster and reproduce more than larger animals. A 220-pound caribou female will produce one 14-pound calf each year, equivalent to 6

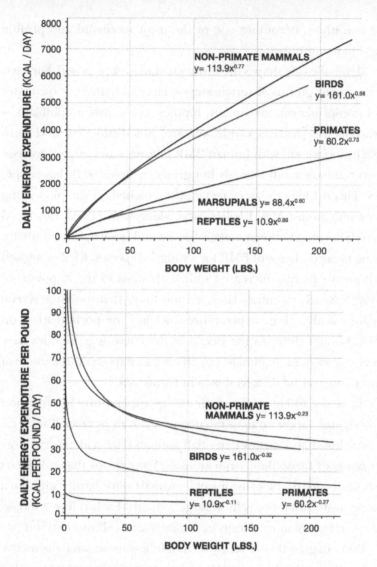

Figure 3.3. Daily energy expenditure across non-primate (NP) mammals, birds, primates, and reptiles. Birds and non-primate mammals burn much more energy each day than primates, marsupials, and reptiles. Larger animals burn more energy each day (top panel). But smaller animals burn far more energy per pound than large animals (bottom panel), following Kleiber's law. Species with greater energy expenditure per pound tend to grow faster, reproduce more, and die at earlier ages than those with lower expenditure per pound. Primates (including humans) burn much less energy each day than other mammals, which corresponds with primates' slow life history schedules and long lives.

percent of her own body weight. In that same amount of time, a 1-ounce female mouse will produce about five litters of seven pups each, equivalent to 500 percent of her body weight. The difference corresponds fairly well with the mouse's ten times higher rate of cellular metabolism. Growth rates compare the same way. Mice grow to thirty times their birthweight in just forty-two days; caribou grow to fifteen times their birthweight and it takes them nearly two years. Metabolic rates aren't the only thing determining rates of growth and reproduction, but they sure seem to set the broad framework.

One Billion Heartbeats

Metabolic rates also seem to determine how much time we get on this earthly plane. When we look around at the dogs, cats, hamsters, and other animals in our lives, we notice a lot of variability in life expectancy among species. Hamsters are lucky to get three years; a cat might live into its teens. We humans can reasonably hope for eighty or more. None of us has a prayer of reaching two hundred years old, a typical life span for a bowhead whale. Instead, even if we avoid accidents and disease, we'll inevitably succumb to "natural causes." But why is it *natural* to die, and why is it *natural* for some species to live for centuries while others get only months?

The biology of death is an area of intense and active research, but researchers have long been aware of an apparent connection to metabolism: the slower a species burns energy, the longer it tends to live. It's an ancient observation. Aristotle, writing *On Longevity and the Shortness of Life* in 350 B.C., compared life to a burning candle and observed that "the nutriment, to wit the smoke, which [a small flame] takes a long period to expend, is used up by the big flame quickly." Since the cells of smaller species burn energy more quickly, the link to metabolic rate also helps to explain why they tend to have shorter life expectancies. Aristotle noticed that as well, writing that "it is a general rule that the larger live longer than the smaller." He was wrong on the mechanism (he thought animals aged because they dried out), and of course had no idea about Kleiber's law, but the early inkling that death was inherently linked to metabolism was there.

Max Rubner, a giant in the science of metabolism in the late 1800s and early 1900s, was the first to put the pieces together into a coherent theory of metabolism and aging. Comparing the metabolic rates and life spans of guinea pigs, cats, dogs, cows, and horses, Rubner observed that the total energy expended per gram of tissue over the life span of the animal was nearly constant despite the enormous differences in body size and metabolism. Rubner proposed that cells had some intrinsic limit on lifetime energy expenditure. When they used up their lifetime allotment, they died, like a candle running out of wax. This "rate of living" theory was further developed and championed by the American biologist Raymond Pearl, an early pioneer in the study of aging, in the 1920s.

Rubner's rate of living theory was insightful and fit the early data but ultimately fell out of favor. We know now, with the benefit of lots more metabolic and life history data, that species with similar metabolic rates often have very different life spans. And faster metabolic rates don't inevitably mean a shorter life. Small birds, for example, tend to have faster metabolic rates than mammals of the same body size, but generally live longer.

A more promising explanation for the apparent link between longevity and metabolism came in the 1950s, with the free radical theory of aging. First proposed by Denham Harman, an American researcher with degrees in medicine and chemistry, the free radical theory proposes that aging is the accumulation of damage caused by toxic by-products of oxidative phosphorylation. In the electron transport chain, the end process of making ATP in the mitochondria (Chapter 2), oxygen molecules are occasionally transformed into free radicals (also called reactive oxygen species), which are oxygen molecules that have lost an electron. These mutant oxygen species are voracious, and they rip electrons from surrounding molecules, causing damage to DNA, lipids, and proteins. Harman argued that aging is the accumulation of damage (sometimes called oxidative stress or oxidative damage) from these free radicals. Since free radicals are an unavoidable by-product of making ATP, it follows that our cells' metabolic rates (which are also their rates of ATP production) determine how quickly we age and die.

The free radical theory could also account for many instances where metabolic rate and longevity diverge. There are a number of evolved mechanisms to neutralize free radicals and repair the damage they cause. But, like every physiological task, these counterstrategies require energy—nothing is free. Depending on their evolved niche, species might evolve to invest more or less energy into repairing oxidative damage. A mouse, under constant threat of falling prey to any number of predators, might be evolved to channel more energy into reproducing now and less into repairing oxidative damage for a future that may never come. A sparrow, on the other hand, might have a similar metabolic rate, but because it's better equipped to evade predation, it could be evolved to channel more resources into maintenance and repair in order to reap the benefits of a longer life span.

The free radical theory of aging has its problems. For one, studies of antioxidant consumption in humans and other animals don't always show the expected effects on life span. The difficulties in finding clear, strong links between metabolism and longevity have left some researchers lamenting whether such links exist at all. For all its grim certainty, death has proven to be a surprisingly slippery subject in biology. Definitive answers remain at large.

Still, the similarities in metabolic rate and longevity are difficult to ignore. Lab studies in monkeys, mice, and other species have shown that reducing their metabolic rate by reducing how much they're allowed to eat leads to longer life spans, and similar calorie restriction studies in humans show promising results. Variation in life expectancy among mammals, birds, and reptiles fits with what we'd expect from size-related differences in metabolic rate. Cells in mice burn energy ten times faster than the cells in a caribou, and their lives are about ten times shorter (even when they die of "natural causes"). As we discussed in Chapter 1, primates burn only half as many calories each day as other placental mammals (Figure 3.3), which accounts nicely for the long lives that humans and other primates enjoy. Other low-energy species live long lives as well. Cold-blooded Greenland sharks can live four hundred years. Just as with the rates of growth and reproduction, metabolism isn't the only factor affecting life span across animals, but it seems to determine the broad patterns.

Whether the relationship between metabolism and mortality is simply coincidental or (as I suspect) there's a deeper connection, something strange and wonderful emerges from the way that life span and metabolic rate change with size and across animal groups. Since the heart has to pump enough blood to all tissues in the body to meet the demand for nutrients and oxygen, heart rates (beats per minute) match the cellular metabolic rates: they are faster in small species and slower in large species. But since small animals also die earlier than large animals, the total number of heartbeats in a lifetime are the same across species, from the tiniest shrews to the mightiest whales. We all get about one billion heartbeats.*

---

* Give or take a few hundred million. And no, you can't stave off death by rationing your heartbeats. In fact, elevating your heart rate by exercising is one of the most surefire ways to live longer (Chapter 7).

The Devilish Arithmetic of Daily Energy Expenditure

With the costs of walking, running, digesting, breathing, reproducing, and everything else so well studied, you might think that calculating your total daily energy expenditure was a straightforward arithmetic problem: calculate your BMR and add the costs of the day's activities. You would be in very good company, but you would still be wrong. In fact, daily energy expenditure is surprisingly tough to pin down, and after more than a half century of trying, we still get it wrong. The problem, as we began to discuss in Chapter 1, is that our bodies are not simple machines. Our metabolic engines are dynamic, adaptive products of evolution. Daily expenditure is not simply the sum of its parts.

The simple armchair engineer view of metabolism dates back to the postwar era in the United States and Europe. With the widespread starvation and other atrocities of World War II fresh in their minds, researchers were interested in figuring out humans' daily nutritional requirements. They had a ton of data on human energy expenditure at their disposal; people like Frank Benedict and his colleague J. Arthur Harris had been amassing large datasets since the early 1900s. But, crucially, no one had any measures of total daily energy expenditure—the data they really were after—because no one had figured out how to measure it. Instead, they had measurements of BMR. Everyone knew that BMR was just one component of total daily expenditure, but the remainder was a mystery. So scientists did what anyone would do in that situation: they tried to make a good guess.

Using lab measurements of the energy costs for various activities, nutritionists at the World Health Organization built a framework for estimating daily expenditure. First, you estimate a person's BMR from their weight, height, and age, using equations similar to those above. Next, you figure out what a person does all day: how much sleep they get, the hours spent walking, sitting, working, and doing other tasks. Each task is assigned an energy cost, expressed as some multiple of BMR, called a physical activity ratio, or PAR. PARs are essentially the same as MET values in Table 3.1. Combining the daily schedule of activities with the energy costs of each, you get an average daily level of expenditure expressed as some multiple of basal metabolic rate. For example, if a person spent twelve hours sleeping (1.0 PAR) and twelve hours doing laundry and other light housework (2.0 PAR), their average twenty-four-hour expenditure would be 1.5 PAR, or one and a half times their basal metabolic rate. Multiply 1.5 by their estimated BMR and you've got their estimated daily energy expenditure.

This approach, called the factorial method, was crude, but it seemed to give reasonable results. And it remains alive and well today: it's still used by the World Health Organization to figure out daily caloric needs for populations they work with, and it's the math behind every online calculator that estimates your daily calorie needs from some combination of height, weight, age (all used to estimate your basal metabolic rate) and your level of physical activity (used to assign an average daily PAR value).

Decades after its development, the factorial method remains just what it was always meant to be: a good guess. Factorial estimates of daily expenditure are in the right ballpark because BMR is predictable from body size and age. BMR makes up most of the energy burned each day, so if you have a good estimate of BMR, you'll end up with a reasonable estimate of total daily expenditure.

But the reasonable estimates you get from the factorial method hide its fundamental flaw. It assumes that daily energy expenditure is simply BMR plus the costs of physical activity and digestion. That view has become so accepted and widespread that it's hard to imagine any other perspective. It's what every student in nutrition and metabolism is taught, what every aspiring doctor learns in medical school, and it's the guiding faith of every exercise weight-loss program. As we'll discuss in Chapter 5, it's not that simple—not by a long shot. The bottom line is that your daily activity level has almost no bearing on the number of calories you burn each day.

Don't Bother Asking

The next big innovation in determining energy expenditures was, like many big innovations, a total failure and a huge step backward. It started with an even simpler premise than the factorial method: if we want to know how much food people eat each day, let's just ask them! It seemed reasonable enough (you can remember what you ate yesterday, right?) and the data could be collected for millions of people with hardly any effort. No need to get heights, weights, and ages, monitor daily activity, calculate PAR values, or anything like that. Just have people fill out a survey.

The idea isn't completely absurd. Since most people are in energy balance most of the time (the calories they take in matches the calories they expend each day), getting solid data on food intake should, in principle, provide a good measurement of daily expenditure. But, like most schemes that depend on human honesty and self-awareness, it was doomed from the start.

It turns out people are shockingly bad at keeping track of what they eat. When you give someone a dietary recall survey and ask them about their diet, the answers aren't reliable. It's like asking people how many times they've had impure thoughts about Brad Pitt: everyone underreports. In a recent study of 324 men and women across five countries, adults underreported actual food intake by 29 percent on average. That's the equivalent of forgetting an entire meal *every day*. Reported energy intake didn't track expenditure whatsoever. Diet surveys are just random number generators, and the data they provide on daily calorie consumption are useless. The only way to make them *worse* than useless is to treat them like real data and base a nutritional program on them.

So in 1990, the U.S. Food and Drug Administration based the nation's public nutrition program on diet surveys. New regulations were being implemented that would require nutritional labels on food packaging, and the FDA wanted some benchmark for daily energy intake to include on the labels. Using surveys from the massive National Health and Nutrition Examination Survey, they found that women reported food intakes of about 1,600 to 2,200 kilocalories per day, while men reported intakes of 2,000 to 3,000. That would leave a rough average for all adults of somewhere between 2,000 and 2,500 kilocalories per day. To discourage overconsumption, and to have a nice round number to work with, they rounded down to 2,000, and that's the number that stuck. Now you know who to blame if you thought that the typical American eats a 2,000-kilocalorie diet.

The Ballad of Nathan Lifson

In the 1950s, around the same time researchers were developing the factorial method, Nathan Lifson, a physiologist at the University of Minnesota, was exploring a very different approach for calculating daily energy expenditure. Lifson was a Minnesota native, born in the Gopher State in 1911. He spent nearly all his adult life at the University of Minnesota, earning his bachelor's degree in 1931, his PhD in 1943, and, other than a two-year stint in San Diego (where he apparently learned to hate sunshine and warmth), staying on at the University of Minnesota for his entire fifty-plus year career. His graduate training coincided with the big developments in metabolic science by Kleiber and his contemporaries, and so perhaps it makes sense that Lifson was eventually drawn to the challenge of measuring daily energy expenditures.

To understand Lifson's breakthrough, we need to start with the observation that the body is essentially a big pool of water (about 65 percent of you is H_2O). In fact, our body water is like a lake, with an inflow and an outflow. The hydrogen and oxygen atoms in our body water pool are in constant flux, entering the body water in our food and drink and leaving the body as urine, feces, sweat, and the water vapor in our breath.

In his early work, Lifson figured out that the oxygen atoms in the body water pool have an alternative way to leave the body. When carbon dioxide (CO_2) is formed during the metabolism of some carbon-based molecule (see Chapter 2), one of the oxygen atoms in the new CO_2 molecule is taken from the body water. That oxygen atom is then exhaled in the CO_2 that we breathe out. The bottom line is this: hydrogens leave the body only as water; oxygens leave as both water and CO_2.

Lifson realized that if he could track the rate of hydrogen and oxygen atoms leaving the body, he would be able to calculate the rate of CO_2 production. And since you can't burn energy without making and exhaling CO_2, Lifson knew that if he could measure the rate of CO_2 production, he could measure energy expenditure. Best of all, the subjects wouldn't have to be trapped in a metabolic chamber. As long as he could track their rates of hydrogen and oxygen flow with the occasional urine sample, the subjects could do whatever they liked.

The tricky part was tracking the hydrogen and oxygen atoms in the body water. Lifson hit on the idea of using isotopes, which are atoms that have the normal number of protons but an unusual number of neutrons. For example, normal oxygen has eight protons and eight neutrons, whereas the isotope oxygen-18 has eight protons and ten neutrons. Deuterium is an isotope of hydrogen that has one neutron (normal hydrogen doesn't have any neutrons). There are trace amounts of these isotopes in the water you drink every day. They aren't harmful. (Only some isotopes are radioactive, giving off harmful radiation as they decay into other types of atoms.)

Working with mice, Lifson used those isotopes to track the flow oxygen and hydrogen atoms as they left the body. The isotopes acted just like normal oxygen and hydrogen atoms in the body, but he could use them as tracers. If 10 percent of the hydrogens in the subject's body water were deuterium on Monday, but only 5 percent of them were deuterium on Wednesday, he would know that half of the body water from Monday had been flushed out and replenished with normal H_2O. He then could use those measurements to calculate the rate at which hydrogen atoms were lost. The same approach would tell him the rate of loss for oxygen atoms. The difference between those two rates had to reflect the rate of CO_2 production. Lifson's mouse studies showed that isotopic measurements matched the CO_2 production measured by the metabolic chamber perfectly.

Since you can't burn calories without making CO_2, Lifson's method provided a precise and accurate measurement of daily energy expenditure. The best part was that subjects didn't need to sit in a chamber: as long as they provided urine or blood samples every few days to measure their isotope levels, they could go about their lives doing whatever they wanted. He had invented the impossible: a reliable means of measuring daily expenditure during normal life.

There was only the small matter of price. The amount of isotope needed for the measurement is proportional to body size. That made studies in mice or other small animals relatively cheap, but posed a challenge for human work. In 1955, the amount of isotope needed for a 150-pound human would cost more than $250,000 in today's dollars. By the 1970s, some creative researchers in animal physiology, like Ken Nagy and Klaas Westerterp, were using Lifson's method in birds and lizards in the wild. Nagy even partnered with primatologist Katharine Milton to measure daily energy expenditures in wild howler monkeys. But other than a handful of studies in small species, Lifson's method didn't catch on.

It would take another decade of advancements in the production and measurement of isotopes to get the cost of human studies into a more manageable range. By the 1980s, deuterium and oxygen-18 were cheap enough to measure an adult human for just 1 percent of what it would have cost in the 1950s or '60s. The 1980s were also the early stages of the global obesity pandemic, and researchers were keen to have a method for measuring energy expenditure outside the lab. Dale Schoeller, then at Argonne National Laboratory in Chicago, stumbled upon Lifson's work while researching a study using oxygen-18 to measure the body water pool. Realizing that technology and costs had changed enough to make the method cost-effective, Schoeller went about adapting Lifson's method to humans. Schoeller published the first doubly labeled water study in humans in 1982. A new field in human metabolism was born.

Soon it was clear that much of what was thought to be known about energy expenditure was wrong. Lifson's method had pushed the science of human metabolism into a new era. By that time, nearly thirty years after his initial publication on the method, Lifson was an emeritus (semiretired) professor, too late in his career to join in the era of discovery. But he lived long enough to see his contribution spark a revolution in metabolic research and garner some of the recognition it deserved. Schoeller had telephoned Lifson in early stages of the first human study, and he was an enthusiastic supporter, happy to hear his idea was taking flight. In 1986, Andrew Prentice at Cambridge convened a British Nutrition Society symposium on the doubly labeled water method, with Lifson as the guest of honor. The following year, Lifson was awarded the prestigious Rank Prize in nutrition for his discovery. He died two years later.

The Doubly Labeled Water Revolution

With Lifson's method—more commonly called the doubly labeled water method—we finally have accurate and reliable measurements of daily energy expenditure for people during normal daily life. These days, labs like mine can measure a person's daily energy expenditure using doubly labeled water for about six hundred dollars. In the three decades since Schoeller adapted the method to humans, the field has measured thousands of people around the world and across the life span. So what's the bottom line? How many calories do we spend each day? It depends, of course—but not on the factors you might think.

The biggest predictors of daily energy expenditure are the size and composition of your body. Bigger people are made of more cells, and more cells doing more metabolic work burn more calories each day. And as we saw above, some of our organs and tissues burn more calories than others. Most important, fat cells burn a lot less energy each day than lean tissue, the cells that make up our muscles and other organs. If fat cells make up a larger proportion of your body weight, you will burn fewer calories each day than a person who weighs the same but is leaner. Since women tend to carry more body fat than men, women tend to burn fewer calories each day than men who weigh the same.

I compiled data from hundreds of doubly labeled water measurements of men, women, and children into a plot of daily energy expenditure against body weight for men and women (Figure 3.4). As you can see in those plots, daily energy expenditure (in kcal per day) increases with body weight (which is in pounds) in a curved manner, similar to the Kleiber's law scaling of energy expenditure and size across species (Figure 3.3).

The equations in Figure 3.4 provide reliable estimates of daily energy expenditure for all humans, from infants to elderly, skinny to stout. You can plug your body weight into the appropriate equation and calculate an estimated daily energy expenditure. Notice, though, the *ln* function in each equations. That means you need to take the natural logarithm of weight before multiplying the result by 786 (females) or 1,105 (males) and subtracting the appropriate intercept value. If your math skills are a little rusty, you can also just find where you fall on the plots in Figure 3.4 to figure out your estimated daily energy expenditure. A 140-pound woman has an estimated daily energy expenditure of 2,300 kcal per day. For a 160-pound man, expected daily energy expenditure is 3,000 kcal per day.

The effect of body size on expenditure is striking. The shape of the relationship with size is similar to the diminishing Kleiber's law curve we see among species (Figure 3.3). Daily expenditure rises steeply with body size in children. Their cells burn much more energy each day than larger, older people. If you've ever held a baby close and felt her heartbeat thrumming in her tiny chest, you have a sense of how hard her body is working. Each pound of a typical three-year-old kid burns about 35 kcal per day. That number steadily declines through childhood and adolescence, flattening out at around 15 kcal per pound each day in our early twenties.

The curved relationship between body weight and daily energy expenditure means that we need to be thoughtful when we compare energy expenditures among individuals. Often, people (including researchers and doctors, who ought to know better) simply divide energy expenditure by weight as a way of comparing metabolic rates among different-sized people. The assumption underlying that approach is that energy expenditure per pound ought to be the same for everyone. But that's not how it works. Because the relationship between size and expenditure is curved the way it is (Figure 3.4), smaller people *inherently* burn more energy per pound (or per kilogram) than larger people. That's just the way the

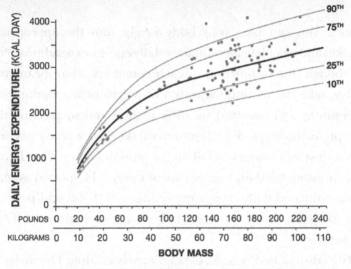

MALE: DAILY ENERGY EXPENDITURE = 1,105 x *LN*(WEIGHT) - 2613

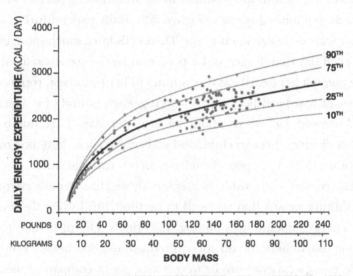

FEMALE: DAILY ENERGY EXPENDITURE = 786 x *LN*(WEIGHT) - 1582

Figure 3.4. Human daily energy expenditure (kcal per day). The heavy curved trend lines and equations give the expected daily energy expenditure for a given body weight. To determine your estimated daily expenditure, find your weight on the horizontal x-axis and track straight up, vertically, to the trend line. Then track horizontally left to the vertical y-axis to find your estimated expenditure. You can also use the equations. For children less than twenty pounds, use the Female panel. Each gray dot represents the average weight and expenditure for one of the 284 doubly labeled water study populations used to compile this figure. The amount of variability is substantial. It's not uncommon for an individual's daily expenditure to deviate from the expected value by ±300 kcal per day. The lighter lines show the 10th, 25th, 75th, and 90th percentiles for expenditure.

biology and the arithmetic work. If we compare daily energy expenditures (or BMRs, for that matter) by simply dividing metabolic rate by body size, we will get the mistaken impression that little people and big people are wildly different, when in fact they are all adhering to the same fundamental relationship.

A better way to ask if a person or a population has a particularly high or low metabolic rate is to plot them on a chart like Figure 3.4 and see how they compare to the trend line. This is the same approach that pediatricians use when they plot a child's height or weight on a growth chart. The chart (or in our case, Figure 3.4) allows the doctor to see if the child falls above or below expectations.

The small gray dots in Figure 3.4 are the population averages from 284 male and female study populations. The heavy black curved line is the trend line for energy expenditure: the average daily energy expenditure for any given body size. As with any average, half of the populations fall above that trend line and half of them fall below. We can say that the populations falling above the trend line have higher than expected daily energy expenditures; populations that fall below have lower than expected daily energy expenditures.

One thing to notice with Figure 3.4 is the amount of variation in daily energy expenditures, even after we account for body size. Many populations fall above or below the trend line—their *expected* daily expenditure—by 300 kcal per day or more. This is the dirty little secret of online BMR and daily expenditure calculators: there is a ton of variation in metabolic rates even after we account for body size and gender. When you plug your info in and get a daily expenditure or BMR back—or find your expected daily expenditure using Figure 3.4—you need to take that number with a large pinch of salt. It could easily be off by a few hundred kilocalories. The idea that some people have "fast" metabolisms while others' are "slow" is not diet magazine hooey. It's reality.

• • •

We used to think we understood why people differed in their daily energy expenditure. Surely, we thought, one could simply add up the kilocalories spent on physical activity, organ function, growth, thermoregulation, digestion, and the rest, and calculate a person's daily energy expenditure. And it's true, of course, that daily expenditure must include all of those costs. But the doubly labeled water revolution has provided a wake-up call, a surprising reality check. Rather than simply adding up like the grocery bill at checkout, all the pieces of daily expenditure—activity, immune function, growth, and the rest—interact and affect each other in dynamic and complex ways. Daily energy expenditure isn't just the sum of its parts.

The New Science of Human Metabolism

The long history of metabolic science gives the field a sense of familiarity and certainty. It stretches back more than two centuries to the visionary work of Lavoisier and his Enlightenment contemporaries. The golden era of discovery by pioneers like the two Maxes (Rubner and Kleiber) and others is nearly a hundred years old. The most common methods used to estimate energy expenditures—the factorial method and dietary surveys—have been around for decades. It's easy to think we know everything there is to know about how our bodies burn energy.

But there is an incredible amount of metabolic diversity among individuals, populations, and species that the established ideas about energy expenditure can't explain. There's much more to metabolic variation among species, including our own, than Kleiber's law. People and populations vary in the energy they burn every day, but the simple arithmetic of the factorial method doesn't capture what our bodies are doing.

Why do humans burn around 2,500 to 3,000 kcal per day? Why do some of us burn more energy each day than expected for our size, while others burn less? How does our metabolism affect our health and longevity? And how does our lifestyle, our daily routines of physical activity and diet, affect our energy expenditure and metabolic health?

The rest of this book tackles these big questions. With a solid understanding of how our body's metabolic machinery works from these last two chapters, we launch into the new era of discovery in the science of human metabolism. We start in an unlikely place, a tiny village in the Republic of Georgia, in the foothills of the Caucasus Mountains along the Ancient Silk Road.

CHAPTER 4

How Humans Evolved to Be the Nicest, Fittest, and *Fattest* Apes

Early on a cool, dewy July morning I awoke in my little tent and gingerly worked my way out of my sleeping bag and through the damp zippered door. The confines of the yellow nylon dome opened out to a panoramic view of dark forested hills and pale green pastures. My tent and several others were scattered about the scruffy lawn beside the dig house, a two-story dormitory and kitchen for our crowded team of archaeologists, geologists, and paleoanthropologists. We were midway through our annual field season, excavating stone tools and fossils of *Homo erectus.*

Somewhere far below me, too distant to hear, the Pinasaouri River rushed past the ruins of old bathhouses that once welcomed travelers and traders along the Ancient Silk Road. Across the valley, the collapsed stone tombs of Mongol invaders dotted the fields on the distant hillside. Above them, perched on a high point along the ridge, sat the remains of a proud medieval city. And in the soil beneath those ruins were the 1.8-million-year-old fossilized bones of ancient near-humans. The entire landscape was a layer-cake monument to our impermanence. Wave upon ceaseless wave of ambition and folly.

Something began to rise within me, a dark and churning tide.

I stumbled toward the edge of the small clearing and puked all over the bushes. The hand of some vengeful god gripped my body and squeezed violently to exorcise the evil within. Hands on knees, eyes watering, I spewed hot, frothy garbage. The initial eruption was followed by diminishing aftershocks of convulsion. Retching heaves wracked my body; it felt like my eyeballs might pop from their orbits and dangle helplessly by the optic nerves. And then finally, mercifully, it was done. Wrung out and crumpled like an old tube of toothpaste, I wiped my mouth with the back of my hand and slowly straightened myself up.

There is a deep and perfect calm that follows such abominations, a brief respite from the headache, nausea, and sense of impending doom of a truly horrific hangover. In those moments of clarity, I considered my position. The unlikely circumstances and accidents of history that had made this magical place. My incredible good fortune in somehow finding myself here. Ah, but I had been ungrateful. Spoiled. It hadn't been enough just to be here. I had overindulged, letting the first glass of wine at last night's dinner turn into a drunken party under the stars. I wasn't alone. I turned to walk toward the long communal table on the dig house porch and saw a few of my fellow revelers, bleary-eyed, begin to bravely face their tea and bread.

As I slowly walked over to join them, I had a vague notion of turning things around, of using this moment to grow and mature and leave such self-destructive foolishness behind for good. With battery acid breath I mouthed the silent prayer of idiots everywhere: *Next time will be different.* This wasn't my first rodeo. I knew the long odds against real reform, but as I stood there in the calm eye of the hurricane I was optimistic. We were a clever crew, after all—budding scientists pursuing our PhDs at prestigious academic institutions from around the world. We had the intelligence and temperament to earn competitive spots in top-tier graduate programs and to work our way here, one of the most exciting fossil sites on the planet.

Surely we had enough good sense to be careful and moderate, to ensure our own self-preservation. True, none of us had demonstrated any talent for self-restraint, but c'mon. Surely we could enjoy the fruits of our evolved human intelligence and collective effort without letting curiosity and hedonism destroy us . . .

The thought disintegrated like a cloud, unfinished. It was time to try to have some breakfast. There were fossils to be discovered, and they weren't going to excavate themselves. I slumped down onto the long bench next to the others at the table, grabbed a slice of bread with unsure hands, and slathered on some butter and honey. I took a sip of tea. Already I could sense my hangover returning, like the distant hoofbeats of a Mongol horde.

It was my annual pilgrimage to the Lower Paleolithic site of Dmanisi in the Republic of Georgia. Every summer during grad school I'd take a break from treadmills and metabolism and make the trek out to the tiny farming village of Patara Dmanisi in the foothills of the Caucasus Mountains. Month-long detours from thesis work aren't exactly recommended for success in grad school, but it was too interesting and too fun to miss. What I didn't appreciate at the time was how connected the site was to my research in human energetics, and how it crystallized a critical period in our metabolic evolution. Our departure from the world of apes, the first evolutionary steps toward something much more human, are captured here. And the secret sauce that made it all work were changes in the way we acquired food and burned calories—changes we're still grappling with today.

An Unlikely Place

Dmanisi is an unassuming location for one of the most important sites in human evolution. All of the other hominin fossil sites from this period, around two million years ago, are found in the dry, gravelly badlands of East and Southern Africa, familiar to anyone who's ever thumbed through a *National Geographic*: Olduvai Gorge, the Great Rift Valley, the cave sites of South Africa. Dmanisi, in stark contrast, is green and leafy, and Georgia, a gorgeous and proud country with a rich history, is distant and obscure to most people outside the region. Yet its geography is precisely what makes Dmanisi so important.

The human lineage split from that of chimpanzees and bonobos roughly seven million years ago (Figure 4.1). But for the first five million years, our ancestors remained in Africa, restricted to a particular set of habitats where their apelike strategies were effective. Then around two million years ago, we hopped the ecological fence. Hominins (species on the human branch of the ape family tree) became smart and adaptable enough to thrive anywhere. Populations grew and spread across Africa and then into Eurasia, stretching from South Africa to Morocco to Indonesia. This was the radical break from an apelike past and into something much more human. Dmanisi is the earliest grainy snapshot we have from this critical period. At 1.8 million years old, it's the earliest hominin fossil site outside of Africa. The stones and bones beneath the soil there capture the first evolutionary inklings of what makes us human. And the key evolutionary advantage that made these hominins so successful, fueling their global expansion, was a change in the way they acquired and burned energy.

My first trip to Dmanisi began as a conversation with Ofer Bar-Yosef, a gray-haired and inscrutable Harvard professor of Paleolithic archaeology, most famous for excavating Neanderthal burials in the Mideast. As a fresh-faced and eager first-year PhD student, I was told I had to track him down if I wanted to do archaeological fieldwork the following summer. I found Ofer one afternoon leaving his office in the Peabody Museum of Archaeology and Ethnology. He invited me to join as he walked to Harvard Square to pick up some photos (these were still the days of print film). "Vee'll valk and talk. No one vastes any time," he offered in his Israeli accent. Of course I agreed.

On the walk, he explained he had connections at two sites where I'd be welcome to do fieldwork: a Neanderthal cave site in the South of France, and Dmanisi. The French site was a bigger operation, more organized, and much easier to get to. "And zee food is better in France," he added. But the work in Georgia sounded more interesting. Two fossil skulls had been discovered there only a year before, and the site was shaking things up in the field of human evolution. After a bit of discussion, Ofer agreed to make the necessary arrangements. I asked if there was anything in particular I should plan to bring, anything I'd need for Georgia that wouldn't be on the typical packing list for a summer of fieldwork. Ofer stopped, turning to face me and sizing me up through thick glasses.

"Maybe an extra liver."

Strangers in a Strange Land

Precisely 1.85 million years ago, a massive volcano erupted in a cataclysm that would have shaken the ground and blackened the skies many miles away, in the low hills that would someday hold the village of Patara Dmanisi. Lava flowed for miles down the nearby Mashavera valley, filling it and obliterating the Mashavera River. As it flowed past the Pinasaouri, a small tributary, it backed up into the side valley and blocked that river, too. The lava cooled into a black basalt, a hundred feet thick in parts. A lake formed as the Pinasaouri River backed up behind its new basalt dam.

As years stretched into millennia, at least two other eruptions filled the skies with ash. The animals that roamed the landscape—a menagerie that included now-extinct species of ostriches, giraffids, horses, gazelles, saber-toothed cats, wolves, bears, and rhinoceroses—

must have choked on the ash and wondered, to the extent that they could, what the hell was going on. These ashfalls blanketed the landscape, including the narrow promontory squeezed between the basalt-filled Mashavera River valley and the Pinasaouri lake. This ash became the soil.

Through it all, plucky bands of *Homo erectus*, early members of the human genus, lived out their lives in the rolling woodlands around the Pinasaouri lake. They were an invasive species, the bleeding edge of an expanding population that had been bubbling out of Africa and spilling out into the rest of the Old World for thousands of years. But none of them would have had the slightest notion of their African origin, or indeed of an origin from anywhere other than right there. With a brain only half the size of ours, they probably thought little about such academic matters at all.

At five feet tall and 110 pounds, the Dmanisi hominins would have been tempting targets for the hyenas, wolves, and saber-toothed cats that prowled the forests. They held their own, though, relying on their wits and simple stone tools. And they were more often predators than prey. The bones of other animals at the site bear the unmistakable gouges and scrapes of stone tool butchery. The Dmanisi hominins and their ilk were not the apelike vegetarians that came before, confined to the African woodlands. They were hunter-gatherers.

They would have been lucky to live into their thirties or forties. Most surely died much younger. Occasionally, the rain would wash their bodies into a nearby gulley, alongside the chewed and scattered remnants of other dead animals. Eventually the gulley would fill with sediment, encasing their remains a few feet beneath the surface.

As eons wore on, the Pinasaouri and Mashavera Rivers cut their way through the thick basalt, reclaiming their valleys and leaving a thin spit of ridgeline once again perched between them. The

Dmanisi hominins were long gone at this point, replaced by waves of later hominins. It's likely that later, larger-bodied populations of *Homo erectus* inhabited the area, though we've yet to find their bones. Stone tools tell us that Neanderthals set up camp a few miles down the valley around forty thousand years ago. Modern humans swept in some time after that. In the early centuries of the Christian Era, a stone church was built atop the promontory. A stone-walled medieval city grew up around it, and the people thrived. Then came the hordes of invaders. Starting around 1080 A.D., they overran the city every couple hundred years like some brutal Mongol time-share. By the fifteenth century the once-proud city was abandoned, and the area was left to the peasant farmers in the valley below.

The initial discovery of the fossil site of Dmanisi was a happy accident. In 1983, archaeologists excavating the medieval city dug into the surrounding soil and pulled out a fossilized rhinoceros molar. Realizing they had stumbled upon the remains of a lost ancient world, they alerted their colleagues at the national museum in Tbilisi. A team of Georgian paleontologists began working the site, focused on the fossils. Stone tools were found a year later, and the first hominin fossil, a jawbone, was excavated in 1991. Paleoanthropologists around the globe were intrigued but skeptical. Then, in 2000, the Georgians reported two new skulls along with solid dates for the Mashavera basalt. They had the oldest hominin site outside of Africa, and the site was producing beautiful, complete fossils. Humanity's first foray across the globe was captured here, at this little site in the foothills of the Caucasus Mountains. Suddenly, Dmanisi was the center of attention in human evolution.

When I showed up mid-season in the summer of 2001, a small crew of Georgian researchers and volunteers, European and

American graduate students, and leading international scholars in human evolution, archaeology, and geology were working to dig the site and reconstruct what life was like for the Dmanisi hominins. The main excavation was a rough rectangle, about five hundred square feet of exposed earth, painstakingly carved flat and level with trowels and brushes. Like every dig everywhere, the site was overlaid with a grid of 1-by-1-meter squares. I spent my days in my assigned square, scraping away claylike sediment with a trowel and a brush while keeping a sharp eye out for the first white flash of fossil.

I was hardly a veteran archaeologist when I showed up, but I had done enough to expect days of finding nothing. Even at an exciting site, most dirt is just dirt. But Dmanisi was different, with rich veins of fossils and stone tools. Rhinos, lions, gazelles, horses; complete skulls and other bones, not the scrappy fragments you learn to cherish on most digs. You'd realize that the person digging in the square next door had gotten awfully quiet and look over to find them absorbed in the ticklish work of wresting some behemoth from the ground, its curved and intricate skull emerging from the surface like Excalibur. The fossils were often softer than the surrounding dirt, and extracting them from the sediment without destroying them was a delicate art.

We found *another* skull—the third from Dmanisi and the most complete cranium of *Homo erectus* ever recovered anywhere—at the end of my first season. It emerged from the sediment upside down, its palate facing the sky. Most excavation teams never recover a major hominin find; isolated molars and fragments of skull are celebrated like holy relics. The great Louis and Mary Leakey spent nearly thirty years scouring Olduvai Gorge before finding a hominin skull. The Dmanisi crew had uncovered three skulls in three years. This most recent one, likely from a male in his late teens, was so perfectly complete that the paper-thin, crenulated bone of the upper palate and lower orbits was still intact. The entire team walked around for days with smiles that wouldn't wear off. Traditional Georgian feasts were held on the long dig-house table, late into the night. Men broke into haunting polyphonic Georgian folk songs.

I was hooked. I knew I'd be back every season for as long as I could. And for the five summers of my grad school career I carved out the time to make the trek to Dmanisi. Every year we found hominins and celebrated (not always in that order). Wine, vodka, and chacha, a grape-based Georgian moonshine, were had in terrifying amounts. And every year I'd find myself yakking into the bushes, ringing in the annual cycle like some putrid combination of Old Faithful and Stonehenge, whispering the same empty promises of reform into the morning air. Ofer was right: I could have used an extra liver.

My second summer at Dmanisi, the crew uncovered yet *another* skull, the fourth from the area. Its most prominent feature was what it lacked. The U-shaped arcade around the perimeter of the palate that should have held teeth was smooth and rounded. All the teeth were gone. And they had been lost while the individual, probably a male in his late thirties or early forties, was still very much alive, the sockets healing over and filling with bone. Whether from disease or advanced age, this poor guy had lost every tooth in his head and somehow managed to survive, choking down food with pulpy, painful gums while he recovered. The resorption of the tooth sockets was so advanced that he must have lived for years without teeth.

The discovery raised an obvious question. *How did he manage to survive?* Wild plants and game are nearly all hard to chew; you need teeth. Few wild foods are easy to harvest, particularly if you're frail. How did he persist for so long?

He owed his life, I believe, to the quintessential human adaptation, the trait that most sets us apart from our ape relatives. It's a behavior so ingrained that we rarely give it a second thought. Yet it revolutionized the human lineage, changing the way we get our food and altering the way our bodies burn energy. The Dmanisi hominins shared.

Selfish, Lazy Vegetarians

Humans are part of the ape family, a subset of the primate order of mammals. The primate bough of the mammalian family tree first emerged as a green twig roughly sixty-five million years ago, in the wake of the asteroid impact and massive extinction that wiped out the dinosaurs. The K-T Mass Extinction event, as it's known, left vacant landscapes into which primates and other mammalian groups bloomed.

Early primates were scrappy, squirrel-sized animals who made their home in the trees. Like primates today, including us, they had dexterous, grasping hands tipped with fingernails instead of claws. One persuasive theory of primate origins is that early primates co-evolved with flowering plants, which also got their evolutionary start after the dinosaur extinction. In this scenario, primates adapted to eating fruits of these plants, unintentionally providing them with a means of dispersing their seeds throughout the forest in their poo. Plants with more attractive (i.e., more energy-rich) fruits were dispersed more effectively and had better reproductive success. An evolutionary partnership was formed, with plants selected to produce fleshy, sugary fruits and primates adapted to seek them out and eat them.

But we owe more than our hands and love of sugary fruits to these distant ancestors. As was discussed in Chapter 1, my colleagues and I discovered that primates burn only half as many calories as other mammals. It's so widespread throughout primates today that this metabolic shift must have occurred very early, at the base of the primate radiation. These early primates were playing the long game. Reduced daily energy expenditure meant slower growth and reproduction, but also longer lives. Rather than concentrating all their reproductive effort over a few short years (where a bad year could wipe out most of your fragile offspring), primates had longer reproductive careers that lowered the consequences of encountering a poor season or two. Slower growth also meant more time for learning during development, with more opportunities for innovation and creativity. As I write this, I'm sitting across the kitchen table from my four-year-old daughter, who is dexterously eating her cereal and apple slices while chatting about preschool and the years of school ahead. Our modern human lives have very deep roots.

The primate metabolic strategy was incredibly successful. Over millions of years, they expanded into a diverse group with two main branches: the lemurs and lorises on one side, and monkeys on the other. Around twenty-one million years ago, a new shoot sprouted from the monkey branch: the apes. The apes, or hominoids, as the group is technically called, grew to be a successful lot. For fifteen million years, they proliferated and expanded across Africa, Europe, and Asia. There were dozens of species.

Then, for reasons that remain obscure, their fortunes changed. The bushy ape bough was pruned to just a few branches. By six million years ago we lose nearly all trace of apes in the fossil record. Only a handful of hominoid species persist today: chimpanzees, bonobos, and gorillas in equatorial Africa; orangutans, and several species of gibbons ("lesser apes" in the casual condescension of primate taxonomy) in the rain forests of Southeast Asia.

The only other ape lineage to survive was ours, the hominins. Around seven million years ago in Africa, a population of apes gradually split in two. One of the resulting populations would become the founding stock of the chimpanzee and bonobo lineage (those two species didn't split until much later; Figure 4.1). The other population was the founders of our lineage, the hominins. There are at least as many ideas about why this split occurred as there are drunk paleoanthropologists, but little consensus. From the fossil record, we know that the earliest hominins walked on two legs and had stubby, less lethal canine teeth. Otherwise, they were very apelike: chimpanzee-sized bodies and brains; long arms, long fingers, and grasping feet for scrambling high up in the trees.

This first chapter of hominin evolution lasted from seven to four million years ago. At least three different fossil species are known from this period, all in Africa. Only one, *Ardipithecus ramidus* from Ethiopia (Ardi to its fans), is well characterized, with dozens of fossils and a nearly complete reconstructed skeleton, from ape-sized head to long, grasping toes. Others are less complete. The oldest, *Sahelanthropus tchadensis* from Chad, is known only from a skull and some scrappy fragments of the body. *Orrorin tugenensis* from Kenya has the opposite problem, with only pieces of the limb bones and some loose teeth recovered.

This might lead to you to ask, "How do the scientists know that these fragmentary finds are different species? Or even that they are hominins at all, and not members of some other lineage?" Congratulations, you've just invented the field of paleoanthropology. The gory details of paleoanthropological research are the topic of another larger book, but suffice to say it's hard work, requiring a keen eye and an encyclopedic knowledge of the morphological signatures of different taxonomic groups. Uncertainty is the norm. Paleoanthropologists routinely work themselves into a lather over the anatomical minutiae that distinguishes one fossil species from another, or get into shouting matches at highbrow academic conferences trying to make the case that *their* fossil species is a direct ancestor to living humans, while someone else's pet species is just a side-branch dead end (or *gasp!* not even a hominin at all). If you want to ruin a paleoanthropologist's day, suggest that the fossil hominin species that he discovered, named, and has dedicated his life's work to, is in fact just a local variant of some other, previously described species.

The second chapter of the hominin lineage, from about four to two million years ago, is known from a much more complete fossil record. This is the era of the genus *Australopithecus*, including the famous Lucy and her kin, *Australopithecus afarensis*. Several species come and go in the fossil record throughout this period, each with their own anatomical distinctions. Still, there are common trends. The grasping foot of earlier hominins like Ardi is gone, morphed into a foot much more like ours with the big toe in line with the others. This, along with changes in the pelvis, suggests these species were more proficient on the ground, burning fewer calories to walk and perhaps venturing a bit farther each day than either living apes or the earliest hominins. Teeth get larger, the enamel much thicker. One strange and specialized side group of species, assigned to the genus *Paranthropus*, take this dental inflation to the extreme, with molars five times larger than ours and massive cheekbones to anchor equally massive chewing muscles.

There is even some evidence for increased cognitive sophistication. Brain size ticks up a bit in *Australopithecus*, from just under half a quart to just above (but still only about a third the size of ours). We used to think that hominins from this period weren't able to make stone tools, but in 2015 researchers reported large, rudimentary stone tools from a 3.3-million-year-old site in northern Kenya. We don't know what these cumbersome tools were used for, or whether they represent a widespread phenomenon or just a short-lived, early experiment. Regardless, they suggest that at least some *Australopithecus* species were a bit more clever and resourceful than living apes, who use rudimentary tools to fish for termites or crack nuts but aren't known to manufacture stone tools.

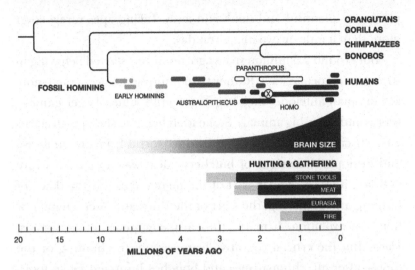

Figure 4.1. The human family tree. Our lineage, the hominins, is one branch of the ape family, and includes over a dozen known fossil species, several of which are shown. The X in the circle indicates the position of the Dmanisi hominins. Hunting and gathering begins with the genus *Homo*, and brings with it increased brain size and changes in diet and behavior (gray: early debated evidence; black: strong and continued evidence). Note the change in timescale at five million years. (Adapted from H. Pontzer [2017]. "Economy and endurance in human evolution." *Curr. Biol.* 27: R613–21.)

And yet, for all the anatomical diversity and hints of creativity, these hominins were most likely apelike in terms of their metabolism. We can be confident in that assessment because, like the living apes today, species from the first two chapters of hominin evolution were essentially vegetarians. Sure, they may have hunted small game occasionally or looted termite mounds for some yummy protein, as chimpanzees and bonobos do. But a look at their teeth and their tree-climbing adaptations tells us Ardi, Lucy, and the others were getting the vast majority of their calories from plant foods. An apelike, plant-based diet, in turn, tells us these species didn't need to walk very much to find food. It's a general rule of ecology that plant-eaters don't travel very far each day, because plants are plentiful and don't run away. Living apes rarely cover more than a mile or two in a given day.

But around 2.5 million years ago, hominins started behaving in strange, un-apelike ways. Rather than hunting the occasional monkey or small antelope, they began targeting much larger game— zebras and other big animals. Stone tools begin to show up all across East Africa in large numbers, and animal fossils from sites in Kenya and Ethiopia show signs of butchery. Meat was no longer a rare delicacy, it was a regular part of the menu. This was the dawn of hunting and gathering, the start of the third and latest chapter of hominin evolution. It marks the early emergence of our genus, *Homo*. But the crucial cognitive leap was not the hunting or the tools—after all, chimpanzees and bonobos hunt and make tools, and it hasn't led to any radical departure from their ape-ish ways. The big dietary innovation that would change our metabolism and our evolutionary destinies wasn't the food these hominins ate, it was the food they gave away.

Human the Sharer

The first Hadza words I remember learning are *amayega* and *mtana*, the back and forth of the basic Hadza greeting. The third word I learned was *za*.

I'm not sure when I first noticed it. My first trip to the Hadza was a flood of new sights and sounds, and the early days are a bit blurred in my memory. If you've ever spent time in a foreign city where you didn't speak the language, at a café or park, you know how the voices around you can form a sort of abstract sonic tapestry, rich in feeling but devoid of meaning. But at some point, my mind caught on to a repeated, simple command, "*za*." Soon I was noticing it everywhere. Two kids hanging out eating a snack, "*za*." Grandma feeding berries to her grandson, "*za*." A man bumming honey from a friend, "*za*."

I asked Brian what it meant, though it should have been obvious. *Za* means "give."

What I couldn't understand was why there was no counterpoint. Nothing was ever said in return, the item in question was simply handed over. Where were all the extras I grew up with, the *magic words*: "please," "thank you," "you're welcome"? To my utter disbelief, I learned that they didn't really have them. They have the concepts, of course; there are Hadza words for requesting help and for expressing gratitude. But the "please" and "thank you" drilled into kids across the Western world is absent from the small-scale exchanges that dominate the day. What kind of language doesn't have the *magic words*?

The more I saw, the more I understood. Giving—sharing—isn't a nicety among the Hadza. It's the rule. Just like you don't go around saying "Thank you for not spitting in my face" to everyone who doesn't spit in your face, the Hadza don't bother saying "please" and "thank you" for sharing. It would imply that the person is doing something beyond simply living up to the societal contract. You need the magic words only if there's a chance the other person might reasonably refuse, but that's not how it works with the Hadza.

To be Hadza is to give. Everyone shares with everyone, all the time. That's the rule. All you have to say is "*za*."

In the 1950s and '60s, researchers in human evolution (nearly all men, it's worth noting) began synthesizing the available data from the hominin fossil record, field studies of living primates, and ethnographic research in living hunter-gatherer populations. It was an exciting time to be asking, *What makes us human?* These fields were still young, but enough work had been done, enough fossils found, to move beyond the mere speculation of previous generations and begin synthesizing holistic, evidence-based reconstructions of our evolutionary past.

The movement was codified in the landmark 1966 "Man the Hunter" conference, which generated a book of the same title. The

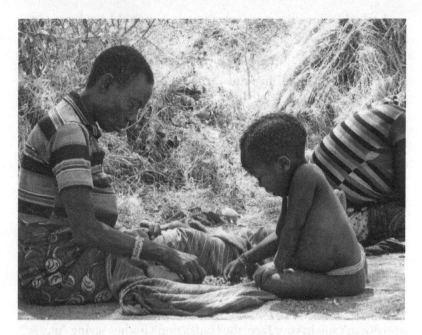

Figure 4.2. Hunting and gathering means sharing. A Hadza grandmother shares berries with her grandson after returning to camp with the day's harvest.

casual chauvinism of the era is obvious from the name. I don't think it was intended, though that hardly matters. Researchers (again, nearly all men) were struck by what they saw as the major differences between humans and other apes: our proficiency in and dependence on hunting and tools. They saw all the major traits that make humans unique as downstream evolutionary consequences of these key innovations. It was a very influential perspective, even if it wasn't entirely new. Darwin himself had speculated humans owed our "pre-eminent success in the battle of life" to hunting, arguing it would "have been advantageous to the progenitors of man . . . to defend themselves with stones or clubs, to attack their prey, or otherwise to obtain food."

The feminist movement of the 1960s and '70s and the glaring omission of women in the "Man the Hunter" paradigm led to a predictable and much needed correction. In 1981, anthropologist Frances Dahlberg edited a collection of essays titled *Woman the Gatherer*, highlighting women's essential contributions in hunter-gatherer populations. In addition to their irreplaceable roles as mothers and grandmothers, women in foraging cultures invariably provide food and goods that are needed for the community to succeed. In many cultures, women's foraging provides well over half of the calories. Moreover, by the late 1960s it was clear that chimpanzees occasionally hunted and used tools. If hunting and using tools weren't uniquely human behaviors, it was hard to argue that hunting and tool use propelled our unique evolutionary trajectory.

Frankly, I think that focusing solely on men's or women's contributions misses the crucial point. Men and women *both* make essential contributions in hunting and gathering societies, but *neither* is enough on their own. What makes hunting and gathering so successful isn't the *hunting* or the *gathering*, it's the *and*. More than just *man the hunter* or *woman the gatherer*, we are *human the sharer*.

In stark contrast, the living apes hardly ever share. Sure, mothers of all ape species will occasionally share some food with their infants or young children. Orangutan mothers in the wild share food with their young kids about one out of every ten meals, usually foods that are difficult to obtain—not exactly "mother of the year" behavior, by human standards. Sharing among adult apes is even less common. Gorillas have *never* been observed sharing food among adults in the wild. Adult chimpanzees in the Sonso community in the Budongo Forest of Uganda share food about once every two months, and much of what passes for "sharing" is more like tolerated theft. Bonobos share the most, but even they fall well short of the human norm. At the site of Wamba in Congo, Japanese researcher Shinya Yamamoto found that adult bonobos (mostly females) share a particular fruit, the large and fleshy junglesop, about 14 percent of the time.

Apes, despite their intricate, lifelong social relationships, live lives of dietary solitude. When it comes to food, they are on their own. Consequently, they are compelled to go for the sure thing, to make certain that they get enough food each day to keep from starving. And there's little upside to pursuing big game or gathering more than they need; anything they can't shove in their mouths *right now* will go to waste or be pilfered by beggars, who are unlikely to ever return the favor. It's telling that the most commonly shared foods for chimpanzees and bonobos are monkeys and duikers (a kind of small antelope) they hunt or the large junglesop fruits at Wamba. These items aren't huge, but they're more than a mouthful. The lucky hunter typically keeps as much as he can manage, "sharing" scraps to quiet the begging and pestering horde. Even bonobos share junglesop only if a friend begs.

Humans are social foragers. We routinely bring home more than we need, with the intention of giving it away to our community. That means we have one another as a safety net; if someone comes home empty-handed, they won't go hungry. This allows us to diversify and take risks, to develop complementary foraging strategies—hunting and gathering—that maximize the potential for big gains while limiting the consequences of failure. Some group members hunt, and will occasionally bring home a big game bounty of fat and protein. Others gather, providing a stable, dependable source of food to get through the days when the hunters are unlucky. It's an incredibly flexible, adaptable, and successful strategy. And the foundation of it all is the inviolable, ironclad, unspoken understanding that we will share.

Sharing is the glue that binds hunter-gatherer communities together and provides the fuel that makes them run. It radically changed the hominin metabolic strategy. Sharing meant more food, more calories, more energy for growth, reproduction, brains, activity . . . all of it (Figure 4.3). As my colleagues and I discovered in our doubly labeled measurements of apes and humans (Chapter 1), we burn about 20 percent more energy every day than chimpanzees and bonobos. Our energetic advantage over gorillas and orangutans is even greater. Those extra calories fuel our big brains, active lifestyles, and big families—the traits that set us apart from the other apes and define our lives. And it began with hunting and gathering, with early members of our genus, *Homo*, foraging for more than they needed for themselves and giving the surplus away. That extra energy propelled hominins armed with primitive stone tools and ape-sized brains across the globe, from Durban to Dmanisi and beyond.

The Metabolic Revolution

We often discuss evolution in terms of physical traits, the appearance of new anatomical features or changes in their shape and size. After all, it's the physical traits that are usually preserved in the fossil record. But behavioral changes are often the true instigators. New behaviors arise and the body adapts. Fish started feeding in the muddy shallows of the water's edge, and those with the strongest fins and best primitive lungs to navigate those puddles had the best reproductive success; the evolutionary transition to land and legs followed. Horse ancestors with unremarkable teeth switched from eating soft leaves to more abrasive grasses. Those with taller teeth survived longer, as it took longer for the teeth to wear out. After millions of years, long teeth became the norm for horses. (Which is why you can tell the age of a horse by looking in its mouth, to see how worn down its teeth are—a savvy move if you're buying the horse, but rude if it's a gift.) Polar bears started swimming and diving to hunt, then evolved webbed feet. Behavior leads, form follows.

It would have taken a very particular set of circumstances for sharing to prevail in the hominin lineage: the costs of acquiring more food than you could eat had to be lower than the benefits of giving it away. Foraging for extra food means less energy for yourself, more for someone else—not the sort of thing that natural selection, Darwin's amoral accountant, usually favors. To the extent that the recipient is related to you and shares the same genes, their reproductive success is partly yours. But the discounting is steep: even your child shares only half your genes. The costs of acquiring extra food would need to be low, and the payoff to the receiver really high, for sharing to be worth it. It's easy to understand why no other apes—in fact, hardly any other species at all—have hit upon sharing as a successful strategy.

Despite the long odds against it, in a population of ape-brained hominins some two and a half million years ago, somewhere in eastern Africa, the right combination of conditions, diet, and behavior aligned. Sharing became the norm. Sadly, the details of its origins may be too fine-grained to be caught in the rough sieve of the fossil record. (Though if you buy a round at the next human evolution conference, you'll be regaled with any number of nuanced and complex scenarios.) The earliest hard evidence for sharing comes from cut-marked bones on large animals like zebra. No hominin could eat a zebra by himself, no matter how hungry. And targeting a zebra, dead or alive, would require teamwork, either to hunt it or to push other hungry carnivores off the corpse. Teamwork pays only if there's an agreement to share the spoils. Perhaps hominin sharing grew from apelike hunting, with some individuals giving more than the limited, grudging scraps we see with chimpanzees.

Or perhaps hominin sharing grew from the sort of fruit-sharing behavior we see among female bonobos at Wamba. A strong case can be made that wild tubers, the distant cousins of the potatoes and yams in our supermarkets today, were an important shared food early on. Tubers are a dietary staple for the Hadza and other hunter-gatherer populations around the world. And they are calorific starch bombs, hard for small kids to dig from the ground but easy enough to harvest in surplus for adults. Just as orangutan mothers tend to share foods that are hard for young offspring to get, hominin mothers (or fathers) could have made a habit of feeding tubers to their kids. Perhaps older females, past their childbearing years, began to channel their maternal efforts into sharing food with their daughters and grandchildren.

Whether it was meat, plant foods, or some combination, this strange act of foraging for others had profound consequences for hominin evolution. Sharing meant more energy for life's essential tasks. Survival and reproduction, the currencies of natural selection, improved. The sharing hominins and their kin outcompeted their less generous neighbors.

We are the descendants of these early, sharing hominins. Over time, hominin physiology responded to this new behavior, ramping up metabolic rates to take advantage of the extra calories. This was the Metabolic Revolution (Figure 4.3), and it has shaped the evolution of our genus, *Homo*, ever since.

Positive Feedback and Virtuous Cycles

Just as your metabolism reflects the orchestrated activities of all of your body's systems working together, the Metabolic Revolution changed every aspect of our physiology. Since calories don't fossilize, it's difficult to dissect which changes came first. The first sign of metabolic acceleration that we see in the fossil record is an increase in brain size. Brains are metabolically expensive organs, as we discussed in the last chapter. By two million years ago, not long after the earliest cut-marked bones, we find fossil hominins with brains nearly 20 percent larger—consuming 20 percent more calories—than their *Australopithecus* predecessors.

The fact that evolution favored channeling those extra calories

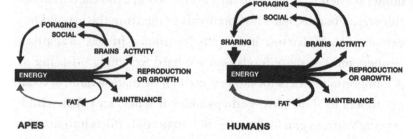

Figure 4.3. The Metabolic Revolution. Like all primates, apes use their metabolic energy for life's essential tasks, including growth or reproduction, maintenance (e.g., immune function, tissue repair), and physical activity. They are smart, social animals that invest in brains for navigating their complex social worlds and finding food, but they feed only themselves. Humans combine social and foraging efforts, sharing surplus food energy with other members of their group. Sharing increases the energy available for all tasks including reproduction and maintenance, leading to longer lives, larger families, larger brains, and increased activity. Humans burn more energy each day than other apes to fuel these traits. Greater energy expenditure also favors directing extra calories to fat (far more than in other apes) to survive periods of energy shortage.

into expensive brains says a lot about the metabolic strategy of our genus. Normally, we'd expect evolution to favor spending those calories directly on survival and reproduction. After all, reproductive success—the number of surviving offspring produced—is the only measure that natural selection pays attention to. There's no evolutionary benefit to investing resources in brains or any other feature unless it pays off in more babies. The caloric investment in brains tells us that cognitive sophistication was so critically important for those hominins that it was worth spending precious calories on more brain power.

Physical activity must have increased substantially as well. Relying on meat for a good portion of the diet requires a lot of work each day to get food. Compared to plant foods, game animals are spread thin on the landscape and are much harder to hunt down. Modern carnivores on the African savanna typically cover four times more ground each day than the herbivores they're after. The transition to hunting early in our genus would have required a similar increase in the daily distance traveled. And it might have meant more than just a lot of walking. Dan Lieberman (my PhD advisor at Harvard) and Dennis Bramble have made a compelling case that early members of the genus *Homo* were adapted for endurance running, wearing down their prey under the hot African sun until they collapsed. Regardless of how they hunted, hominins had embarked on a high-energy strategy, hunting and gathering, spending lots of calories on intellect and effort with the expectation of even greater, shared returns.

The strategy worked. Populations grew and ranges expanded. *Homo erectus*, the first hominin species to go global, appears in East Africa nearly two million years ago and quickly spreads out across the Old World. Within 100,000 years, its range extended from southern Africa, through central Eurasia, and all the way to East Asia, with stone tools recovered in China and fossils as far away as Indonesia. Hunting and gathering had hit its stride. Incredibly, unfathomable eons hence, their descendants would pluck the remains of a handful of these hardy pioneers from the soil of Dmanisi.

Sharing, smarts, and stamina, the key ingredients of hominin cooperative foraging, were a potent combination. Greater brainpower improved our ancestors' capacity to locate and procure the best fruits, tubers, and game, while simultaneously improving their abilities to plan and scheme together. Greater endurance allowed them to cast a wider net, hunting down prey and exploiting the bounties of a much larger home range. And sharing, like the Big Lebowski's rug, tied it all together. With the newfound capacity to acquire more food than they needed, and the social contract to share the surplus, hominins found themselves awash in energy.

It was such a winning strategy that the only way to beat it was to do it better. Each generation, there would be variation among individuals in their cognitive ability, social sophistication, and physical endurance. In each generation, the smartest, fittest, and friendliest individuals were the ones who tended to survive the best and reproduce the most. An arms race developed within the hominin lineage, the early, incipient changes snowballing into an ever more grotesque species, with big bulbous heads, delicate faces, and hairless, sweaty bodies—species more and more like us.

The increase in intelligence is the easiest to track in the fossil and archaeological record. Fossilized skulls like those at Dmanisi enable us to track the growth in brain size—a rough, though reasonable, measure of intelligence when we compare across species. In less than two million years, brain size *triples* in the genus *Homo*, steadily expanding like muffins in the oven (Figure 4.1). Stone tool sophistication increases in parallel. The early tools, from places like Dmanisi, are simple, broken cobbles, with all the beauty and sophistication of a first grader's clay flower vase for mom. By one and a half million years, hominins were making symmetrical, tear-shaped "hand axes," which are tricky to make (I can't do it, but my buddies who are into stone tools can). By 400,000 years ago, hominins were using complex, multistep "Levallois" processes to make long, thin blades and other incredible tools—stuff so complicated that you have to be a Level 7 archaeology nerd with years of experience to make it today. Tools get only more intricate from there, their sophistication growing in an unbroken chain of innovation from Paleolithic obsidian blades, to the bow and arrow, to the smartphone in your pocket.

It's not only the tools, of course. By 500,000 years ago, hominins are controlling fire. (This breakthrough may have come a good deal earlier. Debate on the subjects is . . . heated.) Language abilities must have been developing throughout this period as well, though it is fiendishly difficult to track its evolution. By the time our species, *Homo sapiens*, emerges in Africa around 300,000 years ago, trade networks for highly prized raw materials stretch for miles, and natural red pigments are being used for decoration and perhaps symbolic art. By 130,000 years ago, if not earlier, humans along the coast of southern Africa were harvesting shellfish on an annual schedule, paying attention to the seasons and the tides to get the best catch. Our species expands out of Africa and into Eurasia around 120,000 years ago, echoing the earlier waves of *Homo erectus*, bringing art and innovation wherever we go. By 40,000 years ago, we're painting lurid murals on cave walls from Bordeaux to Borneo.

Reconstructing hominin cognitive evolution is relatively easy because brain size and the tools, art, and the other stuff we make leaves a trail of bread crumbs in the fossil and archaeological records. It's more challenging to track the pace of evolutionary change in fitness and friendliness, because neither leave much definitive hard evidence behind. What we can say with certainty is that humans today are far and away the best endurance athletes among all of the living apes. Our VO_2 max, a common measure of peak aerobic power (see Chapter 8), is at least four times that of chimpanzees'. We carry more muscle in our legs (though less in our arms) than other apes, and we have a much greater proportion of fatigue-resistant "slow twitch" muscles. Our blood holds more hemoglobin to ferry oxygen to working muscle. And our naked, sweaty skin (by far the sweatiest on the planet) keeps us cool, protecting us from overheating even when exercising in hot conditions.

All of this allows us to go farther and faster than any of the other apes. Chimpanzees travel less than two miles per day, on average. Other apes are even lazier. Humans, particularly hunter-gatherers like the Hadza, walk five times farther each day. People run marathons for *fun*. We are built for intense, all-day activity. Many of the anatomical traits that help make us such prodigious walkers and runners, like our long legs, the springy arches in our feet, and our short toes, are present in early *Homo*, suggesting our endurance abilities were present fairly early in our genus and have been honed by evolution as part of the hunting and gathering strategy over the past two million years.

It's a similar story for sharing. Hard evidence of butchered zebra and other big game at sites like Dmanisi tells us that sharing was established early in our genus. In fact, as I've argued above, sharing is probably the key behavioral innovation that sparks the evolution of our genus, *Homo*. But it's difficult to track the degree or amount of sharing, as it changes over time from then until now. Still, there are some suggestive clues. By at least 400,000 years ago, tool technology and hunting techniques were quite sophisticated. In addition to deadly stone tools, they were making well-balanced spears with fire-hardened tips, and regularly taking down wild horses and other big game. Such dedication to crafting tools and developing hunting strategies indicates, perhaps, that some community members specialized in hunting while others focused on gathering, similar to most hunter-gatherer populations today. Division of labor like that needs a strong commitment to sharing to make it work.

Brain size and behavioral complexity offer another clue about sharing. Enormous brains and a behavioral strategy dependent on learning means that we come into the world at birth as helpless, useless, damp bundles of pudge. We can't walk, talk, feed ourselves, or keep out of danger for *years* after we're born. Instead, we are completely reliant on others—on sharing—for the food, attention, and safety we desperately need. We spend the first decade or two of our lives soaking up the shared resources of generous community members, learning (one hopes) to be a functioning, productive adult. Our brains burn so much energy on learning, building, and pruning neural connections as information floods in that our body's growth slows down during the early elementary school years. In hunting and gathering societies like the Hadza, people don't become self-sufficient—acquiring enough food to feed themselves—until late in their teenage years.

The payoff for all this waiting and learning is incredibly high adult productivity. Adult hunter-gatherers, both men and women, can easily bring home thousands of extra food kilocalories per day, far more than they need for themselves (see Chapter 9). This is the extra energy that fuels our faster metabolic engines and greater daily energy expenditures. The extra energy is shared with children, as well as with their moms and other caregivers. In fact, because the energetic burden of reproduction is shared, with moms getting lots of help, mothers in hunter-gatherer societies typically have a kid about every three years, a much faster pace than that of ape mothers who do all the work themselves. (Average interbirth intervals for chimpanzees, gorillas, and orangutans are five years or longer.) It's the human life history paradox: each kid takes longer to grow up, but we still manage to reproduce faster than our ape relatives. And it's our commitment to sharing and unique metabolic strategy that make it work.

Brain size creeps up into the low end of the modern human range by about 700,000 years ago, in a species called *Homo heidelbergensis* that is found throughout Africa and Eurasia. Their big brains and technological sophistication suggest that long childhoods and super-productive adult foraging was established well before our particular species, *Homo sapiens*, evolved in Africa. Likewise, their big, expensive brains and hunter-gatherer lifestyles tell us they likely had the same accelerated metabolic rates that we see in humans today, burning more energy than their *Australopithecus* forebears. But even if the essential human metabolic strategy was in place before we got here, it might be our unique twist on sharing that kept us from going extinct.

As our *Homo sapiens* ancestors expanded throughout Africa and across the globe, they found they weren't alone. The world was already full of strange and wonderful humanlike species, their evolutionary cousins: Neanderthals in Europe, Denisovans in central Asia, relict populations of *Homo erectus* in Asia, an *erectus*-like species in southern Africa called *Homo naledi*, and a miniaturized species called *Homo floresiensis*, nicknamed the Hobbit by paleoanthropologists, in the islands of Indonesia. The modern science fiction fantasy of meeting some almost-human in a distant realm, communicating, living with them, played out again and again in Paleolithic wilderness.

Some of these species, like *erectus* and *naledi*, are helpful reminders that evolution has no momentum. These species evolved slightly larger brains than *Australopithecus* and were among the earliest hunter-gatherers. But at some point early on, natural selection stopped pushing them toward ever larger brains and more complex foraging. The vagaries of their particular habitats and ecologics didn't favor it. The costs of bigger brains and the risks of increased generosity were greater than the benefits. So with no pressure to change, they kept their modest brain sizes and early *Homo* habits for hundreds of thousands of years, even as hominin populations in other parts of the world kept changing. Evolution isn't trying to get anywhere. Just because brain size increased steadily for a million years doesn't mean it will continue. We were not inevitable.

Other species, like the Denisovans and Neanderthals, tell us we were not particularly special. These species were smart, adaptable, resourceful, just like us. In fact they were so much like us that we interbred, raising hybrid families and wondering, no doubt, why the in-laws always seemed a bit peculiar. We find bits of their DNA in our chromosomes today, a few scattered bricks of a lost civilization recycled into modern construction.

Why *they* went extinct and *we* persisted—why we're the only hominins left on the planet today—remains one of the great mysteries. It's often been argued that we were simply smarter or more creative, but it's not at all clear that was the case. Neanderthals had brains a bit larger than ours and were making cave art, playing music, and burying their dead long before we showed up. Perhaps it was just dumb luck, a cosmic roll of the dice where chance happened to favor us. Perhaps we brought new diseases into Eurasia with us as we expanded across the globe, wiping out the Neanderthal and Denisovan populations in the same way that European diseases devastated Native American populations after contact.

One compelling explanation is that humans persisted because we were friendlier. Richard Wrangham at Harvard University, as well as Brian Hare and Vanessa Woods, my colleagues at Duke, have argued that *Homo sapiens* became hyper-social through a long process of self-domestication. In this scenario, individuals (particularly men) who tried to get their way through violence and intimidation were ostracized (or in Wrangham's telling even executed) by members of their group. Over time, friendliness and the gene variants that promoted it were favored; mean people didn't have as many kids. Humans took the sharing behavior of earlier *Homo* species to the next level. Our communities began to function as hyper-cooperative superorganisms, like beehives or ant colonies. In this scenario, our greater social cohesion was our key advantage over Neanderthals and Denisovans as we spread into Eurasia. When we found ourselves on the same landscapes as Neanderthals and other hominins, our hyper-cooperative strategy won out.

Whether humans were unique among hominins in our propensity to work together, it's clear that our extreme sociality, huge brains, and capacity for physical activity are the key traits that set our species so fundamentally apart from the other apes. And we owe it all to our two-million-year legacy of hunting and gathering, stretching from Dmanisi to today. Our complex social worlds and empathy, our ability to explore the galaxy and split the atom, our ability to endure, our willingness to share lunch—*all* of it is literally part of our DNA. And *all* of it is fueled by our high-energy metabolic strategy. Our metabolism—the way we get our energy and the way we spend it—was essential to our radical evolution.

Did I mention there's a downside?

The Downside

I grew up in the rolling, remote hills of the Appalachian Mountains of northwest Pennsylvania, in a little town called Kersey. Like yours, my childhood was filled with daily lessons and constant reminders of my social identity. I was a Pontzer, a Catholic, a public school student, a Kersey kid, a Steelers fan (even if I rarely watched a game). Each of those layers meant something. It defined who my friends were and who was inherently suspect (private school students, kids from St. Mary's). None of these identities was stronger than being a Penn State fan.

My parents, older sisters, and many aunts, uncles, and cousins had all gone to Penn State. We watched few televised sports in my house growing up, and neither my mom nor dad cared much about sports, but if we were home on a Saturday in autumn, Penn State football was on the TV. My senior year of high school, I applied to exactly one college: dear old Penn State. I honestly couldn't imagine going anywhere else. Penn State was my tribe.

The ultimate tribal ritual—the ecstatic rite of passage of my freshman year—was attending a Penn State football game. For a true believer, it's a religious experience. Perched on the steep aluminum bleachers with 115,000 rapt fans, all adorned with the colors and other signifiers of the tribe, we cheered on the gladiators below. It didn't matter that we didn't know one another. Anyone in the stadium (aside from the small, brave-faced contingent in the visitors' area) was an instant friend. And in full voice we'd shout the defining Penn State cheer, a deafening call-and-response across the stadium. *WE ARE . . . PENN STATE!* It was nearly as intoxicating as the sleep deprivation, freedom, and alcohol that defined my freshman year.

An integral part of being hyper-social, sharing apes is our insatiable need to belong to a group. From childhood we are keenly aware of who our tribe is. We pick up the language, the appearance, the signifiers of our group, and we adopt them. We want to belong. This makes a good deal of sense when we consider the evolutionary importance of sharing. Without our group, we're dead. And we need to know who to be nice to. The social contract demands that we are generous with those in our community.

Just as important is understanding who is *not* in our group. Sharing with outsiders is an enormous risk. If they aren't part of our tribe, they might not reciprocate. Even worse, they might be hostile. Come to think of it, they seem to have an awful lot of resources, things our group could really use. *Look at them!* Just sitting there with all their stuff. The smug jerks. I mean, it's practically criminal of them to keep it all to themselves. I say we go over there and *strongly recommend* that they give us what is *rightfully* ours. After all, *We are Penn State . . .* and *they* are not.

You see how this sort of thing can get out of hand.

Sharing made us incredibly generous to our fellow group members, but also gave us the capacity to be frighteningly callous and evil to those who are not. It's part of what Brian Hare and Vanessa Woods describe in their book *Survival of the Friendliest.* Hundreds of thousands of years of evolution for sharing and friendliness within our tribe has made daily life a miracle of peace, harmony, and collaboration for most of us. We volunteer, donate our time and money, coach kids' soccer or organize the school bake sale. We can watch a tense movie in a crowded theater with hundreds of strangers and no one bats an eye. A theater full of unfamiliar chimps would be a bloodbath before the opening credits. But the flip side is that we are generally indifferent and even hostile to anyone we deem an outsider. We divide our world into an in-group and an out-group. Penn State and Pitt, Steelers and Patriots, Republicans and Democrats, citizens and immigrants, my race and yours, Tutsi and Hutu, Muslims and Christians . . . ad infinitum. It matters very little whether the groups are defined by something meaningful or completely arbitrary. Members of our group are family for life. Outsiders might even not rate as human.

So many of the atrocities that scar our history and shake our faith in humanity today—genocides, slavery, human trafficking—are born from our evolved ability to view outsiders as less than human. In the past, this horrific behavior was often sanctioned, even required, by religion or the state. Biology and evolutionary science were coopted in this effort in the 1800s and 1900s, with appalling and wrongheaded "science" used to justify racist policies and behavior. The slimy tendrils remain today in the "intellectual" arguments for racism (in fact, there is no evidence whatsoever that the minute genetic differences among ethnic groups today affect behavior, intelligence, or anything else that we value in our fellow humans). It's chilling to see these themes rising again in our increasingly tribal politics, in countries that are supposed to be civilized enough to know better, dehumanizing people we disagree with and anyone seen as an "other."

The crucial argument of our time is, *Who is part of our group?* Who counts as one of us, and who doesn't? Of course, the only morally acceptable answer to that question is *everyone.* Everyone counts. We are all people. We are all part of the same human tribe.

To win this argument, which we must, we will need to overcome our suspicion of outsiders, the evolutionary price we pay for our incredible willingness to share.

The other downside of our evolved metabolic strategy is our evolved propensity for metabolic disease. Obesity, type 2 diabetes, and heart disease don't evoke the same moral horror as genocide, but they kill more people globally each year than violence. These diseases aren't inevitable. The Hadza don't get them. They are what people in public health call "diseases of civilization," the unintended consequences of development. And they have come to the forefront even as, by some accounts, human societies globally have become less violent. We have graduated as a species from brutally killing each other to mindlessly killing ourselves.

The problem isn't simply our built environments. It's deeper. The faster metabolism and greater daily energy expenditures of the hominin metabolic revolution put our hunter-gatherer ancestors at an increased risk of starvation. Greater daily energy needs mean sharper consequences when food is in short supply. Of course, sharing helps mitigate most of this risk. But there are many potential threats to our energy supply, from prolonged illness wiping out our appetite to unpredictable weather wiping out local plants or game. With a faster metabolism demanding a continuous supply of calories, selection to buffer us against energy shortages led to a second, complementary solution: more fat.

When Steve Ross, Mary Brown, and I conducted doubly labeled water measurements in dozens of apes living in zoos around the United States and compared them to humans, we found differences in more than just energy expenditure. We also found that apes are incredibly lean. Chimpanzees, bonobos, gorillas, and orangutans idling away in zoos and sanctuaries don't get fat, at least by human standards. Chimpanzees and bonobos put on less than 10 percent body fat in captivity, on par with elite human athletes in training.

Even active hunter-gatherers like the Hadza put on more fat than that. And for sedentary people in modern cities (the equivalent of zoo-living apes), the sky is the limit. Men can easily carry 25 or 30 percent body fat, and women more than 40 percent.

Raise an ape in a zoo, with lots of food and limited exercise, and they get big but they don't get fat. Their bodies use the extra calories to build more lean tissue, bigger muscles, and other organs. As a result, zoo apes weigh considerably more than they do in the wild, but they stay lean. In contrast, hominins like us evolved to store a lot of those extra calories away as fat, a rainy day fund to survive future food shortages, prolonged illnesses, or other disruptions in our energy supply. In our modern-day built environments, those rainy days never come. Too many of us end up with far more fat than our bodies need, and the negative health consequences that come with it.

Our hominin bodies are also evolved to support, and in fact *depend on*, the high levels of daily physical activity that were the norm throughout the past two million years of hunting and gathering. We have evolved to require daily exercise. Without it we get sick. The World Health Organization puts the worldwide number of deaths each year from inactivity at 1.6 million. The number of healthy years lost as people struggle with heart disease, diabetes, and other consequences of a sedentary lifestyle is far greater. And it is a uniquely human problem. Apes in zoos, with modest amounts of exercise each day, don't develop high blood pressure, diabetes, humanlike heart disease, or the host of other maladies that plague the developed world.

Modernization has brought an incredible amount of good into the world, from modern medicine and global connectivity to warm houses and sanitary indoor plumbing. But its unintended consequences have grown increasingly scary (and we haven't even touched on climate change, habitat loss, the threat of nuclear annihilation . . .).

Our species is only 300,000 years old. If we're going to survive another 300,000, or even enjoy the next three hundred, we've got to start building better human zoos.

Our one hope is our enormous, intelligent, creative brain. A long evolutionary history as hunter-gatherers has given us the cognitive capacity to shape our world. We have been smart enough to tame fire, build incredible machines and send them to distant planets, create new species, and piece together our own evolutionary history. Are we smart enough to take control of our future? Or are we destined to stumble, to give into temptation and fall short, puking into the bushes yet again and suffering needlessly from self-inflicted misery? Will our distant ancestors pluck our fossils from the soil and marvel at our genius or shake their heads at our inability to avoid disaster?

To figure out how to set things right, we need to figure out what's gone wrong. How did we get so off track, and how do we get back? It's time to head back to Hadzaland and see what they can teach us about living well and staying healthy.

CHAPTER 5

The Metabolic Magician: Energy Compensation and Constraint

I f the quintessential Hadza outlook on life were to be boiled down to its fundamental essence, it would have to be *hamna shida. No problem.* There's rarely a conversation with a Hadza man or woman that doesn't end with this catchall upbeat assessment. Want to stay in our camp for a few weeks and hang out? *Hamna shida.* You'd like to measure our food and follow us around? *Hamna shida.* Wondering about the hyena that's been lurking around camp? *Hamna shida.* Within a day or two in Hadzaland, Brian Wood, Dave Raichlen, and I are saying it to one another. It becomes shorthand for flexibility and adaptability. When things gets tough, we try to stay *hamna shida.*

I envy the Hadza for their bottomless reserve of resilience, and I've often pondered how they come by it. Perhaps, in a world full of things you can't control, from elephants to malaria to green mambas in your blankets, a solid *hamna shida* outlook is the only way to face your day with a smile. Hungry? Tired? Still ten miles of hard walking from home? *Of course you are!* Do those look like lion prints to you? *Yep!* Wondering whether that growing abscess in your thigh will go away on its own or explode and go septic? *Us, too!* But what's the use in worrying? It'll probably be fine, and getting worked up won't do you any good anyway. *Hamna shida.*

To thrive in a tough, unpredictable world as the Hadza do, you've got to be flexible, adaptable. You've got to be *hamna shida*.

So I was trying very hard to be *hamna shida* about everything as Dave and I stood there wondering how to avoid being engulfed in flames. We had been hanging out in camp that morning, a gorgeous blue-sky day in the Tli'ika Hills, setting up a track around camp to measure walking costs (Chapter 3). It was the dry season, and the savanna was a tinderbox, the dry golden grass three feet tall and aching to combust. We lit our morning cooking fires with a handful of it, stuffing it into the fire ring and tossing on a single lit match. The grass would instantly ignite and quickly catch the kindling. We had seen brush fires in the hills around camp a couple of days earlier in the field season, but figured (for no good reason) that they wouldn't advance into camp. We had discussed those fires a bit with our Hadza friends, but got the predictable response: *hamna shida*.

I'm not sure if Dave or I noticed it first. In the relative quiet of the vast savanna, the unmistakable crackle of fire drifted into camp on the breeze. We snapped to attention, looking at each other with the same incredulous expression. *That isn't what it sounds like, right?*

We walked toward the crackling to investigate. Soon we could smell the smoke. Then, through the low acacia trees not too far off, we could see it: a wall of fire at least a hundred yards wide marching steadily for camp, pushed by the languid breeze. Orange-yellow flames leapt six feet into the air, licking at the low branches of the acacia trees. We were adrift in a vast undulating ocean of golden grass, and the ocean was on fire.

Dave is a Southern California guy, an easygoing Jimmy Buffett character with a fondness for barbecue. He keeps a razor-sharp intelligence well hidden beneath layers of sarcasm and an easy smile. Dave is very *hamna shida*. When things look grim, he doubles down on nonchalance, humming "Margaritaville" and carrying on. As we walk back to camp, I look over at him to gauge my own anxiety. Maybe I'm overreacting? But no, it seems Dave is not feeling very *hamna shida* at this particular moment. Like me, he seems to be wondering if we're truly as screwed as it seems.

Here was the problem: We'd spent two years of our professional lives getting funding and permits to measure daily energy expenditures among Hadza adults—the first doubly labeled water measurements in any hunter-gatherer population. Then we'd spent a summer sweating it out in Dar es Salaam (the Cleveland of East Africa), meeting every few days with bureaucrats from the Tanzanian government in hours-long conferences, pleading for official permission to do the work. We had returned this summer with a small laboratory of equipment, including a tank of liquid nitrogen to store urine samples, that we crammed into two Land Cruisers and trundled out to the middle of Hadzaland. We were damn near done, only a couple of weeks to go. The culmination of three years of work—the computers, notebooks, tank of liquid nitrogen with all our samples, not to mention all of our camping gear, tents, and two Land Cruisers—now sat in the path of certain fiery destruction. Judging by the pace of the fire, we had about ten minutes to figure out a solution.

It would have been nice to have Brian in camp. He's also Californian, but from the north up near Davis. He's got an unpretentious shaggy mane of hair, clear eyes, and a penchant for busting out old country tunes on a guitar he keeps in camp that gives him a young Willie Nelson vibe. Brian has lived years of his life in Hadza camps and he's seen it all. Brian is *hamna shida* to the core. No doubt he'd have a good solution. Too bad he was out of camp on a foray, following along with a couple of Hadza men searching for a giraffe one of them had shot with his bow a couple days before.

Here's what Dave and I came up with. We piled all the tents, food, and other camping gear into the circle of bare ground that served as our kitchen and dining area. There was enough bare perimeter that we figured that stuff (probably) wouldn't burn. Then we took all of the precious, irreplaceable science equipment, including the tank of liquid nitrogen and pee samples, and hurriedly shoved it into the Land Cruisers. We started them up and headed for the only place on the landscape that we figured couldn't burn: on the *other side* of the fire, where everything had already burned. All we had to do was drive *through* the fire to the other side, and we'd be fine. Did I mention the back of one of the Land Cruisers was soaked in diesel fuel from a leaky spare tank?

We crept toward the fire in the Land Cruisers, picked a gap in the fire line, and punched it. Success: we didn't die. Dave and I stepped out of our Land Cruisers onto the blackened moonscape where the fire had just passed and exchanged the uneasy smiles of survivors walking away from an airplane crash unscathed. The plan had worked nicely. *Hamna shida.*

And what about the Hadza in camp? They couldn't simply pick up and move their grass houses out of the path of the fire. There was no fire department to call for help. Instead, the women and kids had a dance party. They cut boughs from the bushes around camp and used them to beat down the fire, pushing it around camp as the wind swept it along, singing and smiling and laughing the entire time. Dave and I helped and sang along, learning how to stare down destruction the Hadza way, with some hard work and a song.

The fire passed by camp, and after a break to settle down, Dave and I got back to work on the trackway. The women and kids in camp went back to their usual business. But a couple of hours later, when no one was paying close attention, tragedy struck. The wind shifted and the fire returned. It sneaked into camp from the other direction, too strong and too fast to be pushed away. Dave and I stood there sick to our stomachs as Hadza houses went up in flames, round bonfires of burning grass. We all watched helplessly. There was nothing to do but let them burn.

When the fire had passed, Dave and I walked over to the women to ask how they were doing and offer our condolences. Three of them had lost houses. Amazingly, they were already back to their normal routine, chatting and joking while they tended to the usual daily chores around camp.

"I'm so sorry about your house," I said to Halima, one of the unlucky ones.

She gave me a confused look. "What are you sorry about?"

"Your house. I'm sorry about the fire," I offered.

"Oh, *that*," she said. She shrugged, and turned back to her conversation with her friend.

She had gotten the important stuff—clothing, her family's few belongings—out of the house long before the fire got to it. Sure, it was annoying to lose your house in a fire, but no reason to get upset. There was always more grass to build another one. *Hamna shida*.

I walked away dumbfounded at how adaptable, resilient—how completely *hamna shida*—the Hadza can be. After weeks in camp I still couldn't quite wrap my mind around it. What I could never have guessed—what no scientists understood at that moment, what would have sounded not just incredible but *impossible*—was that their physiology was just as adaptable. And it wasn't just them. The Hadza had something fundamental to teach us about how our bodies burn energy.

Hard Living

The one thing we knew for certain going into the Hadza energetics project was that life as a hunter-gatherer is tough. Like other hunter-gatherers, and like all people prior to twelve thousand years ago, the Hadza have no crops,* no domesticated animals or plants, no machines or cars or guns, no modern conveniences to help them get by. Every morning, they wake up with the sun and set out into the wild savanna for the day's food. Women typically go in groups, relying on their encyclopedic knowledge of the plants around them and the latest info on what's in season to find productive groves of berries or tubers. Several species of wild tubers form the core of the Hadza diet, and a woman can spend two or three hours on any given day digging them out of the hard rocky soil with a sharpened wooden stick. They can easily cover five miles or more on a foray, often with a child in a sling on their back and loaded down with twenty pounds of hard-won tubers on the return trip. Back at camp, they're often busy tending to kids, preparing food, or collecting firewood.

Men usually leave camp alone, preferring to hunt by themselves to improve the odds of sneaking up on a zebra, baboon, antelope, or anything else unlucky enough to cross their path. They aren't picky; just about everything except snakes and other reptiles are on the menu. Hadza men make powerful bows with giraffe-sinew strings, and add a glob of poison to the shaft of their arrows, just below the sharp iron tip—poison strong enough to kill a zebra with a single shot. Men regularly break from hunting to collect wild honey, climbing thirty feet into the crown of massive, ancient baobab trees and hacking into the giant, hollow limbs to plunder an angry hive (Chapter 6). They'll bring the game or honey back to camp, covering ten or fifteen miles round trip, to share with the community.

It's utterly exhausting. Men occasionally spend a day in camp to

---

* Hadza households in some camps, nearest the surrounding villages, do a small amount of farming. We work in remote bush camps where no one farms.

make arrows and rest, but women rarely skip a day of foraging. We've quantified the amount of physical activity that Hadza adults get each day, and the results are staggering: both men and women average more than two hours of hard work each day, roughly ten times more than the average American. That's in addition to the walking. They get more physical activity in a day than the typical Westerner gets in a week. The kids and old folks are active, too. Kids are often tasked with fetching water, which can be half a mile from camp, and men and women in their sixties, seventies, and even eighties are out most days foraging like they did in their prime.

This impressive amount of physical activity isn't unique to the Hadza. All hunter-gatherers lead lives that would make Westerners melt. And while you wouldn't know it from our cushy, urbanized existence today, this extreme level of physical activity was the norm for *all* humans only a few thousand years ago. Our ancestors—all of them—were hunting and gathering only a few hundred generations ago, the blink of an evolutionary eye. We are a hunting and gathering species from hunting and gathering stock (see Chapter 4).

In the industrialized human zoos that we've built for ourselves in the United States, Europe, and other developed societies, we have become much, much more sedentary. Modernization has brought with it a number of important innovations that improve and extend our lives, from indoor plumbing to vaccines and antibiotics. But by several measures we've also become much less healthy. Obesity, type 2 diabetes, heart disease, and the other major killers in the developed world are virtually unheard of among hunter-gatherers and subsistence farmers. Many in public health believe that these diseases of civilization are due in part to a reduction in daily energy expenditure resulting from our sedentary modern lifestyles. In this scenario, our slothful ways reduce the amount of calories we burn each day, and those unspent calories accumulate as fat, leading to obesity and cardiometabolic disease, the catchall term for diabetes, heart disease, and many of the other common maladies of modern life.

That is why we were in Hadzaland that season, measuring daily energy expenditure. We knew the Hadza were incredibly active. Because of that, we believed like everyone else that the Hadza burned an incredible amount of energy each day. No one had actually measured energy expenditures in a hunter-gatherer population before. We wanted to be the first to document their impressive metabolisms and, by comparison, the pathetic, reduced expenditures of the industrialized world. We wanted to understand how the human body functions as a hunter-gatherer.

Things Get Weird

I was new to measurements of daily energy expenditure back in 2009 when we started the Hadza energetics project. I had measured walking and running energy expenditures in humans and a range of other species in my graduate school days, but had done only a bit of work with doubly labeled water. Luckily, I had great colleagues to work with who were expert in the area: Susan Racette at Washington University in St. Louis (where I was working at the time) and Bill Wong at the Baylor College of Medicine. Bill is an internationally recognized leader in doubly labeled water research. He was one of the first scientists to work with the method back in the early 1980s when the technique was first being applied to humans, and has been running one of the best doubly labeled water labs in the world ever since. He also happens to be an incredibly nice guy.

Bill and Susan oversaw the doubly labeled water protocol we developed for the Hadza study, making sure we had properly sized doses and a rock-solid sampling regime. When I got home from

Tanzania after the Hadza field season, I carefully packaged up all the urine samples and shipped them off to Bill's lab. Then I waited. It took a few months for Bill's lab to work through the samples, carefully measuring the isotope enrichments in each one using mass spectrometry.

Then one day late in the fall, far removed from the heat and dust of Hadzaland, an e-mail arrived from Bill. The Hadza results were attached. I was ready for data but not prepared for what they had to say.

I had prepared for the Hadza data by putting together a big comparative dataset of daily energy expenditure measurements for adults from industrialized populations. Anyone who knows anything about energy expenditure (including you, unless you skipped Chapter 3) knows you have to account for body size. Bigger people burn more calories because they have more cells toiling away. So I started my analysis of the Hadza data with a plot of daily energy expenditure and body size for well over a hundred men and women from the United States, Europe, and other industrialized countries. Specifically, I plotted daily energy expenditure against fat-free mass, since fat mass contributes very little to metabolic rate. Then I overlaid the Hadza data—we had measurements for seventeen women and thirteen men. I expected the Hadza data to form a cloud hovering well above the United States and European data. Everyone *knew* that the Hadza had exceptionally high energy expenditures because they were so physically active.

Except they didn't. The Hadza data sat right on top of the measurements from the United States and Europe (Figure 5.1). Hadza men and women were burning the same amount of energy each day as men and women in the United States, England, the Netherlands, Japan, Russia. Somehow the Hadza, who get more physical activity in a day than the typical American gets in a week, were nonetheless burning the same number of calories as everyone else.

I couldn't believe it. *I must be missing something.* I went to work, using increasingly complex statistics to try to account for other factors that might be obscuring the expected result and to tease out the high Hadza expenditures that I *knew* must be there somewhere. I controlled for age. Sex. Fat mass. Height. But none of it mattered. The results were clear and robust. Hadza men and women had the same daily energy expenditures as you and me and everyone else. They were far more active every day, but they didn't burn more calories. What the hell was going on?

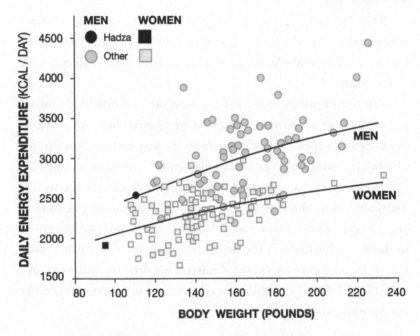

Figure 5.1. Daily energy expenditures for Hadza men and women are the same as adults in industrialized populations. Each point represents average daily expenditure and body weight for an adult male or female cohort (same data as Figure 3.4). Black lines are trend lines for men and women from industrialized populations. Hadza men and women fall on or below those lines, indicating that they burn the same number of calories per day as other populations, accounting for body weight.

Constrained Daily Energy Expenditure

Results from the Hadza seemed to fly in the face of the factorial approach to estimating daily energy expenditure (Chapter 3), which assumes that daily energy expenditure increases in response to daily physical activity (Figure 5.2). This is the dogma, the armchair mechanic's view of how the body's metabolic engine burns calories: the more active you are, the more energy you'll burn each day. The factorial approach is so intuitive and pervasive that it seems indisputable. But it couldn't explain what we were seeing with the Hadza.

Somehow the Hadza were adapting to their strenuous lifestyles in a way that kept the total number of calories burned each day in check. Their metabolic engines were flexible and resilient, very *hamna shida*.

The implications extended far beyond Hadzaland. Humans are all one species. Around the globe, despite our fantastic cultural diversity and superficial differences in the way we look, our bodies all work the same way. The metabolic flexibility we were seeing with the Hadza was a capacity that all of us shared, all over the world. The Hadza were showing us a new way of understanding ourselves. Daily energy expenditure wasn't simply responding to differences in daily activity. Instead, the body seemed to be maintaining daily energy expenditure within some narrow window, regardless of lifestyle (Figure 5.2). I call this view of metabolism "constrained daily energy expenditure."

Of course, if the Hadza results were a fluke, we could have dismissed them. Overturning a big, established, and comfortable way of thinking like the factorial model takes more than one study. But in fact, there's a large and growing body of work in human and animal energetics all pointing to constrained daily energy expenditure. Some of it was out there well before our Hadza work, hiding in plain sight.

Since the Hadza project, my colleagues and I have measured daily energy expenditures in other hunter-gatherer and farming populations, with similar results. Sam Urlacher, a postdoc in my lab, spent months with the Shuar population living in the remote Amazon rain forests of Ecuador. Like the Hadza, the Shuar live an incredibly active lifestyle, hunting, fishing, and gathering plant

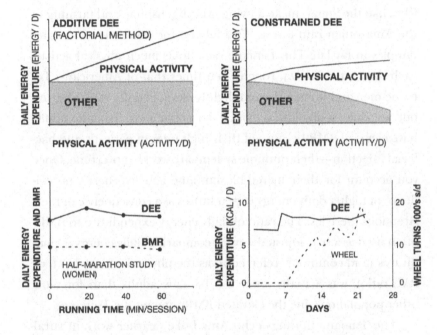

Figure 5.2. Top row: Traditional "armchair engineer" models of metabolism are Additive, and assume daily energy expenditure increases directly with daily physical activity. In the Constrained model, the body reduces energy spent on other tasks (shaded area) as physical activity increases, keeping daily energy expenditure within a narrow range. **Bottom row:** When humans (left), mice (right), and other animals increase their daily physical activity, daily energy expenditure does not increase with activity but plateaus. **Left:** Women from Westerterp's half-marathon study. **Right:** Mice kept sedentary (days 1–7), then allowed access to a wheel (days 7–28). Daily expenditure adjusted initially with wheel access but then remained steady as daily wheel activity climbed.

foods from the wild. They also farm a bit, using hand tools and a lot of hard work to grow and harvest starchy staples like manioc and plantain. Sam measured daily energy expenditures among five- to twelve-year-old Shuar kids and compared them to kids from the United States and U.K. The Shuar kids were more physically active, and they also had elevated BMRs due to higher levels of parasites and other infection (Chapter 3). Nonetheless, their daily energy expenditures were identical to those of U.S. and British children.

Further south, in Bolivia, Mike Gurven and his team measured daily energy expenditure in men and women among the Tsimane, who, like the Shuar, make a living hunting, fishing, and farming in the Amazonian rain forest. We analyzed the doubly labeled water samples in my lab. The Tsimane rack up as much physical activity each day as the Hadza, roughly ten times that of Americans. Tsimane men and women showed slightly elevated daily expenditures, but not due to physical activity. Like Shuar kids, Tsimane adults have elevated BMR because of their high rates of parasitic and bacterial infection—their immune systems are working overtime. Once you account for their incredible immune activity, there's no evidence of higher daily energy expenditures as a consequence of their strenuous lifestyles. The ratio of daily energy expenditure to BMR, often used as a size-adjusted way for comparing daily energy expenditures (and commonly referred to as the physical activity level, or PAL ratio), was actually lower for Tsimane adults than for most other populations due the elevated BMRs among the Tsimane.

The Tsimane findings echo Amy Luke's earlier work in rural Nigeria. Amy is an expert in metabolism and cardiometabolic disease, and has been studying the health effects of the increasingly sedentary American lifestyle for over two decades. In the early 2000s, she led a team of researchers measuring (among other things) daily energy expenditures in black women from Maywood, Illinois, and rural Nigeria. Like the Tsimane, the Nigerian women, many of them farmers, had elevated BMRs compared to their U.S. counterparts. Daily energy expenditures (adjusted for differences in body size) were slightly elevated as well, reflecting greater BMRs. But there was no difference in activity energy expenditure, the portion of daily expenditure that's left when you subtract BMR and the costs of digestion. The PAL ratio of daily energy expenditure to BMR was the same for Nigerian and U.S. women despite clear differences in lifestyle.

The list goes on. Lara Dugas, a postdoc working with Amy Luke at Loyola Medical School, analyzed daily energy expenditures reported for ninety-eight populations around the globe. There was a good deal of variability in daily energy expenditure—some were high, some were low. But the populations in rural farming communities, who work hard each day to make a living, had the same daily energy expenditures as pampered urbanites in the industrialized world. Even among industrialized countries, there's no correspondence between measured physical activity and daily energy expenditure, activity energy expenditure, or PAL ratios. People who work harder don't necessarily burn more calories.

Constrained daily energy expenditure is what we see when we look *within* populations as well. I teamed up with Amy Luke, Lara Dugas, and their team to analyze daily expenditures for 332 men and women in five different countries. We pooled everyone together and adjusted their daily energy expenditure to account for the effects of body weight, fat percentage, age, and other characteristics, and plotted their adjusted expenditures against daily physical activity. There was a ton of variability among people even after accounting for body size and body fat (see Chapter 3). Still, we were able to pick up a weak signal from physical activity—a whisper in a football stadium of noise—showing a slight uptick in daily expenditure in more active people. But not only was the effect of activity weak, it petered out at higher activity levels. People who were moderately active burned about 200 kilocalories more, on average, than total couch potatoes, but there was no difference between moderately active adults and those with the highest levels of physical activity. Just as the constrained model predicts, daily energy expenditure plateaued. And the variation in daily expenditure among couch potatoes was far greater than the difference between the average couch potato and the average high-activity adult.

All of these comparisons so far have been between people with different levels of habitual physical activity. What happens if we change someone's lifestyle by enrolling them in an exercise program? There are lots of these types of studies, and while there's some variability in results depending on the duration and intensity of the exercise program, they generally point toward a constrained daily energy expenditure model. Here's my favorite: Klaas Westerterp and colleagues in the Netherlands enrolled men and women who never exercised into a year-long program to train them to run a half-marathon. Three of the women and four of the men had their daily energy expenditures measured before starting the program and then at week 8, 20, and 40, which corresponded to stages in the training protocol. In the beginning, subjects were running 20 minutes per day, 4 days a week. By the end, sessions were 60 minutes long, and subjects were running roughly 25 miles per week.

Unsurprisingly, with all this training, the women gained muscle, about four pounds of it. In addition, they were burning around 360 kcal per day running, based on their body weight and mileage. If the factorial model were correct, we'd expect their daily energy expenditures to be at least 360 kcal per day higher by the end of the study, and closer to around 390 kcal/day if we factor in the calories consumed at rest by their increased muscle mass (Chapter 3). Instead, at week 40, their daily energy expenditure was only about 120 kcal higher. These women went from never exercising to running 25 miles per week, fit enough to run a half-marathon, and their daily energy expenditure was essentially the same as when they started (Figure 5.2). Men in the study showed similar results.

The duration of the Westerterp study is worth noting. In the world of research, it's considered an ambitious, long-term study, lasting a full year. But twelve months isn't *that* long. As we'll see below and in Chapter 7, adjustments to new lifestyles can occur over years. Populations like the Hadza have years and years—literally, entire lifetimes—to adjust to their high levels of physical activity. They are the ultimate long-term study populations. Perhaps we shouldn't be surprised, then, that researchers often find no evidence of elevated daily energy expenditure in traditional populations.

And it's not just humans. Constrained daily energy expenditure seems to be the rule among warm-blooded animals. Several laboratory studies in rodents and birds have measured daily energy expenditures while increasing daily physical activity—not so different from Westerterp's half-marathon study. Again and again, we see the same result: daily energy expenditure doesn't change even as the animals work harder and harder. The juggling act that our bodies do to keep daily expenditures within a narrow window is apparently an ancient and widespread evolutionary strategy.

Which brings us to the zoo. As we discussed in Chapter 1, my colleagues and I have spent the last few years measuring daily energy expenditures in apes, monkeys, and any other primates we can get our hands on. Just as the constrained model would predict, we've found that zoo-living primates have the same daily energy expenditures as those in the wild. Same goes for kangaroos and pandas. Each species maintains its evolved metabolic rate whether it's struggling for survival in the jungle or chilling out at the zoo; lifestyle has little effect. Ring-tailed lemurs have the same daily energy expenditure whether they're eking out a living in the forests of Madagascar or lounging in the comfortable enclosures of the Duke Lemur Center. No wonder humans burn the same amount of energy whether we're living off the land as hunter-gatherers or cooped up in the industrialized zoos we've built for ourselves.

Our metabolic engines shift and change to make room for increased activity costs, ultimately keeping daily energy expenditure within a narrow window. As a result, physically active people—whether it's hunter-gatherers living today or in our collective past, or people in the industrialized world who exercise regularly—burn the same amount of energy as people who are much more sedentary.

Trying to Outrun Obesity

The realization that daily energy expenditure is constrained changes the way we think about the modern obesity epidemic. First, the fact that hunter-gatherers burn the same amount of energy as urbanites in the developed world means that daily energy expenditure is likely unchanged from our Paleolithic past to the computerized present. The modern explosion in obesity and all its downstream effects can't be blamed on decreasing energy expenditures in industrialized countries. Doubly labeled water studies in the industrialized world, which stretch back to the 1980s, seem to confirm this: daily energy expenditures and the PAL ratio have stayed the same in the United States and Europe for the past four decades, even as obesity and metabolic disease have skyrocketed.

Second, constrained daily energy expenditure means that increasing daily activity through exercise or other programs will ultimately have little effect on the calories burned per day. This realization should change the way we tackle obesity. Weight change is fundamentally about energy balance: if we eat more calories than we burn, we gain weight; if we burn more than we eat, we lose weight. Those are the rules of physics and, as established by Lavoisier, Atwater, Rubner, and the pioneers of metabolic science, humans and other animals play by the rules (see Chapter 3). The widespread evidence that daily energy expenditure is constrained tells us that durable, meaningful changes in daily energy expenditure are extremely difficult to achieve through exercise. If the energy burned is *really difficult* to budge no matter how much we exercise, we'd be better off battling obesity by focusing on the amount of energy we eat.

Exercise is still essential for health! You still need to exercise! If you want to reassure yourself that the gym membership you just purchased was a smart move, go directly to Chapter 7, where we discuss all the important benefits of exercise. As we'll see, the constraint on daily energy expenditure is actually an important reason *why* exercise is so good for you. Exercise will keep you healthy and alive. It just won't do much for your weight.

Now, if you're paying close attention to the numbers, you might be asking why the small changes in metabolic rate that exercise can induce aren't important for battling obesity. After all, the women training to run a half-marathon might have ended up burning a lot less energy than we'd expect, but still . . . 120 kcal per day is still *something.* Lots of exercise programs show *some* lasting increase in energy expenditure, even if it's small. Over time, even small effects can add up. And even if your metabolism eventually adjusts to accommodate the new exercise regime, at least there's the weeks or months during the adjustment period where daily energy expenditure is higher than before (see below). Those increases in daily expenditure will lead to weight loss, right?

Don't count on it.

If our bodies were simple machines, small increases in daily energy expenditure would eventually lead to weight loss. But our bodies aren't simple machines. They're dynamic products of evolution built over hundreds of millions of years to be agile and flexible and respond to changes in activity and food availability. Our bodies—or more to the point, our brains—manipulate both our hunger and metabolic rate in ways that make it awfully hard to maintain weight loss. Our metabolic engines are exquisitely tuned to match the energy we burn each day with the energy we eat, and vice versa. (In fact, that's probably why animals evolved constrained daily energy expenditure in the first place: to match expenditure to the amount of food available.) Even transient increases in daily energy expenditure are met with increases in energy intake. When we burn more, we eat more.

Take the Midwest Exercise Trial 1 study conducted in the United States in the late 1990s. Young adults who were sedentary and overweight were randomly assigned to either an exercise group or a control group. Exercisers worked their way up to doing about 2,000 kcal of exercise (the equivalent of running twenty miles) every week for sixteen months. At 2,000 kcal a week for sixteen months, the exercisers should have lost forty pounds. Instead, the men lost ten pounds, and nearly all of the weight loss occurred within the first nine months. They stopped losing after that even though they kept exercising. If that sounds grim, consider the women in the exercise group: they lost *nothing*. They weighed exactly the same after sixteen months of supervised, strenuous exercise as they did when they showed up on day one (Figure 5.3). Perhaps they took some comfort in knowing that women assigned to the control group, who didn't exercise at all for sixteen months, tended to gain a couple of pounds.

In the wake of those disappointing results, the researchers tried again with a more demanding workout regime in Midwest 2. Men and women were assigned to either 2,000 or 3,000 kcal of supervised exercise per week. That's an incredible amount of exercise, equivalent to running twenty or thirty miles per week for a 150-pound person (Chapter 3). Only 64 percent of enrolled subjects completed the ten-month study, perhaps because it was so strenuous. For those who completed the study, daily energy expenditure increased just 220 kcal/per day on average, well below the 285 to 430 kcal/day increase we'd expect from their exercise regime. Average weight loss was around ten pounds, not much different from men in the easier Midwest 1 study, and far less than we'd expect from so much exercise. And there was no difference in average weight loss between the 2,000 and 3,000 kcal/week exercise groups, further suggesting the dose of exercise had little effect on weight. Even more surprising, for thirty-four of the seventy-four men and women who completed the study, average weight loss was zero. These poor souls, labeled "non-responders," exercised like mad, even managed to push their daily energy expenditure up a bit, and still lost nothing.

The Midwest 1 and 2 subjects were not an anomaly. All studies that try to achieve weight loss through exercise show the same pattern: the longer the study lasts, the less that weight loss meets expectations (Figure 5.3). For the first couple of months in a new exercise program, results are all over the place. People generally lose weight, but there's a huge amount of variability in how they respond in the short term (some people even gain weight). But after a year, even with someone watching them exercise so they don't skip or cheat, the average amount of weight lost is less than half of what's expected. By two years, the average amount of weight lost is less than five pounds, and many, as we see with the Midwest studies, will lose nothing.

In other words, if you start a new exercise program tomorrow and stick to it religiously, you will most likely weigh nearly the same in two years as you do right now. You should still do it! You'll be happier, healthier, and live longer. Just don't expect any meaningful weight change in the long term from exercise alone.

•••

Such disappointing weight-loss results are due in part to the sort of metabolic compensation to increased activity that we discussed above, but constrained daily energy expenditure isn't the whole story. The other important change is that exercising drives us to eat more. Our brains are exceptionally good at adjusting our hunger levels so that we make up for any increase in expenditure by increasing intake, something we'll discuss more below.

The tight coordination between eating and expenditure also explains a curious and counterintuitive fact of human metabolism: burning more energy doesn't protect you against gaining weight. As we discussed in Chapter 3, there's a great deal of variation in daily energy expenditure among people, even after we account for differences in body size and fat percentage. Some people burn more energy each day, some burn less. (Two people of the same size, age, and lifestyle can easily differ by 500 kcal per day.) Occasionally we even see high daily energy expenditures in some groups (we've measured elevated daily expenditures in a small sample of Shuar men, for example). But there's no relationship between having a fast metabolism and being thin. Obese people burn just as much energy each day as thin people, after accounting for differences in body size and composition (in fact, if you don't correct for body size, obese people tend to burn *more* calories each day simply because they're larger; see Chapter 3 and Figure 5.1). And daily energy expenditure, high or low, doesn't predict anything about your likelihood of gaining weight. In Amy Luke's study of Nigerian and U.S. women, for example, there was no relationship between a woman's daily expenditure and her weight gain over the following two years. Studies of children have shown the same result. People who burn more don't weigh less. People who burn more, eat more.

So to lose weight, we just need to eat less, right?

Turns out that's complicated, too.

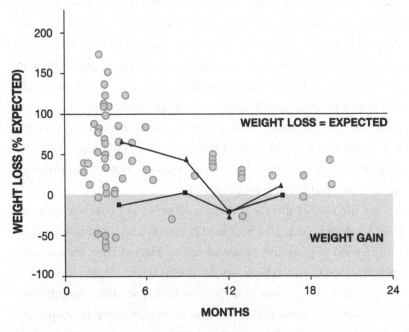

Figure 5.3. Weight loss with exercise. Each dot shows the average weight loss for one exercise study: 100 percent weight loss means subjects lost exactly as much weight as expected for the amount of calories burned in exercise, while 0 percent means subjects lost no weight. The longer the study, the less weight loss is observed. Weight changes for Midwest 1 study men (triangles) and women (squares) are plotted over the course of that study.

We Are All the Biggest Loser: Metabolic Responses to Overeating and Undereating

The Biggest Loser is reality television for viewers who don't want to choose between voyeurism and sadism. The premise is straightforward: Sixteen people with extreme obesity, somewhere north of three hundred pounds and desperate to turn things around, are sent away to an isolated weight-loss boot camp for thirteen weeks.

There they are put through an outrageous program to lose weight. They exercise for four and a half hours each day under the stern eye of a militant trainer. They starve themselves, eating less than half the calories they were eating before entering the competition. Occasionally, for the enjoyment of viewers, contestants are tormented with their favorite foods or the chance to call home. Every week or so, they are weighed in public like deli meat. The person who loses the fewest pounds is sent home, usually in tears. Watching people suffer in this particular manner is apparently something that humans across the world enjoy. Like the obesity epidemic itself, the show began in the United States (of course), but it has spread to more than thirty countries worldwide.

It's the sort of spectacle that you'd never get past a human research ethics board. The workload is brutal, and intentional public humiliation is generally frowned upon. Even if they let you start such a project, the crying would surely be cause for shutting it down. But for a curious and clever scientist studying metabolism and obesity, the show presents a unique opportunity. If people are going to endure this insanity anyway, why not use it as an opportunity to see how the body responds to massive amounts of exercise and extreme dieting?

So in 2010, Kevin Hall led a group of researchers from the National Institutes of Health and Pennington Biomedical Research Center to study metabolic changes among *Biggest Loser* contestants. They measured BMR, daily energy expenditure, and hormone levels in addition to tracking changes in body weight and body fat. Much like the Hadza energetics project, Hall's work showed just how flexible our bodies can be.

First, the good news: the contestants all lost a lot of weight. By week 6 of the competition, they'd lost an average of thirty pounds. By week 13, those who hadn't been sent home had lost *another* thirty to forty pounds. And by the big TV finale, a homecoming of sorts at week 30, where the contestants are flown back to the ranch for a final weigh-in after four more months of self-policed dieting and exercise, the contestants had lost an average of 127 pounds. They had burned off the equivalent of an entire normal-weight adult human. There were other health benefits as well. Contestants' fasting glucose levels (their blood sugar) went down, as did their insulin resistance, reducing their risk of developing type 2 diabetes. The amount of circulating triglycerides in their blood was lower, too, which is good for cardiovascular health.

Now the not-so-great news: their bodies were in starvation mode. By week 30, their BMRs had dropped nearly 700 kcal per day, or about 25 percent. The reduction in BMR wasn't just a function of weighing less; it was far greater than expected from weight loss alone. The change was deeper. Their cells had reduced their metabolic rate, working and burning energy more slowly. And the changes weren't temporary. When Hall and colleagues checked in with the contestants again six years after the show, their BMRs were *still* lower than expected. From a public health perspective, this seems perverse. Why were their bodies working against their efforts to burn off unhealthy weight? But from an evolutionary perspective, it makes all the sense in the world.

As the products of hundreds of millions of years of evolution, we should expect our bodies to be extremely sensitive to the amount of food in their environment and the amount of reserve energy we have stored away as fat. All organisms need energy for life's essential tasks, and in general, the more they can burn, the better (Chapter 3). Burning more energy means more growth, maintenance, and reproduction. But it's a Darwinian game of blackjack: going over is *bad*. Burning more energy than you eat—what researchers refer to as negative energy balance—requires consuming your own body. You can eat into your fat stores for a while (that's what they're for), but it's not sustainable indefinitely. Eventually you'll starve to death.

Not surprisingly, there are ancient, evolved responses to negative energy balance in humans and other animals. When our bodies sense that we're not eating enough to meet our daily energy requirements, we start throttling things down. The body struggles mightily to balance its energy budget so that expenditure doesn't exceed intake. Our thyroid gland, the body's master controller of metabolic rate, reduces the amount of thyroid hormone produced, which is like taking your foot off the gas pedal. Our cells slow down, which lowers BMR and daily energy expenditure. At the same time, the hormones and brain circuitry that control hunger increase our drive for food. We become ravenous, fixated on food as our body directs our mental energies toward finding something—*anything*—to eat. This is the evolved starvation response, also known as dieting.

The starvation response is well studied. Some of the earliest work measuring metabolic rates, in the late 1800s and early 1900s, focused on changes during starvation in humans and other animals. One of the first thorough studies was conducted in 1917 by Francis Benedict and colleagues, in the midst of World War I. The aim of the study was to better understand and treat the victims of starvation from the war. Twenty-four college-aged men were fed half of their normal amount of calories for several weeks until they had lost about 10 percent of their weight. Their size-adjusted BMR dropped 10 to 15 percent, and they grew irritable and lost their interest in sex.

The most famous and thorough starvation study was done in 1944 and '45, in the waning months of World War II (apparently the lessons of World War I, both for international diplomacy and the physiology of starvation, had not sunk in). As the atrocities and deprivations of World War II came into focus, researchers were eager to improve treatment for starvation. Ancel Keys and colleagues at the University of Minnesota took thirty-two young men, conscientious objectors whose pacifist beliefs kept them from serving in the war, and put them on a semi-starvation diet for twenty-four weeks. The men ate just 1,570 kcal per day, less than half of their estimated daily energy expenditure at the start of the study. They lost 25 percent of their body weight. Unsurprisingly, their irritability and moodiness increased, while their interest in sex and other activity fell. They were constantly hungry, obsessed with food. Eating literally haunted their dreams. BMR dropped 20 percent below that expected for their body weight.

All of these changes went away when the men were allowed to eat again. As their weight came back, their bodies called off the alarm. Unlike the *Biggest Loser* contestants, their BMRs returned to normal, as did their mood and interest in sex and other hobbies. They were no longer in starvation mode.

Notably, the men overshot their initial weight when they regained after the study, putting on a couple more pounds of fat than they had had at the start of the study. The same thing had happened to the men in Benedict's study during World War I. The overshooting phenomenon isn't as well studied, but it makes evolutionary sense. Experiencing a period of starvation is a reasonably good indicator that you're in a poor, unpredictable environment. In that case, storing a bit more fuel for next time is probably a good idea. Still, it's impressive that their bodies "knew" what their normal weight was supposed to be and returned them to it, more or less, calling off the alarm when they'd hit their pre-study size. Clearly, the mechanisms that shape our metabolism and hunger are quite specific about the body weight and composition they work to defend.

The *Biggest Loser* contestants regained weight, too, despite their best efforts. When Kevin Hall and his group checked in with fourteen of the contestants six years after the show, all but one had regained a considerable amount of weight. Three were back to their initial weight before the show; two others had overshot and were heavier than when they started. And how were metabolic rate and BMR reduction related to weight regain? The traditional view of energy expenditure—the armchair engineer's view—is that contestants with higher metabolic rates and less BMR reduction would be protected against regaining weight. In that case, there should be a negative relationship between BMR reduction and weight regain. Contestants with higher BMRs should have regained less.

Instead, Hall and colleagues found the opposite: six years after the show, contestants with higher BMRs had regained the *most*. That's a surprising result if we expect higher BMR and daily expenditures to be protective against weight gain, but it makes sense if we understand metabolism from an evolutionary perspective. BMR and daily energy expenditure don't *dictate* weight change, they *respond* to weight change. The *Biggest Loser* contestants were in starvation mode during and after the competition. Their lower BMRs and daily expenditures were a desperate, evolved strategy to keep expenditures in line with their severely reduced intake. In the years following the show, contestants who ate the most and regained the most weight gave their bodies the strongest signals that the danger of starvation had passed. Their BMR and daily expenditures rebounded along with their body weight.

The Brains Behind the Operation

With all of the evidence that our bodies respond dynamically to changes in physical activity and diet, we need a new way of thinking about our metabolic engines. The current consensus in metabolism—the armchair engineer's view—assumes the body is a simple machine: the more work it does, the more energy it burns, and the more energy it burns, the less fuel (fat) it will carry. As we've just seen, that's not how it works. The body is clever and flexible in how it burns energy. It does things that simple engines cannot. We need a better metaphor.

To make sense of metabolism, we need to think of the body like a business. This business is the product of evolution and therefore has only one real goal: reproduction. But like any big business, it has lots of operations in support, organized into various organs and physiological systems. There are 37 trillion employees, the cells, hard at work each day doing their part. Calories are the currency for all transactions. Energy comes in with the food we eat and is allocated to each of the support systems and their employees as needed. If there's any extra, it's deposited into a checking account for quick access (glycogen), or into savings (fat).

A strict and heartless Darwinian manager keeps an eye on the budget, watching energy coming in and energy going out. More energy coming *in* than going out is generally a good thing; it keeps the coffers full and allows the manager to allocate more energy to systems that can use it. More energy going *out* than coming in is cause for concern. If a deficit is too severe or persists too long, the manager will take action and change how energy is spent. In general, keeping a balanced budget means keeping daily energy expenditure equal to the amount of food energy that is dependably available from the environment.

Most of the time, in the industrialized world, the body isn't directly involved in reproduction (sex, pregnancy, nursing), but that hardly matters. The business needs to be ready, and so the support systems need to be kept humming. Just keeping all 37 trillion of your employees fed and functioning is a major undertaking. Interacting with the outside world requires the coordinated efforts of your muscles, nerves, brain, heart, and lungs. Defense and repair are never-ending, with your various systems wearing out a bit each day and the constant assault of viruses, bacteria, pollutants, and parasites. And of course the reproductive system itself needs to be maintained and ready to go. All of this requires energy, and your brain and digestive system work together nonstop to acquire a steady supply of food and turn it into useful nutrients (Chapter 2).

The Darwinian business manager juggling all these tasks is a product of our evolution. When it's twelve P.M. and you're starving for lunch, that's the manager responding to your empty stomach, low blood sugar, and other cues by activating the hunger circuitry in your brain. When you're fighting the flu, lethargic and running a fever, that's the manager shifting energy away from physical activity and toward immune activity. When you demolish a cheesecake by yourself, it's the manager's job to direct all those calories to the systems that can use it and store the rest in your fat cells.

The metabolic manager isn't just a metaphor or a cartoon, it's your brain. Specifically, it's your hypothalamus, a nondescript lump of neurons sitting dead center on the bottom of your brain like a wad of gray chewing gum. The hypothalamus is the control center for your metabolism and a host of other housekeeping functions that keep your body alive. In concert with your brain stem, the hypothalamus senses energy coming in by monitoring the blood for factors like glucose and leptin (a hormone secreted by fat cells when they're storing energy from a recent meal), and neural signals from the taste buds, stomach, and small intestine that relay information on the size and macronutrient content of a meal. The hypothalamus can also sense when we're in negative energy balance, monitoring levels of ghrelin (a hormone produced by the stomach when it's empty), leptin (which decreases when fat cells are depleted), and other cues. In response, the hypothalamus can crank our metabolism up or down by controlling the activity of the thyroid gland and the production of thyroid hormone. It can also change our hunger levels, adjusting the amount of food we need to eat to feel full.

You can think of the actions of the hypothalamus like the algorithms we interact with every day online. Google, Facebook, and every other site we interact with uses hundreds of pieces of data—our age, gender, location, the type of device we're using, the time of day, our previous browsing history—to tailor the stories and advertisements we see. It all happens automatically, instantaneous and unseen. The nature of the algorithm is the same for everyone, but the results are tailored to us and our particular situation. The same is true for the internal algorithms that manage our metabolism. The variables (leptin, ghrelin, blood glucose, stomach fullness, food flavors) are the same for everyone, but our immediate environment, genetics, and past experience shape the way the system weighs each variable and responds. For example, lower leptin levels generally push the hypothalamus to activate the hunger response, but the *precise* threshold at which leptin will trigger *your* hunger response will have a lot to do with your genes, eating habits, and the typical levels of leptin circulating in your blood.

Evolution shapes the metabolic algorithms for each species, determining the "normal" ranges for BMR, daily expenditure, hormones, body fat percentage, blood glucose levels, circulating triglycerides, and the rest. "Normal" is what emerges when the hypothalamus and its evolved metabolic algorithms are able to keep things under control, managing the flow of calories in and out. (The general term for keeping all of your systems running and stable is homeostasis.) But what's normal isn't the same for all species. For example, as we read in the last chapter, humans have a faster metabolic rate than other apes, but we also put on body fat much more readily. That's because our hypothalamus and its metabolic algorithms have evolved: they keep a heavier foot on the gas pedal and are a bit quicker to store extra energy away as fat.

Chimpanzees and other apes burn energy more slowly, but are apt to burn off extra calories or convert them into lean tissue.

Our evolutionary legacy also shapes the way we respond to challenges like reduced food availability or increased activity. When we're in starvation mode, the hypothalamus acts quickly. The objective is to survive the lean period to reproduce sometime in the future when conditions improve. Within days, thyroid hormone, the main control hormone for our metabolic rate, plummets. BMR goes way down, as we saw in the Minnesota starvation study and with the *Biggest Loser* contestants. If food restriction is severe and lasts for a long time, our organs will actually shrink. But not all organ systems are hit equally hard. We know from careful studies of the bodies of victims starved to death in war and famine that the brain is spared. The spleen, on the other hand, shrinks dramatically. Our Darwinian manager is making tough decisions, picking winners and losers, preserving brain function but letting some of our immune function slide.

The hypothalamus controls nearly every system in the body, from stress response to reproduction, and can manipulate specific functions. For example, humans are quick to put reproduction on the back burner when times are tough. Subjects in starvation experiments lose their interest in sex. Women often see a decline in estrogen levels and, if the food restriction is sufficiently severe, will stop ovulating. Putting off reproduction when times are bad makes good evolutionary sense in a species like ours, where life is long and each kid costs a fortune in time and calories. But in a short-lived species, delaying reproduction means you might never get the chance. That's why male mice faced with starvation maintain two organs above all else: their brain and their testicles.

Metabolic response to increased exercise, the phenomenon we see with physically active groups like the Hadza or in Westerterp's half-marathon study, is less well studied but seems to follow similar logic. With the muscles demanding a much larger share of the business's energy and draining fat reserves, the Darwinian manager acts to rebalance the budget. In the immediate term, hunger is increased in order to match intake to expenditure. If high levels of daily activity persist for weeks or months, though, other changes are made. Other systems, including reproduction, immune function, and stress response, are suppressed, making room in the budget for greater activity costs. (Interestingly, these metabolic changes don't always show up in BMR where we might expect them, something we'll discuss in Chapter 8.) Behavior may change as well, inducing us to rest more and fidget less. We should expect these responses to follow an evolutionary logic, cutting nonessential tasks first and prioritizing our long-term reproductive success. In three to five months we'll be acclimated to our new exercise regimen. Daily energy expenditure will be nearly the same as before we started. Our metabolic business and its 37 trillion employees will have adjusted to the new conditions.

All of the tricks our bodies play to modify energy expenditure and hunger in response to exercise and diet make it sound as though our weight should never change. Maintaining the same weight without really trying seems an impossible dream to most of us, but it's far more common than you think. At least, it used to be. Hadza men and women, for example, are incredibly weight stable across the life span; body weights and BMIs hardly change from early adulthood to old age. Ponder that for a moment. In the face of seasonal changes in food availability, through good years and bad, and despite the fact that men and women in their twenties and thirties (usually with young children) work a bit harder than older adults, their weight doesn't change. Presumably, this sort of effortless weight management was the norm in our hunter-gatherer past. In hunter-gatherer environments like those in which we evolved, our bodies are perfectly capable of managing our weight by adjusting our metabolism and hunger to suit the conditions. *Hamna shida.*

Even in the industrialized human zoos we live in today, with unlimited delicious food always at our fingertips, our hypothalamus does a remarkably good job matching energy expenditure to intake. When we eat more calories than we burn, our metabolic rate increases as our body tries to make use of some of the surplus. When we burn more calories than we eat, hunger increases and expenditure goes down. Sure, day to day, there's some mismatch between calories in and calories out—record your body weight every morning for a month and you'll see those fluctuations for yourself. But over the long term, our energy balance is incredibly precise. Today, in the grips of an obesity epidemic, the average American adult gains about half a pound per year, an error of around 1,750 kcal. That's only about 5 kcal per day, or less than 0.2 percent of daily energy expenditure. In other words, without thinking much about it, we match our daily energy intake to within 99.8 percent of our daily expenditure (and vice versa).

A Smarter Way of Thinking About Metabolism and Obesity

It is absolutely and inescapably correct that obesity results from eating more calories than we burn. There is no other way to gain weight. And the mounting evidence that daily energy expenditure is hard to budge strongly points to diet as the primary culprit. If our bodies keep daily energy expenditure in check regardless of lifestyle, energy imbalance and weight gain must come primarily from eating too many calories.

But that doesn't mean that obesity is a simple matter of gluttony. Sure, in some cases, the causes of unhealthy weight gain might be clear—a daily cheesecake habit, for example, is probably a bad idea, and people do tend to gain weight around the holidays from all those cookies and feasts. But the slow rate of weight gain that most of us experience, waistlines inching out year by year, is much more insidious. The modern obesity epidemic reflects a breakdown in metabolic management. Our evolved algorithms have adapted reasonably well to recent changes in the foods available and the ways we use our bodies (or don't), but for many of us they bring in too much food. Our Paleolithic brain is overwhelmed by our modern environment. Rather than perfectly matching intake to expenditure, we have a tendency to overeat—not by much, usually, but the error is consistent and it adds up over time as fat. Like moths mistaking a porch light for the moon, we are responding poorly to novel environments—environments *we've* built—doing things that feel good but ultimately lead to trouble.

When we blame our metabolism for our struggles with obesity, or we rely on exercise to increase daily expenditure and lose weight, or we fall for the latest metabolism-boosting scam, we are making a fundamental mistake about the way metabolism works. The global obesity epidemic cannot be a problem of energy expenditure. For one thing, as we see with the Hadza, daily energy expenditures are the same today in the industrialized world as they were in our hunter-gatherer past. Our bodies are incredibly adept at responding to changing activity levels to keep daily energy expenditures within a narrow window. But more crucially, blaming obesity on slow metabolism gets the cause and effect of weight change completely backward. Our metabolism doesn't *dictate* energy balance, it *responds* to energy balance.

To return for a moment to the metaphor of our bodies as engines: the traditional armchair engineer's view has us in the driver's seat of a sports car, revving the motor. We can decide how hot to run the engine and when to stop for gas. It's an appealing vision, but it gives us far more control over our metabolism than we actually have. At best, we're backseat passengers in a peculiar metabolic taxi. Our hypothalamus is in the driver's seat with its foot on the gas pedal, a steady eye on the fuel gauge, and an array of tricks to keep the engine running steady and avoid running out of gas. We can dictate the route and harangue our Darwinian driver to speed up or slow down, but we don't have much real control over the engine or how often we fuel up.

It's still the case that obesity is fundamentally a problem of taking in more fuel than our engines burn. But rather than pretending we're in the driver's seat, we should be asking why the evolved mechanisms that normally match intake precisely to expenditure are failing in our industrialized world.

Calories In, Calories Out, and the Metabolic Magician

When we published the Hadza daily energy expenditure results in 2012, we were unprepared for the response. We figured there would be *some* interest in the work (we certainly hoped there would be) because it was the first energetics measurement from a hunter-gatherer population, and because the results were surprising and held big implications for tackling obesity. Hadza men and women were far more physically active than people in the United States and Europe, yet they burned the same number of calories (Figure 5.1). We argued that to fix the obesity crisis we needed to focus on diet and the energy we take in, rather than on energy expenditure, which seemed to be constrained and hard to move. We expected a handful of science journalists and colleagues might contact us to discuss the project.

Instead, we had journalists from around the globe calling to talk about the work. The study found its way into *Time* magazine and the BBC. The *New York Times* asked me to write a piece on the study for the Sunday paper. Scientists from other labs e-mailed to ask about the results. It was fun and exciting to discuss the project and its implications. To date, the article has been viewed a quarter of a million times online. Not exactly Beyoncé or cat video numbers, but a lot more attention than the usual scientific study receives.

As you can imagine, not all the response was positive. Big believers in the power of exercise to cure all of society's ills, including some exercise researchers in public health, absolutely hated the suggestion that exercise isn't the solution to obesity. It didn't help that obesity research has gotten a bit tribal over the years, with different factions arguing about the importance of diet versus exercise. It also didn't help that many of the news articles about the study ran with misleading clickbait headlines that our results meant that there was no reason to exercise. We made a point of saying in the article itself, and to any journalist we spoke with, that exercise was still vitally important for health, even if it's not the best tool to battle obesity.

None of the e-mails and phone calls were as baffling or as animated as those from people arguing that *calories don't matter! Didn't I know I was wasting my time?* Energy balance—calories in and calories out—has no effect on body weight, they argued. Sure, that sentiment seemed to violate the laws of physics, but as one helpful stranger wrote, "The human body is NOT a steam engine. The second law of thermodynamics does not apply." These folks weren't angry so much as worried that I just didn't understand how metabolism *really* worked. (I suppose it was a small victory for gender equality that I was mansplained by nearly equal numbers of men and women.) Didn't I know that calories were meaningless? *Hadn't I read Gary Taubes?!*

In fact, Taubes was one of the first to reach out via e-mail after the study came out. He was very generous and thoughtful (and explicitly dismissed the idea, often attributed to him, that weight gain somehow violates the laws of physics). We had a great discussion over e-mail about the implications of the Hadza work for understanding the role of diet in obesity. Of course I knew his work. Taubes is famous in diet circles for arguing that carbohydrates (especially sugars) are the main cause of obesity due to their particular effects on insulin and fat accretion, something we'll delve into in the next chapter.

While Taubes doesn't reject the laws of physics, he has argued extensively that calories aren't important in tackling obesity. In his view, the calories we eat have no meaningful effect on body fat and weight gain *unless those calories are carbohydrates.* Taubes is a leading voice in a movement that rejects calories as a useful measure. A quick stroll around the Internet, the Twitterverse, or the health and fitness section of the local magazine stand reveals what seems like an anti-calorie political revolution. Even the venerable Weight Watchers, the preeminent school of calorie accounting for decades of dieters, has rebranded itself, focusing its diet plans on the quality of food eaten, rather than the quantity.

In its purest form, the argument that calories don't make you fat makes as much sense as the argument that money doesn't make you rich. It's magical thinking. As we discussed in Chapter 2, every gram of tissue in your body, fat and lean, is made from food you ate, and nothing else. Every calorie of fat you carry is a calorie you ate and didn't burn off.

The Hadza energetics study, however, and all the other research we've covered in this chapter highlights how pointless it can seem to count calories: our bodies do such a good job of adjusting to the calories we eat and expend that it can feel like calories aren't real at all. Our hypothalamus is a master of metabolic sleight of hand, altering our energy expenditure and hunger when we're not looking. Without the tools of modern metabolic science, keeping track of calories is a fool's errand, like trying to follow a magician's cards as they vanish and reappear.

Energy balance is the only thing that alters our weight. That's the inescapable reality of physics. The problem is that we're atrocious at keeping track of the food we consume (Chapter 3), and our evolved metabolic trickery makes it nearly impossible to keep track of energy we expend. No wonder many otherwise rational people are driven to magical thinking when it comes to calories.

Is a calorie a calorie? Yes, of course it is, by definition. But that's not to say that all foods will have the same effect on our bodies. The hypothalamus and its evolved algorithms are constantly assessing and responding to both the quantity *and* the quality of the foods we eat. A lot of exciting research over the past few decades has revealed how different foods and the nutrients in them affect the way our bodies manage our metabolism. Much of this work has been wrapped up in Paleo diet arguments about what foods are "natural" for humans to eat. We'll delve into this work in the next chapter. With the Hadza as our guides to what a real hunter-gatherer diet can look like, we'll discuss the evolved human diet and the ways that different foods might promote or defend against obesity.

Exercise is still vitally important for health. The metabolic tricks our bodies play on us don't change the fact that daily physical activity is absolutely critical for avoiding disease. Constrained energy expenditure and metabolic compensation make exercise a poor tool for weight loss (Figure 5.3), but nearly every other aspect of our health relies on regular activity. In fact, as we'll discuss in Chapter 7, constrained energy expenditure and the metabolic changes our bodies make in response to exercise are a big reason that exercise so important for our health.

First, though, it's time to figure out how diet affects energy expenditure and energy balance. Let's head to Hadzaland and see what's for dinner.

CHAPTER 6

The Real Hunger Games: Diet, Metabolism, and Human Evolution

We were half a mile from camp when our small party left the sandy dry riverbed we'd been following and began to climb. A couple, Mwasad and Halima, with their first child, had graciously agreed to let me tag along for a day out. We walked silently, Mwasad in the lead, Halima in the middle, me trailing in the rear. Halima had two-year-old Stefano wrapped in a sling on her back and a digging stick in her hand. Mwasad carried the typical Hadza man's tool kit: his bow and arrows, a small axe, and a quart-sized container.

Without changing pace, Mwasad bent our path upward through knee-high golden grass, the rocky ground beneath our feet sloughing under the weight of each step. Burrs from the grass burrowed into my shoes, and I wondered when I might steal a minute to dig them out, or if I was doomed to a day of itchy, prickly feet. Up on the hillside, out of the shade of the riverbed, we were hit by the full force of the equatorial sun, pressing hot against our backs. The air crackled and hummed like a high-voltage transformer. Acacia leaves danced in the faint breeze as they drank in the light. It was seven o'clock in the morning.

As we crested the ridge, Mwasad began to whistle. Liquid and melodic, his whistle split the air. The short, plaintive phrase was followed by a few minutes of silence, then repeated. His whistle wasn't some sighing, absentminded daydream. It was an announcement, broadcast into the canopies of the ancient copper-gray baobab trees that towered overhead. The sound seemed to hang in their branches. As the morning wore on, Mwasad's whistle became part of our sonic landscape. It felt like a call to the universe. *Anyone out there?*

A little before noon, the universe answered back. Mwasad snapped his head toward a call I'd missed, turning abruptly to follow the sound of a small but remarkable bird, the greater honeyguide. The honeyguide, a drab and solitary creature about eight inches tall, makes a living pillaging the honey and comb from beehives. But it goes about its business in a most peculiar way, recruiting human partners to do the dirty work of ripping into trees and exposing the colonies. It isn't hard to find humans who are happy to help. The Hadza rely on honeyguides to find the biggest hives, which are usually high up in the baobab crowns and hard to spot from the ground. Men like Mwasad often whistle when they're out on a walk, advertising their services. Honeyguides with a fix on a bountiful beehive will answer back, chirping their distinctive *whhrrRIIP err, whhrrRIIP err, whhrrRIIP err* and flitting about, leading the way. The Hadza call the species *tikiliko*. European taxonomists named it *Indicator indicator*.

It's an ancient partnership, far older than our species. DNA analysis shows that the greater honeyguide split from the other species in its family more than three million years ago. As far as we can determine, its ancestors have been guiding our ancestors to honey ever since. We share our love of honey with the other great apes, so presumably it's always been part of the hominin diet. But for the last three million years or more, hominins have been eating enough honey to create an entire niche for another species. Today, honey

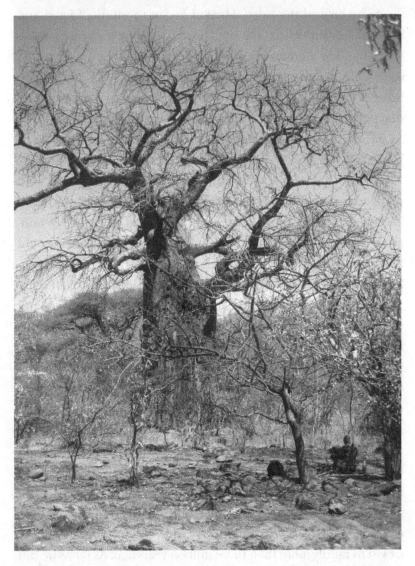

Figure 6.1. Honey. Mwasad (circled) chops into the hollow limb of a baobab tree high above the ground while Halima (underlined) nurses their son and waits for lunch.

remains a major part of the diet for hunter-gatherer and farming populations in tropical and temperate regions around the globe.

The greater honeyguide is found all over sub-Saharan Africa, partnering with people from dozens of cultures. The Hadza consume an incredible amount of honey, accounting for about 15 percent of their calories each day, and much of that is aided by these amazing birds. Brian Wood calculates that 8 percent or more of all the calories the Hadza community consumes are acquired with the help of honeyguides.

Finding his informant high in the canopy of a massive baobab, Mwasad set to work. Using his axe, he quickly cut down a nearby slender tree, about two inches in diameter, and sectioned it into foot-long pegs. He stuffed the pegs into his belt and started up the vertical face of the baobab. With one deft overhead swing he sank the blade of the axe into the baobab's soft, silvery bark. Next he removed the axe and jammed the end of a peg into the gash, then pounded it halfway in with the back of the axe head. The protruding bit of peg provided a hold, and he pulled himself up onto it, eventually balancing atop on one foot. Gingerly he repeated the process, perched on the peg. *Thwack. Jam. Whack whack whack.* Lather, rinse, repeat, peg over peg, three stories up into the crown of the tree.

Mwasad returned to earth to gather a smoldering stick that Halima had lit for him and the small plastic container he'd brought along for just this occasion. Then back up the tree, where he calmly used the stick to blow smoke into the beehive. Then the chopping. *Whack whack whack* . . . It wasn't easy or quick work, and he earned a few stings from the angry bees. (Side note: I was once stung between my shoulder blades by one of these bees that had found its way up the back of my shirt. Had I been high in a baobab at the time rather than safely on the ground I suspect the pain of it would have knocked me off my perch. The intense, hot ache stayed with me for a day. These are not the bees I grew up with in Pennsylvania.) Mwasad stuffed himself with honey and larvae while he worked, then returned to earth with a quart-sized can full of honey and stacked above the rim with comb. Mwasad, Halima, and Stefano drank honey for lunch, and sucked honey, brood, and other goodness from the comb, spitting out clumps of wax as they worked their way through the haul. They kindly offered some to me, I shared a few of the cheap cookies I'd brought in my backpack, and we had a bit of a picnic. The honey was smoky and intense. Glorious.

Mwasad hit at least half a dozen hives that day; I watched the three of them eat more honey than I consume in a year. Halima was plenty busy that day as well, stopping several times on our foray to dig wild tubers from the rocky ground (that's her in Figure 1.2). These wild tubers are the more fibrous cousins of the potatoes, yams, and other domesticated root vegetables in your supermarket. They are the caloric cornerstone of the Hadza diet: energy rich, plentiful, and available year-round. Between the tubers and the honey (and aside from a few larvae), it was an all-carb day.

Hadn't they read Gary Taubes?

More Data, Less Shouting

As we discussed in the last chapter, our metabolism is tightly regulated by our hypothalamus, which constantly monitors the food we eat and the calories we burn to keep our bodies in energy balance. But something—or, more likely, *several* things—about our modern environment is causing the hypothalamus to misfire, leading us to consume more calories than we expend. As our collective metabolic health hurtles like Thelma and Louise toward the abyss, it makes sense to ask if the foods we're eating are part of the problem. How are the foods that we eat today different from the foods our bodies evolved to eat, and how do those differences make us fat? If we could just get back to the diets our bodies are built for, surely we'd be healthier.

The problem is that it's hard to tell what hominin ancestors ate with any real precision. The evidence is hard to come by and doesn't usually tell you want you really want to know: What was on a typical week's menu for Paleolithic humans? My fellow anthropologists are often hesitant to say too much, because we know how much uncertainty there is. Into the void left by cautious academics leap a mix of diet-promoting charlatans, hobbyists, and condescending medical professionals who got an A in their freshman "Intro to Human Evolution" course (or are certain they would have) and are happy to explain the anthropological data to the anthropologists. The people most certain about diets our hunter-gatherer ancestors ate are people with little training or expertise.

Overconfident interpretation by shouty people who don't know as much as they think they do has a name in science, the Dunning-Kruger effect. In 1999, David Dunning and Justin Kruger, psychologists at Cornell University, had a brilliant insight that seemed to explain why incompetent people are so annoying: their very incompetence blinds them to how incompetent they are. To test this hypothesis they had dozens of Cornell undergrads take tests in logic, grammar, and (my favorite) the ability to identify humor. Then they asked the students to rate themselves on how well they thought they did. To no one's surprise (but to our collective satisfaction) the worst performers—those *least* knowledgeable—routinely rated themselves as *experts* at what they were doing. This isn't a new problem. Even Darwin complained that "ignorance more frequently begets confidence than does knowledge." (Thankfully, the American public is aware of this issue and elects only smart, fair leaders with proven competence in governing and expertise in world affairs.)

In the hot, crowded ecosystem of competing dietary movements, the loudest voices seem to attract the most attention. Paleo diet evangelists have distinguished themselves by projecting a hard-nosed, steely-eyed view of human nature and evolution. Humans, they assure us, have evolved to eat *meat*, bro. They push high-fat, low-carb diets that send the body into ketogenesis (see Chapter 2), arguing that our ancestral diet was all bison and no berries. Paleo proponents, particularly the self-styled carnivores, reject the notion that vegetarian or (god forbid) vegan diets are healthy or natural, dismissing plant-based recommendations or cautions about fat as politically correct pandering or corporate propaganda. In their view, no self-respecting hunter-gatherer would eat a starchy, carb-rich diet, and they sure as hell wouldn't eat any sugar.

Vegans can be just as militant and annoying. When I lived in Brooklyn and spent my mornings and evenings on the subway, a very energetic and upset woman on the F train used to walk through the cars, haranguing passengers and handing out pamphlets explaining how humans are naturally evolved to eat plants. *"Look at our teeth!"* she'd yell. *"Meat rots in our herbivore guts!"* She may have been a diet vigilante, but she wasn't alone. Those are talking points from PETA.

Happily, we can tune out these diet extremists and have a look at the data ourselves. There are three lines of solid evidence that tell us something about the diets our ancestors ate: the archaeological and fossil record, ethnographies of living hunter-gatherers, and functional analyses of the human genome. The details differ and it's easy to get lost in the weeds, but the overarching message from each is clear: we evolved as opportunistic omnivores. Humans eat whatever's available, which is almost always a mix of plants and animals (and honey).

Archaeology and the Fossil Record

If we go back the full seven million years to our ancestral break with chimpanzees and bonobos, it's clear that our hominin ancestors got their start as apelike plant eaters. For the first four to five million years of hominin evolution, the different species we see in the fossil record (including the famous Lucy skeleton and her *Australopithecus* kin) had molars (cheek teeth) with rounded cusps for eating plant foods. They had long arms and slightly curved fingers as well, which tells us they were climbing into trees often, presumably for fruit and other plant foods. Sure, they probably hunted monkeys or other small game occasionally like chimpanzees and bonobos do today. Insects might have been a regular part of the menu, too, much the same way that chimpanzees target honey and eat ants and termites. But all the evidence from the long early period of hominin evolution points toward a heavily plant-based diet.

One innovation during this period might have been the exploitation of tubers. *Australopithecus* species, which are found in the fossil record roughly four to two million years ago (Chapter 4) have really large molars with thick enamel. Their teeth also preserve scratches that suggest sediment in their food, and the isotopic signature of the enamel is similar to that of wild tubers. Chimpanzees occasionally dig up and eat tubers, but it's rare—unlike in humans today where root vegetables are a mainstay of the diet in cultures around the globe. We aren't yet sure that *Australopithecus* was eating a lot of tubers (it's hard to be certain with fossil data!), but the available evidence suggests our love of potatoes and other starchy vegetables predates our genus.

At around 2.5 million years ago, we see a momentous dietary shift with the origins of hunting and gathering. We detailed the metabolic impact of this change in Chapter 4, but it's worth recapping the effects on the foods our hominin ancestors were eating. As the genus *Homo* began hunting and scavenging more, meat became an ever-larger part of the diet. We see cut marks from stone tools on animal bones starting about 2.5 million years ago, and that continues right up to the present day. At 1.8 million years ago, the *Homo erectus* population we were excavating at Dmanisi was eating antelope and other animals. By 400,000 years ago, *Homo heidelbergensis* was regularly taking down wild horses and other big game. By 100,000 years ago, Neanderthals were regularly eating reindeer and mammoth. The cave floors of Neanderthal sites are often thick with the butchered remnants of their meals, and their position as meat-eaters in the food web is evident from the telltale isotopic signatures of their bones (animals that eat other animals have elevated levels of the isotope nitrogen 15, which gets concentrated as you move up the food chain). Our own species was equally adept at hunting, with charred bones from a staggering number of species found in ancient hearths.

The inclusion of meat in the diet had big effects throughout the body. Eating animals means more energy—particularly fat—in each bite of food, which meant less food was needed to meet daily energy demands. The need for big molars and other digestive machinery was reduced. Natural selection favored smaller teeth and guts, freeing up energy for other tasks. Today, our digestive tracts are 40 percent smaller, and our livers 10 percent smaller, than they would be if our digestive systems were proportioned like our vegetarian great ape brethren. These reductions free up about 240 kcal per day, which we spend on bigger brains and other energetically expensive adaptations (Chapter 4).

Still, it's a common misconception among many in the Paleo crowd that our hunter-gatherer ancestors were somehow *only* hunting. Perhaps this view reflects the inherent biases in fossil and archaeological record. Bones preserve much better than plant foods, as do the tools used to hunt. Hunting technologies often involved stone flakes or points, which don't rot or degrade. As we see with the Hadza, collecting plant foods requires nothing more than strong hands and a wooden stick. Direct evidence for eating plants isn't as readily available in the archaeological and fossil record, but all signs point to a balanced diet similar to that of living hunter-gatherers.

Some of the newest and most exciting research on hominin

diets comes from analyses of food particles trapped in the plaque stuck to the teeth of fossil hominins. Amanda Henry at Leiden University is a pioneer in this burgeoning subfield of human evolution. She and her colleagues have carefully extracted the dental calculus (calcified plaque) from the teeth of Neanderthals at fossil sites all across Europe and into the Near East. Under a microscope, she found grains and starches from plant foods in nearly every sample, despite the fact that she was looking at mere milligrams of material. Neanderthals were the quintessential big game hunters, but they balanced all that meat with carb-rich grains, starchy tubers, sweet fruits, and nuts. Henry has found similar evidence in the fossilized teeth of members of our own species from this period. Our Paleolithic ancestors would no doubt be amused by the widespread notion in today's Paleo diet circles that grains and starchy carb-rich plant foods were off the menu.

Even flour and bread are far older than typically thought. Archaeological excavations in Jordan have recently uncovered an ancient oven and charred bread remnants dated to over 14,000 years ago, thousands of years before the emergence of agriculture. The bread flour was made from wild cereals. While the Jordan find is notable for being the oldest preagricultural site for bread, it's quite likely that similar practices were widespread prior to farming. For example, aboriginal Australian cultures are known to have made breads from wild grains before the introduction of wheat flour from Europe. Hadza women still routinely pound baobab kernels into flour and mix it with water to eat.

Ethnography

It's getting harder and harder to find living populations like the Hadza who still hunt and gather. Globalization and the implacable march of economic development continues to marginalize most of these communities, pushing them into villages or, as we did in the

United States with Native American populations, onto reservations. Still, there are a few proud and fortunate populations, like the Hadza, the Tsimane, and the Shuar, who have kept their traditions alive and managed to fend off the developers. We've also got written ethnographies for hundreds of hunter-gatherer populations from around the globe, collected during the 1800s and 1900s before these cultures were lost. Together, observations of living and recent hunter-gatherer and horticulturalist societies provide a sense of the incredible dietary diversity that marks our species.

In Figure 6.2, I've plotted a rough dietary sketch for 265 hunter-gatherer populations from summaries compiled in 1967 by the anthropologist George Murdock in his *Ethnographic Atlas*. For each society, the *Atlas* lists the proportion of the diet from plants, game, and fish, as well as any foods from domesticated crops or livestock. Unfortunately, the methods used to determine dietary proportions are rarely given, and the quality of the data isn't great. Still, Murdock's *Atlas* is widely used despite its obvious deficiencies. Like the sad hand dryer in a gas station restroom, it's far from ideal, but for most of these populations, it's all we've got.

When we plot the proportion of calories from plants and from meat against latitude (Figure 6.2), two things are immediately obvious. First, there is a *lot* of variation. Within 50° latitude of the equator (that is, south of Winnipeg, Canada, and north of the Falkland Islands), you can find meat-heavy diets, plant-heavy diets, and everything in between. The range of "natural" human diets is vast. People eat whatever is available. And this brings us to the second point. In really cold climates, more than 50° from the equator, populations eat a lot of meat. (It's worth noting, though, that Arctic populations worked to get plant foods wherever they could, even pillaging rodent burrows to steal their stores of wild tubers.) Why do Arctic groups eat a lot of meat? Because plants don't grow there, at least not very well. We eat what's around.

Among the best studied groups like the Hadza, for which we

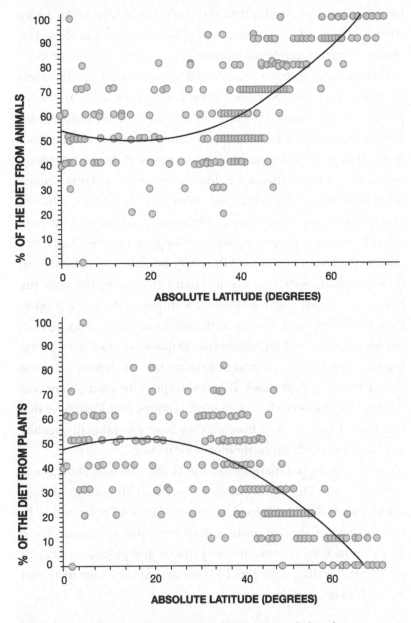

Figure 6.2. Diet breakdown for 265 hunter-gatherer populations from Murdock's *Ethnographic Atlas*. Each population is plotted on both panels. In warmer environments, below 50° absolute latitude, there's a wide variety of diets, and most populations eat a balance of plant and animal foods. Populations in cold, subarctic climates eat a lot of meat.

have modern, high-quality data and don't have to rely on Murdock's *Atlas*, we find a high amount of carbohydrate in the diet. The Hadza, Tsimane, and Shuar populations all get 65 percent or more of their calories each day from carbohydrates (compare that to less than 50 percent for the typical American diet; Figure 6.3). It's not just honey and tubers, either. No wonder we've never observed ketosis among Hadza men and women—their diet is about as far from being ketogenic as one could imagine. Much of this carbohydrate comes from starchy vegetables, like the tubers that Hadza women often bring home. The other big source of carbohydrate is honey, which Hadza men and women consistently rank as their favorite food. There's a tendency among diet bloggers and New Age nutritionists to view honey as healthy simply because it's "natural," but there's nothing special about it. Honey (including the stuff the Hadza get) is just sugar and water, with nearly the same proportions of fructose and glucose as high-fructose corn syrup. In fact, our blood sugar and fat metabolism respond identically to honey, high-fructose corn syrup, and table sugar (sucrose, which is formed from fructose and glucose). If carbs—especially sugar—were particularly bad for you, these high-carb cultures should all have diabetes and heart disease. Instead, they have exceptionally healthy hearts and virtually no cardiometabolic disease.

Diets among populations like the Hadza, Tsimane, and Shuar are also low in fat, which makes up less than 20 percent of their calories each day (the typical American diet is 40 percent fat). In fact, outside of the far north (which we'll discuss below), there aren't any well-documented hunter-gatherer groups (like the Hadza) or horticulturalists (like the Tsimane and Shuar) with diets that are high in fat.

The impressive amount of carbohydrate in the Hadza diet and those of other groups is the mirror image of the 30 percent protein, 20 percent carbs, and 50 percent fat energy mix typically promoted as "Paleo." And some Keto and Paleo proponents have pushed this supposed ancestral mix even further. David Perlmutter, author of the popular book *Grain Brain*, argues—without providing any evidence—that the ancestral diet was only 5 percent carbs and 75 percent fat! Why do so many of today's Paleo diet evangelists insist that the "natural" hunter-gatherer diet is low carb and high fat?

Part of the answer lies with Murdock's *Atlas*. The modern Paleo diet movement was founded in the late 1990s by Loren Cordain, a professor at Colorado State University who wanted to know why hunter-gatherers were seemingly immune from heart disease and other common Western problems. Cordain was trained as an exercise physiologist, not an anthropologist, so he didn't go to the field to observe hunter-gatherer diets firsthand. Instead, he and his collaborators compiled diet summaries for the hunter-gatherers in Murdock's *Atlas*, much as I've done in Figure 6.2. They went to great lengths to translate Murdock's diet scores into precise percentages of fats, carbs, and protein in the diet, and concluded that about 55 percent of calories in the average hunter-gatherer diet came from animal foods. These analyses spawned a number of peer-reviewed scientific papers and formed the basis for Cordain's influential book, *The Paleo Diet*, which launched the movement.

These studies were well intended, but they fall short in some key ways. Most fundamentally, the data from Murdock is simply not good enough to get a precise read on dietary intake. His cultural summaries don't say anything about fats, carbs, or protein. Instead, Murdock assigned a dietary score, 0 through 9, to relay a rough estimate of the contribution of different food types to the diet. For the most part, the methods used to determine those scores aren't described. It's likely, though, that they missed a lot of carbohydrate-rich foods. As we discussed in Chapter 4, anthropologists in the early and mid-1900s consistently overlooked women's contributions, which would tend to underestimate the amount of plant foods. And we know that Murdock's summaries ignored honey, which is a big part of the diet for the Hadza and many other hunter-gatherers.

Another problem with Cordain's analyses is the focus on the average proportion of animals and plants rather than on the enormous diversity of diets across the globe. Focusing on the average suggests that there's one "true" natural human diet, and anything else leads to disease. That makes as much sense as arguing there is one "true" human height, and anyone who deviates from it is pathological. For some measures, the average value isn't very meaningful. All of the populations in Figure 6.2 are equally natural, and as far as we can tell, all of those populations were equally healthy, despite the fact that their diets ran the gamut from mostly plants to mostly meat. Humans can be healthy eating a broad range of diets, and have done so in the past. There is no single Paleo diet.

A third issue is that a lot of the discussion around Paleo diets seems to just make things up (like Perlmutter's suggestion that ancestral diets were 5 percent carbs) or gets important details badly wrong. For example, Stephen Phinney, a doctor, biochemist, and vocal advocate for low-carbohydrate diets, has often argued that populations like the Maasai of East Africa, the bison-hunting Plains cultures of North America, and the Inuit populations in the Arctic are useful examples of our collective past. In reality, it's hard to think of three cultures that are *less* representative of Paleolithic hunting and gathering. The Maasai are pastoralists who herd goats and cattle. Their way of life is old, but not *that* old. The archaeological record shows that pastoralism arose less than 10,000 years ago. It gets going only around 6,500 years ago in Africa, after other cultures in the Near East had already started farming. Similarly, bison-hunting cultures of the Plains weren't established until around 10,000 years ago. Inuit and other Arctic cultures are even a bit younger, about 8,000 years old. In the 2.5-million-year history of our genus (Chapter 4), all three of Phinney's exemplar groups are newcomers, no older or more representative of our past than the early farming cultures that Paleo dieters rail against. In fact, only a small percentage of people alive today can trace their ancestry to Arctic or other meat-heavy cultures. Phinney is probably an excellent doctor and biochemist, and as we'll discuss below, low-carb diets can be really helpful for some people. But he should have hired an anthropologist.

The low-fat content of diets in populations like the Hadza, Tsimane, Shuar, and other small-scale societies is worth noting (Figure 6.3), given its potential role in heart health. The Hadza, Tsimane, and other small-scale societies have excellent heart health, even among elderly adults, and their low-fat diets could be one reason why. We'll discuss heart disease and lifestyle more in the next chapter.

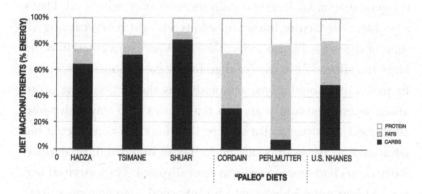

Figure 6.3. Macronutrient breakdowns for the Hadza, Tsimane, and Shuar diets compared to "Paleo" diets reconstructed by Loren Cordain and David Perlmutter. U.S. dietary macronutrients are from the 2011–2014 National Health and Nutrition Examination Survey (NHANES).

Genetics

Pastoralism, Arctic living, and farming may be only ten thousand years old, but that's still a long time. How much have humans around the world adapted to their local environments and foods over the past few thousand years? Recent advances in human genetics have made it possible to look for evidence of natural selection across the human genome, shining new light on the history of dietary adaptations in cultures around the globe. Just as we see with the ethnographic evidence, people everywhere eat what's around and make it work.

Pastoralists like the Maasai offer a great example of a local adaptation to diet. Milk is a large part of the diet in pastoralist cultures, and much of the energy in milk is provided by lactose, a disaccharide sugar made of glucose and galactose (Chapter 2). Like all mammals, we need the enzyme lactase to break lactose into its glucose and galactose during digestion. Infants make lactase in abundance to digest their mother's milk, but in most people, and in all human populations prior to ten thousand years ago, the gene that makes lactase usually shuts off after childhood. That's a problem for lactose intolerant adults who eat dairy, causing all sorts of digestive distress as lactose sugars pass unscathed into the large intestine, where they're digested by gas-producing bacteria. In pastoralist populations, a mutation in the lactase gene arose about seven thousand years ago that causes it to stay active into adulthood. In a pastoralist society, this mutation conferred a big advantage to those who carried it. Those unbloated, unabashed dairy eaters had more calories at their disposal. They survived better and had more kids—kids who inherited their mutant lactase gene. Remarkably, this happened twice, independently, among early pastoralist groups in East Africa and northern Europe. Today, the descendants of these early pastoralists carry the lactase persistent version of the gene that doesn't switch off.

Lactase persistence is hardly the only example of genetic adaptation to diet. Some of our genes reveal both ancient and recent evolution. For example, all humans have more copies of the gene that makes salivary amylase (an enzyme in your spit that digests starch) than other apes, resulting in twice the amount of amylase in our spit and reflecting the importance of starchy foods in the hominin diet. But while all humans living today carry plenty of salivary amylase genes to digest starch, populations vary a bit in the number of gene copies. Cultures with deep traditions of eating more carbohydrate tend to carry even *more* copies of the salivary amylase gene, increasing their levels of salivary amylase even further and improving their ability to digest starch.

There is also evidence for genetic adaptations to farming. A variant of the NAT2 gene, which produces an enzyme involved in several metabolic pathways, is thought to have become more common in farming cultures in response to decreasing levels of dietary folate. Farming in African and Eurasian cultures, and the resulting shift in the types of fatty acids in the diet, appears to have driven changes in the fatty acid desaturase genes (FADS1 and 2), which are important in lipid metabolism. Diet and metabolism are such strong evolutionary drivers that we can adapt to almost anything we have to eat. Indigenous groups living in the Atacama Desert of Chile have adapted to the naturally high levels of arsenic in their groundwater, with natural selection favoring a variant of the gene that speeds up clearance of arsenic from the body. The unlucky ones, without the variant, were lost from the gene pool (they were sickly and had fewer kids).

Arctic populations have also adapted to eating a lot of meat, but not in a way that most Paleo diet proponents would predict. Work with Inuit populations in Greenland and Canada has shown that the FADS genes have changed in these groups as well, presumably in response to the high fat content (particularly omega-3 fats) in their diet, which has traditionally included a lot of seal and whale blubber. With a diet so heavily dependent on meat and fat, these populations are often held up by Phinney and others as great examples of the benefits of a ketogenic diet. But remarkably, most people in these groups can't go into ketosis. Instead, they carry a mutant variant of the gene CPT1A that essentially prevents the production of ketones (the "normal" variant of the gene regulates the ketone production in the mitochondria; see Chapter 2). The non-ketogenic variant was so advantageous among the Inuit and other Arctic cultures that it is ubiquitous among these populations today. Paleo dieters often expound upon the advantages and antiquity of a high-fat, ketogenic diet, but in the populations who have actually lived with these diets for generations, natural selection has pushed back hard.

The archaeological, ethnographic, and genetic evidence clearly shows that humans are an adaptable and flexible species. We are opportunistic omnivores, eating whatever is around. There is no singular, natural human diet, and the typical diet in the past looked nothing like the carnivore Paleo diets of today or their equally restrictive vegan counterparts.

Our evolutionary past is an important guide to how our bodies work today and how to keep them healthy—that is, after all, one of the guiding themes of this book. But the diets of our past aren't necessarily the ones that will keep us healthiest in our strange, modern worlds. Just because we didn't eat a certain way in the past doesn't necessarily mean we shouldn't. We didn't evolve with indoor plumbing, modern medicine, vaccines, or literature, but they undoubtedly make our lives better. Our Paleolithic ancestors didn't play violin or go to the moon, but that doesn't mean we shouldn't. And even if we wanted to return to some version of an ancestral diet, we'd be hard pressed to find the undomesticated plants and animals that we ate in the past. None of the plumped-up, fat, and sugary foods available at the supermarket or farmers market were available even a few thousand years ago. Times have changed, and so have the foods available to us. What *should* we eat today?

Magical Ingredients: Sugar, Fat, and Testicles

"What kind of meat is that?" asked Bagayo. It was a fair question. I was spooning a gelatinous pink cylinder of canned meat into the pasta sauce we were cooking for dinner. Bagayo had come by our cooking area to chat and observe, a fairly regular occurrence. Hadza men and women were often curious about the weird food we brought with us. Our research camp was like a *Seinfeld* rerun; they had seen it all before, but still found it mildly entertaining.

"Snake," I deadpanned.

Bagayo smiled. "Really?" he asked, knowing I had to be joking.

"Oh yeah. Snake. They put a picture of a cow on the can, but it's really snake in there." (Honestly, it could have been true. The only canned foods available in Arusha, where we got our supplies, were produced by unknown companies of uncertain origin. The meat-snot was salty and ground into a pulp. The word *beef* on the label was not reassuring.)

Bagayo chuckled but couldn't hide a look of disgust. "Snake," he muttered, shaking his head, and went off to share the joke with the other guys. There are few things that the Hadza won't eat, but snakes are top of the list. Any reptiles, in fact, are viewed with disgust. They aren't food.

Food has power far beyond its nutritional qualities. The placebo effect is strong, and the cultural weight we attach to many foods (or nonfoods) can affect how we feel regardless of how our bodies digest and metabolize them. For the Hadza, *epeme* meats—the kidneys, lungs, heart, and testicles of large game—are seen as sacred and powerful, and only men are allowed to eat them. Marketers and charlatans develop similar myths in the United States, though they tend to fade away before achieving religious status. We're promised a new superfood every month: acai berry, pomegranate, kale, dark chocolate, eggs, coffee, yak butter, wine. As I write this, Dr. Oz is pushing "detox water," promising it will boost your metabolism 77 percent (spoiler: it won't). Social media is full of people who swear these foods work magic on their health, waistline, mental acuity, libido, and energy levels, without any compelling evidence. No doubt, for some, these foods really *do* seem to work magic. The human brain is a master of self-deception and often finds patterns in noise—the face of the Virgin Mary burned into a slice of toast. We want to believe. And if enough people try yak butter, some of them, somewhere, will convince themselves it's working, and that it's the sole cause of the pounds they're losing or the vitality they feel. Of course the people who fail to see any benefit don't flock to the Internet to rave about it.

Food taboos are equally powerful and usually just as unfounded. Hadza men and women routinely eat undercooked or somewhat rotten meat, but are grossed out by the thought of eating reptiles or fish. I like sushi, raw oysters, roasted grasshoppers, and I've eaten rattlesnake, escargot, and my fair share of squirrel. But I can work myself up to the brink of puking just by thinking about eating maggots. In Sardinia, cheese crawling with live maggots (*casu marzu*) is a delicacy. Americans and Europeans are often horrified that some Asian cultures have traditionally eaten dogs, but I can't see how eating pigs and cows is any different. Devout Jews, Muslims, and Hindus might agree.

Not all food taboos have deep cultural roots. Every market-driven superfood has its evil counterpart, the villains in the fanverse of foods: gluten, trans fats, carbohydrates (especially fructose), milk, coffee, eggs, wine. Some characters are double agents, playing on different teams depending on the episode. The scientific support behind most superfoods or supervillains is as solid as the Hadza rules about snakes and zebra testicles.

When it comes to your metabolism, there are very few foods shown to have any measurable impact beyond the normal costs of digestion (Chapter 3). "Energy-boosting" drinks and supplements, like Dr. Oz's detox water, are universally bullshit. (Same goes for foods that "cleanse" you or cure cancer: bullshit and *dangerous* bullshit, respectively.) "Negative calorie" foods that supposedly take more energy to digest than they contain, like celery and leafy greens, are also a myth, though filling up on low-calorie, high-fiber veggies is a good way to lower your daily calorie intake, as we'll discuss below. Drinking ice water won't change the amount of energy you burn each day. Even for foods proven to ramp up metabolic rates, the effects are usually modest. The 100 milligrams of caffeine in a cup of coffee will increase your daily energy expenditure by around 20 kilocalories, the equivalent of five M&M's. And as we discussed in the last chapter, any increases in daily energy expenditure are more than likely to be offset by increased hunger and food intake.

Fat Versus Sugar

The godfather of food villains in the modern era is fat. As the epidemic of heart disease emerged in postwar America and Europe, no one seemed safe. Even President Eisenhower was cut down with a coronary. Ancel Keys, whom we met last chapter in our discussion of the Minnesota starvation study, spearheaded a massive international research effort in the 1950s and '60s to try and put out the fire. His work showed clear links between heart disease and fat consumption. This science has largely stood the test of time: the best available evidence still points to saturated fats and trans fats as important risk factors for heart disease. Still, vilifying fat led to some unintended consequences. Reducing meat in the diet removes a source of protein, which as we'll discuss below helps put the brakes on overconsumption. The early work also underplayed the potential benefits of unsaturated fats, the kind typically found in fish and fat-rich plant foods like nuts and avocados. Perhaps most important, the war against fat led to a generation of "low-fat" processed foods where the fat calories were replaced with sugars. These foods were promoted as "heart healthy," but we now know that replacing fat with sugar does nothing to lessen the risk of cardiovascular disease. Keys saw it coming. He argued that fatty foods should be replaced with protein-rich complex carbs like beans, even writing a cookbook promoting them, *The Benevolent Bean*, with his wife.

Today, the main front in the current Diet Wars is whether sugar and other carbs aren't just poor replacements for fat but are in fact the true villains. As we discussed in the last chapter, Gary Taubes and many others have argued for years that sugar was the real culprit behind the modern epidemic of obesity and cardiometabolic disease all along. Fat was framed, they argue, and was never the health threat that Keys and others claimed. In their view, public health efforts to wean us off of fat were a catastrophic mistake. We'd be thinner and healthier, they say, if we adopted low-carb diets and ate *more* fat.

It's easy to dismiss these claims as more magical thinking. As with many movements, the true believers leading the charge, pitchforks in hand, are so extreme and fixed in their views that they're far beyond any sort of real scientific discourse. There's no point arguing with someone who is absolutely certain that the laws of physics don't apply to the human body, that "calories don't matter," and that the *only* thing that determines whether you gain or lose weight is the mix of fats and carbs in your diet. The modern Paleo claims that low-carb diets were the norm for our hunter-gatherer ancestors are equally dubious, as we discussed above. And the conspiracy theories that the evidence against sugar has been buried or ignored in some dark money, decades-long global scientific cabal are laughable. I can tell you firsthand that scientists have a hard time organizing a conference lunch, and we all take great delight in challenging one another and the status quo.

Yet at the core of the anti-sugar argument is a plausible mechanism that really could promote obesity, diabetes, and other metabolic disease. Called the carbohydrate-insulin model, it works as follows: eating carbohydrate-rich foods, particularly those high in easily digested sugars, raises your blood glucose levels (blood sugar). In response, the pancreas produces the hormone insulin. Insulin has wide-ranging effects throughout the body, but one important role is to move glucose out of the blood and into cells to store as glycogen or to make ATP (Chapter 2). But there's a limit on how much glycogen our body can hold, and insulin stimulates the conversion of excess glucose into fat and inhibits the pathways that mobilize and burn fatty acids (see Figure 2.1). Consequently, Taubes and other proponents of the carbohydrate-insulin model argue that carbohydrate-rich diets lead, paradoxically, to less fuel circulating in the bloodstream, as the glucose is converted to fat and stored away in our adipose tissue; the body responds as though it were starving, reducing energy expenditure and increasing hunger, promoting overconsumption. In their view, then, the accumulation of fat is the cause of overeating, not the other way around; focusing on calories misses the interplay of carbs and insulin, and therefore misses the point. It's an intriguing idea with a plausible mechanism for the etiology of obesity, fleshed out in many papers and books over the years by Taubes and others, including David Ludwig.

If only it were true.

•••

Low-carb proponents often complain that mainstream science has ignored the carbohydrate-insulin model, but in fact a number of scientists over the last decade or so have sought to test its predictions. Among them is Kevin Hall, a senior scientist at the U.S. National Institutes of Health (he also led the *Biggest Loser* studies discussed in the last chapter). In one study, Hall's team kept men who were overweight or obese in a metabolic ward for eight weeks, the first four on a standard high-carb diet followed by four weeks on a low-carb, high-fat, ketogenic diet that had the same number of calories but less than one-tenth the sugar. The subjects steadily lost weight throughout the study, but the low-carb ketogenic diet was no different than the high-carb baseline diet in promoting fat loss. Daily energy expenditure was slightly higher (57 kcal/d) on the ketogenic diet, but by much less than the carbohydrate-insulin model predicts. And the pièce de résistance? The study was designed in collaboration with Gary Taubes and his Nutrition Science Initiative, who presumably thought the results would vindicate him. It was *precisely* the test the anti-sugar faction wanted to see—just not the results they were hoping for.

In another inpatient study, Hall and colleagues fed women and men who were obese a baseline diet for five days followed by a reduced calorie diet, with 30 percent fewer calories than baseline achieved either through cutting carbs or cutting fat. In that study, subjects had slightly higher energy expenditures on the low-fat diet, and they lost more fat on the low-fat diet as well. The small and conflicting effects on energy expenditure between studies suggests that the effects of low-carb diets on expenditure could just be noise. That would fit with work done three decades ago, before the sugar crusades, by Eric Ravussin and colleagues. They found no difference in daily energy expenditure for subjects eating a high-carb or high-fat diet.

Large-scale real-world studies examining the effects of low-fat and low-carb diets on weight loss generally find that they are equally good (or bad). The DIETFITS study, which was funded in part by Taubes and the Nutrition Science Initiative, randomly assigned 609 men and women to either a low-carb or low-fat diet. After twelve months, both groups had lost thirteen pounds and 2 percent body fat, on average. Resting energy expenditure dropped in both groups, as we'd expect for people losing weight (see Chapter 5), but there were no differences between diets (if anything, average resting energy expenditure trended slightly lower in the low-carb group). Low-carb diets were tested in a large real-world sample, and they fared no better (and no worse) than the traditional low-fat approach.

Epidemiological data on food consumption and obesity in the United States and other countries also challenge the idea that carbohydrates are to blame for the alarming rise of obesity and metabolic disease. In the 1960s and '70s, when John Yudkin, the father and hero of the modern anti-sugar movement, began attacking Keys's research on the role of dietary fat in promoting heart disease, he could point to data showing obesity rates in the United States and Europe increasing right along with increased sugar consumption. But in recent decades, sugar and metabolic disease have been out of sync. Heart disease deaths, while still alarmingly high, have fallen steadily since the 1960s in the United States even as sugar consumption climbed. Cancer deaths in the U.S. peaked around 1990, a decade before the decline in sugar consumption. The amount of sugar consumed (including high-fructose corn syrup) peaked around 2000, but the prevalence of overweight, obesity, and diabetes have continued to climb even as people eat less sugar (Figure 6.4). The disconnect between sugar and metabolic disease is apparent elsewhere as well. In China, the percentage of calories from fats has risen dramatically since the early 1990s and the calories from carbohydrates has fallen, but obesity and diabetes have steadily climbed nonetheless. As obesity and metabolic disease have taken hold in the developing world, economic improvements, access to easy calories, and excess energy intake, not any single macronutrient, explains the rise in weight.

The low-carb warriors are far from done. Taubes and others still maintain that low-fat, high-carb diets are making us sick. A recent study by David Ludwig and colleagues examined metabolic rates in men and women before and after weight loss. They reported that subjects had somewhat elevated daily energy expenditures when eating a low-carb diet during the period after they lost weight. A reanalysis of their data by Kevin Hall challenges this conclusion, and it's likely that the effect, if it's there, is quite small. Regardless of whether the low-carb diet led to somewhat elevated expenditures after weight loss, the results don't do much to

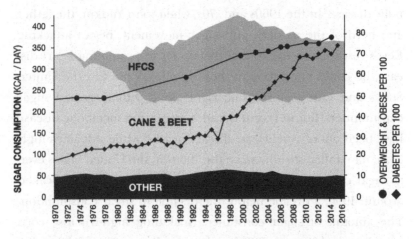

Figure 6.4. Sugar consumption per person in the United States grew steadily from 1970 until its peak in 2000. Rates of overweight and obesity (including extreme obesity) and diabetes continued to climb even after sugar consumption, including the calories from high-fructose corn syrup (HFCS), declined.

resuscitate the carbohydrate-insulin model. For one thing, weight loss was achieved through straightforward calorie reduction, not through carbohydrate restriction. And second, there's no indication that the greater daily expenditures initially reported for the low-carb group made weight maintenance any easier.

When we look at the dozens of studies that have measured metabolic rates on different diets, it's most likely that the ratio of carbs to fats has little or no effect on daily energy expenditure. If there is an effect, it appears to be much lower than the carbohydrate-insulin model predicts, and the potential gains from any metabolic bump seem to be offset by increased intake. There's no clear effect of sugar or other carbohydrates on body fat or metabolic disease beyond the usual dangers of overconsuming calories. Sugar certainly isn't healthy (it holds zero vitamins, fiber, and other nutrients, for a start), and sugary foods are easy to overconsume, as we'll discuss below. But there's little evidence that calories from sugar (including high-fructose corn syrup) are any worse or better for your weight or metabolic health than the calories from fat.

Why Low-Carb Keto Diets (and Others) Succeed

If the carbohydrate-insulin model isn't accurate, why do low-carb ketogenic diets succeed? Stories abound on social media of pounds lost, waistlines slimmed, and diabetes reversed by following a low-carb diet. No doubt most of these online testimonials are heartfelt and real; for a lot of people, the weight loss and improved metabolic health appear to be life changing. But while the results might seem like magic, the reason that low-carb diets work is simple: they reduce energy intake and impart negative energy balance. You burn more calories each day than you eat.

Low-carb diets may be particularly effective in the short term because they force the body to burn through your glycogen. On a very low-carb diet (usually 20 grams or less of carbohydrate per day), the carbohydrate metabolic pathway in Figure 2.1 shuts down. As that happens, glycogen stores are depleted—the last passengers to take the carbohydrate line into the mitochondria. Unlike fat, glycogen holds water. Because the body stores glycogen in its hydrated form, with three or four parts water per glycogen, burning it also leads to water loss and a rapid reduction in body weight.

Once glycogen stores are depleted, the body relies on the fat metabolic pathway to provide energy. You'll start burning your stored fat, but only if your daily energy expenditure exceeds your intake. Here's where the much-touted magic of low-carb diets comes in: *people claim that they lose weight without reducing their calorie intake.* As evidence, they describe all the high-fat, calorie-rich foods they enjoy and claim they never feel hungry. They often make the point that they "don't count calories," but they seem assured— adamant, even—that they're eating just as many calories (or even more!) as they did before.

These weight-loss success stories are great to hear, and if you find a diet that works for you, stick with it. But there's simply no way that anyone is losing weight without consuming fewer calories than they expend, regardless of what those calories are made of. Those are the laws of physics. People on low-carb diets may *feel* like they're eating just as many calories as before, but, as we discussed in Chapter 3, *all* of us are notoriously bad at estimating how many calories we eat each day. It's entirely possible to lose weight without counting calories, just like it's possible to drain your bank account without paying attention to your finances. But it isn't possible to lose weight without eating less than you burn.

Low-carb and ketogenic diets play by the same rules as other diets, and in head-to-head comparisons they perform equally well (or badly). We saw this with the DIETFITS study described above, but broader comparisons investigating a wider range of diets show the same thing. In a 2005 study, Michael Dansinger and colleagues randomly assigned 160 adults living in and around Boston to one of four popular diets for twelve months: Atkins, Ornish, Weight Watchers, or Zone. The Atkins diet is low carb, the Ornish is low fat, and the Weight Watchers and Zone diets fall somewhere in the middle. Not surprisingly, there was a lot of variation in how well people adhered to their assigned diets, but rates were similar among diets (no diet was easier to stick with than any other). Crucially, the type of diet assigned had no effect on the amount of weight lost. Regardless of diet, the people who adhered to them lost weight. All diets work if you stick to them.

Even terrible diets can lead to weight loss and improvement in metabolic health, as long as they reduce calorie intake. So-called monotrophic diets, in which you eat only one food, often lead to weight loss because people get tired of eating the same thing over and over again, and end up eating less. The potato diet is a popular example. The magician Penn Jillette reportedly lost more than a hundred pounds eating only potatoes (which, it's worth pointing out, are full of starchy carbohydrates). Mark Haub, a professor at Kansas State University, followed a junk food diet for ten weeks to make the point that calories are all that really matter for weight, and tracked his progress on Facebook for the world to see. He ate a Twinkie every three hours instead of normal meals, and rounded out the diet with chips, sugar-rich cereal, and cookies. The diet sounds like a health disaster (and I'm not recommending it!), but the key piece of the puzzle was the calories: Haub limited himself to 1,800 kcal per day, well below his daily energy expenditure. At the end of ten weeks, he had lost twenty-seven pounds, went from an "overweight" BMI of 28.8 to a "normal" 24.9, and lowered his cholesterol and triglycerides.

It's possible that low-carb diets are helpful for people with type 2 diabetes, since a large dose of carbohydrates can send blood sugar levels soaring to unhealthy levels in people who lack the usual response to insulin. (Even in people without diabetes, restricting carbs tends to lower blood glucose levels.) In fact, as far back as the eighteenth century, low-carb diets were used to treat diabetes. Virta, a health initiative founded by Stephen Phinney to study the benefits of a ketogenic diet on diabetes, has produced a number of hopeful results. Many of the men and women enrolled in the Virta low-carb program have lost weight and reduced or even eliminated their need for insulin and other diabetes medication. We can't say the low-carb diets have *cured* their diabetes, because their high blood sugars and need for medication would return if they went back to a typical carb-containing diet. But whatever we want to label it, the results are promising and the benefits for those men and women are real.

Still, though, it's not clear that Virta works because it's low carb rather than simply low calorie. The Virta study wasn't designed to compare low-carb diets to others. We know that significant weight loss can reverse type 2 diabetes in overweight and obese adults, and it doesn't seem to matter how you get there. In the Dansinger study, which randomly assigned people to low-carb, low-fat, or mixed diets, men and women who managed to stick to their diet all lost weight and showed improvements in levels of inflammation, the proportion of "good" HDL cholesterol, and insulin sensitivity, three major risk factors for cardiometabolic disease. These health improvements were directly correlated to the amount of weight they lost, not the type of diet they were on. In the DIETFITS study, which assigned large groups of men and women to low-carb or low-fat diets, both groups showed similar improvements in cardiometabolic health. In both groups, thirty-six people who had metabolic syndrome when they entered the study were free of it twelve months later at the study's end. For people who are overweight or obese and dealing with diabetes and other metabolic disease, losing weight improves health.

And it doesn't seem to matter much whether you restrict the calories at each meal or skip some meals altogether. Intermittent fasting, in which you abstain from eating for large portions of the day, has been widely touted for weight loss. The buzz can sound surprisingly similar to that for low-carb diets: eat what you want (when you aren't fasting), don't bother counting calories, it's how our ancestors ate! But as the science has caught up with the hype, the reality is more mundane. In randomized control trials similar to the Dansinger study, people assigned to intermittent fasting diets are no more successful at losing weight and keeping it off than those assigned to traditional calorie restriction diets. Both groups see the same positive effects on insulin, blood sugar, and cholesterol. If you're overweight, restricting calories leads to weight loss and positive cardiometabolic outcomes, no matter how you do it.

None of this advocates for or against any particular diet. If you find a diet that works for you, one that keeps you at a healthy weight and free from metabolic disease, keep with it. Instead, these studies from the front lines of the Diet Wars seem to argue that we're missing the point. All diets work if you stick to them, because all diets reduce calorie intake. But sticking with a diet is often incredibly difficult, because, as we discussed in the last chapter, our evolved metabolic managers typically fight our efforts to lose weight, prodding us until we give in and eat more. Rather than believing that low-carb diets are magic and allow us to break the laws of nature, it's more interesting to ask why some people on low-carb diets can lose weight without *feeling* like they're reducing calories. After all, dieting without feeling miserable is the Holy Grail of weight loss.

Hungry Hungry Hypothalamus

Despite all the abuse that the laws of physics have suffered as collateral damage in the Diet Wars, the available data point to calories as the only real factor determining weight loss and gain. If you eat more calories than you burn, you gain weight. Eat less than you burn, and you lose weight. The mix of carbs, fats, and proteins don't have any special effects on energy expenditure, weight loss, or the health benefits of getting to a healthy weight. So if all diets work the same way, by cutting calories, why are some easier to stick with than others? And if sugar isn't the supervillain mastermind single-handedly making us sick, what is it about our modern diet that leads so many of us astray?

The answer seems to lie in our brains. As we discussed in the last chapter, our hypothalamus—a nondescript nub of tissue at the bottom of our brain—sits at the center of a complex system that regulates both metabolism and hunger. Stephan Guyenet, a researcher in the neural control of appetite and obesity, has written a thorough and engaging book, *The Hungry Brain*, describing this system in detail. Sensory information from your taste buds and guts, along with nutrient contents and hormones circulating in the bloodstream, provides your hypothalamus with a detailed account of the calories coming in and going out. The hypothalamus reacts accordingly, manipulating your hunger and metabolic rate to keep you in energy balance. Normally, this system does an incredibly good job matching intake and expenditure. When we eat enough to meet our needs, we feel full and stop. When we burn our stores of glycogen and fat, we get hungry and eat. If we happen to overeat or starve, our metabolic rate responds appropriately to correct the imbalance. This is why populations like the Hadza live their entire adult lives at the same body weight without giving it a moment's thought.

But the strange and wonderful universe of foods we've developed in the industrialized world have exposed a weakness in the system. For far too many of us, the foods we eat overwhelm the usual checks and balances that moderate intake. In short, our modern diets are too delicious.

We like food for the same reason we like everything: it triggers the reward system in our brains. Like all animals, from the simplest worms to the most complex primates, we have brains that are evolved to reward behaviors that improve our chances of survival and reproduction. Sex, sugar, social connection . . . all the essential, universal cravings are built into us from the beginning. We are prewired with neurons waiting to sense "good" things and release reward molecules like dopamine and endocannabinoids in response, to keep us going back for more. The evolutionary logic is simple: organisms with reward systems that are well tuned to their social and physical environments seek out more food and more sex, and tend to have more offspring that inherit their neural reward systems.

Because we're such complex, cultural animals, we learn a million ways to express these desires and a mind-bogglingly diverse set of associations for each reward. Our brains learn to trigger our reward systems at the mere hint of an impending goodie. We salivate at the sight of a donut or the smell of popcorn, or fantasize over a pair of high heels or a low voice because of the associations our brains make subconsciously. What seems sexy or tasty or socially appropriate can differ completely from Hong Kong to Helsinki, but the underlying reward systems are the same.

The human brain has reward centers that respond strongly to food, particularly fat and sugar. But not all foods are created equal. Some foods, like an unseasoned, boiled potato, hardly budge the reward system. Delicious foods—typically some combination of fat, carbs, and salt—activate our reward system like a symphony orchestra, with dopamine and other reward molecules flooding our brain and making us feel great. Researchers would describe these delicious foods as "highly palatable." In other words, we like to eat them.

Counteracting our desire to eat palatable foods is a set of signals that reduces the reward they bring and makes us feel full. As food is digested and absorbed into the bloodstream, our pancreas releases insulin and our fat cells release the hormone leptin, both of which act in our brain to muffle the reward response to food. Stretch receptors in the stomach and hormonal and neural signals from the digestive tract communicate to our brain that we're filling up. Protein intake is monitored as well, making us feel fuller the more we eat (in fact, there's compelling evidence that we monitor the amount of protein we're eating and don't feel satisfied until we've had enough). All of these satiety signals essentially turn the volume down on the reward signals that food provides and make us feel full, leading us to stop eating, even if the food is delicious.

The push and pull of palatability and satiety are managed by the brain's reward system, which communicates with the hypothalamus. The hypothalamus integrates all of these signals (and others—we've only touched the surface of the system here) to determine hunger and fullness. As we've already discussed, it generally does an excellent job at managing energy balance and body weight, at least in small-scale societies like the Hadza, with traditional diets.

Modern diets overwhelm our hypothalamus and its ability to balance intake and expenditure in two ways. First, we're bombarded with far more variety than our hunter-gatherer ancestors ever encountered. This variety sabotages our ability to judge intake by jumping from one set of reward neurons to another. Our brain shuts down the reward response for flavors it's experiencing but leaves others exposed, a phenomenon called sensory specific satiety. The classic example is getting dessert at a restaurant even though you were completely stuffed from the main course. The main course is usually savory, lighting up the reward neurons for fat and salt. By the time you've finished it, your hypothalamus has successfully extinguished the reward of savory food; you couldn't eat another bite. But dessert is sweet, and *those* reward neurons are open for business. Just the sight of the dessert menu starts the sugar reward circuits firing. Your hypothalamus is helpless. You laugh about having a separate stomach for dessert and order the crème brûlée.

We've known about the waistline-destroying effects of variety for decades. At the dawn of the obesity epidemic, in the late 1970s, researchers found that if you feed lab rats the standard, nutritionally balanced lab diet of chow and water, they will maintain a healthy weight indefinitely. But offer them a "cafeteria" diet of typical Western foods, with lots of tasty options, and they will inevitably overeat and get fat. Since the initial finding with rats, researchers have shown the same phenomenon in a range of species, from monkeys to elephants, and, unsurprisingly, in humans.

The other major problem with modern foods is that they are literally designed to be overeaten. This process began thousands of years ago with farming and the breeding of plants and animals to enhance the palatable aspects of domesticated foods, like sugar and fat, while reducing the elements that make us feel full. Industrialization has taken this process to a whole new level. Much of the food we buy at the supermarket, the canned and packaged foods that my Hadza friends find so amusing, has been engineered beyond anything our ancestors would have recognized. Fiber, protein, and anything else that will make you feel full is removed. Sugar, fat, salt, and other things to tickle your reward system are added. As a result, added sugars and oils are the two leading sources of calories in the American diet today, accounting for fully one-third of the energy we consume. Our evolved reward systems are unprepared for the intensity and breadth of reward signals that these processed foods provide. Our hypothalamus is too slow to shut down our appetite, and we overconsume.

The food companies know exactly what they're doing. Flavor

engineering is a multibillion-dollar industry, with teams of scientists using a mind-boggling array of techniques and additives to make food that is highly palatable without being satiating: foods that always leave you wanting more. These foods are designed to circumvent the brain's evolved system of reward and satiety. In addition to adding fat and sugar, chemical flavorings are focus-group tested until they find a mixture that is irresistible. Wandering the aisles of processed foods at your local supermarket with your Paleolithic food reward system and hypothalamus is like bringing a stone hand axe to a gunfight. "Betcha can't eat just one" might sound like a friendly wager, but the food companies know just how steeply the odds are stacked in their favor.

A recent study by Kevin Hall and his team at the NIH demonstrated just how powerful processed foods can be. In a four-week inpatient study, men and women were fed two sets of meals that were identical in their proportions of carbs, fats, and protein, as well as the amounts of fiber, sodium, and sugar. The big difference was the processing: one set of meals consisted of highly processed foods like hot dogs, prepackaged pasta dishes, and boxed breakfast cereals; the other consisted of relatively unprocessed foods like beef tenderloin, salmon fillets, fresh fruit, vegetables, and rice. Subjects ate one set of meals for two weeks followed by the other (half started with processed foods, half started with unprocessed). They were given no instruction other than to eat whatever they wanted. The results were alarming. Subjects ate 500 kcal more each day on the processed diets, gaining nearly a pound a week.

How Does Anyone Avoid the Obesity Trap?

The increased availability of a wide variety of delicious, processed foods can easily account for the rise in obesity in the developed world over the past few decades. But while the rise in available food calories per person explains the increase in the average weight per person, it doesn't explain the diversity in body shapes and sizes. If the variety of delicious processed foods that surrounds us in the industrialized world is so fattening, why aren't we all obese? Why are some of us able to keep the pounds off despite the temptation?

One important clue is that obesity tends to run in families. It is highly heritable, which means there appears to be a strong genetic component: people who share the same gene variants tend to end up the same weight. Studies of twins in the 1990s helped to show how these similarities play out. If you overfeed people, they'll gain weight (no surprise), but because of the metabolic compensation we discussed last chapter, some will gain more than others. Twins tend to compensate in the same ways, and as a result they gain similar amounts of fat, and in the same places on their bodies. Twins respond in similar ways to underfeeding and weight loss as well.

The revolution in genetic research over the past two decades has uncovered over nine hundred gene variants associated with obesity. Just as we'd suspect, nearly all of these genes are active primarily in the brain, clearly pointing to the brain as the epicenter of dysregulation in obesity. The food reward system is complex and expansive, as are the systems that regulate hunger, satiety, and metabolic rate. The myriad pieces of those systems are built by our genes, and those genes vary a bit from person to person. Some genetic variants make our reward and satiety systems more prone to overeating, others make them more resistant. The hand you're dealt has a lot to say about whether you find it easy to maintain a healthy weight.

But genes aren't destiny. After all, biological evolution is slow. The same genetic variants that get us into trouble in the industrialized world today were there in our great-grandparents' generation, long before the obesity crisis. The same variants can also be found in populations around the globe, including the Hadza, where obesity isn't an issue. Clearly, we can modify our environments in ways that help or hurt us.

One obvious strategy to manage our weight and maintain good metabolic health is to build our diet around foods that are filling and nutrient rich without packing in a lot of calories. Luckily for us, the characteristics of a satisfying, moderate calorie diet have been worked out. A foundational study by Susan Holt at the University of Sydney in 1995 tested thirty-eight different foods to see which ones left people feeling the most full in the two hours after eating a 240 kcal portion. Whole foods, like fresh fruit, fish, steak, and potatoes were the most filling. Processed foods like white bread, boxed cereal, and flavored yogurt were among the least satiating foods, and baked treats like cookies, cakes, and croissants were the least filling of all. The common threads were protein, fiber, and energy density. Foods with more fiber, more protein, and fewer calories per bite were the most filling. Unsurprisingly, palatability was also a factor. Foods ranked as more palatable—meaning they had a greater reward system response—were the least satiating.

Holt's work on satiety provides a solution to the Diet Wars, the terms of a truce for any warriors willing to listen. Diets that work, including both low-carb and low-fat varieties, are effective because they cut out low-satiety foods and help us feel full on fewer calories. Vegetables, fruits, meat, and fish can all be part of a healthy diet, as long as we avoid foods that prod us to overconsume. Low-carb enthusiasts rightly point out that sugary foods are too easy to overeat: they jangle our reward systems without making us feel full. Sugar-sweetened beverages (sodas and sports drinks), fruit juices, and processed carb-rich foods are dangerous because they carry lots of reward response without any of the fiber that make whole fruits and vegetables so satiating. But fatty foods, particularly processed foods devoid of protein, can cause the same problem. That's why low-carb diets typically put the focus on meat and other high-protein foods that reduce calories without sacrificing satiety. Plant-based and mixed diets can be high in fiber as well as protein, reducing energy intake while still being satisfying. The diet that works best for you will depend on your particular reward system and the variety of foods that satisfy you most on the fewest calories.

Even without adopting a particular brand of diet, there are things we all can do to reduce calorie intake without feeling miserable. Getting calorie-rich processed foods out of your house and off your desk at work, and replacing them with protein- or fiber-rich alternatives (like plain nuts, fruit, or fresh veggies), can help reduce the amount of calories you consume each day while still feeling full. Cooking for yourself more often can also help, as most restaurants are in the business of making delicious food that's easy to overeat.

We can also try to lower the stress in our lives. Emotional and psychological stress, as well as physical stress like sleep deprivation, can cause dysregulation in our neural reward systems that can lead to overeating. Our brains can also learn to substitute food reward for the emotional and psychological rewards we crave when we're feeling isolated, scared, or sad. The result is stress-eating, and it's a real thing: even in a laboratory setting, people eat more after a stressful experience. The combination of delicious food and social stress helps to explain why the people in the United States and other industrialized countries gain an average of one to two pounds over the holidays each year. Over a lifetime, chronic stress can have devastating effects on our weight and our health. No wonder that poverty and lack of opportunity are so strongly associated with obesity and cardiometabolic disease in the U.S., particularly in African American communities and others that have to navigate the slings and arrows of structural racism. We'll tackle some of the societal challenges in energetics and metabolic health in Chapter 9.

How to Eat Like a Hadza

Morning in a Hadza camp. Brian and I were making the rounds, going house to house to hand out GPS units (part of our work on landscape use) and ask how things were going. A bit of small talk at each hut, not much else. People were still waking up. Then we got to Manasi.

Manasi had spent the night on a blanket on the ground, under the stars. As is typical of unmarried men when they're passing through a Hadza camp, he hadn't bothered to build a house when he moved in a week ago. But he'd been feeling pretty grim the last couple of days. Hadn't felt like leaving camp. He sat on his blanket and rummaged through the hot ashes of a small cooking fire with his bare hand as he described his issues. Stomach trouble. Cramps. Diarrhea. Oh, and did we want a piece of zebra?

Manasi pulled a thin hunk of blackened zebra meat out of the ashes and began tearing it into three bite-sized pieces. The zebra had been killed five days prior, and the meat had been shared widely across camp: thin strips hung limp and warm in the sun from the tree branches above every house. It was unclear how long this particular piece had been resting in the coals, but I noted, to my dismay, that the inside was bubblegum pink. Manasi handed me and Brian each a piece without breaking from his story of gastrointestinal woe. The Hadza imperative to share is strong, and it would be rude to refuse. Brian and I exchanged sidelong glances: *I guess we're doing this.* I popped it into my mouth before I lost my nerve and started chewing. It had the taste and texture of charred leather. I gulped it down, trying very hard to believe that the ashes had purified both the meat and Manasi's dysenteric fingers.

Part of my job as a scientist is giving public talks about my research, and I'm often asked what the Hadza eat. I wish I could provide a suitably exotic answer. I've sampled a range of Hadza foods, from honey and tubers to several types of berries and meat. It would be satisfying to describe some otherworldly palette of flavors and textures, the complex nuances of warthog, kudu, and baobab. But here's the truth: Hadza food isn't very exciting. Aside from the honey and some of the tangy fruits, it's all quite bland. Spices are unheard of, other than the occasional sparing dash of salt. Nearly all the food is served on its own, either raw, roasted, or boiled. It's not what most Westerners would describe as tasty or even appealing. No food is too bloody, too old, or too unsightly. If you've ever opened your grill the day after a big barbecue to find a cold, forgotten drumstick and a lonely potato blackened on the grate, you've encountered Hadza cuisine.

Adopting the principles of a Hadza diet would have profound health benefits for the industrialized world, but don't hold your breath for a new diet craze. It would be nearly impossible to market in a society awash with highly palatable, processed foods. There are no silver-bullet foods to idolize or avoid, aside from testicles and snakes. The Hadza diet isn't low-carb, ketogenic, or vegetarian, and they don't starve or fast intermittently. Instead, like other small-scale societies, their diet is simple and filling, with plenty of tubers and berries that are high in fiber and meat with lots of protein (the Hadza eat about five times as much fiber each day as a typical American). It's relatively low in fat (although the proportions of saturated and unsaturated fats haven't been studied), which likely helps protect them against heart disease. There is always food available on the landscape (tubers are always in season), but they have to work to get it. They aren't constantly surrounded by a wide variety of delicious foods, much less processed foods engineered to be over-eaten. As a result, the Hadza don't develop obesity and metabolic disease for the simple reason that their food environment doesn't drive them to overconsume.

Bringing these lessons from the savanna into our daily lives means moving beyond the Diet Wars, magical thinking about calories, and conspiracy theories. Humans are opportunistic omnivores, and the available evidence, from Paleolithic and living hunter-gatherers to controlled diet studies like DIETFITS and Hall's work at the NIH, shows us that a wide range of diets can be healthy. As a general rule, we ought to seek out foods higher in fiber and protein that fill us up, and avoid processed foods with added sugars and fats that push our food reward systems over the edge. The diet that works for you is the one that allows you to achieve and maintain a healthy weight without feeling like you're starving. You don't need to count calories (which is hard to do accurately anyway) or sign up for a scientific study to track your intake and expenditure. You just need a bathroom scale. If you're consuming less than you're burn-ing, your weight will go down. If you aren't at a weight you like or on a trajectory to get there, it's time to try different foods.

Diet is still only part of the solution to staying healthy, just half of the metabolic equation. A better food environment will help us regulate our weight and the energy we take in, but it won't af-fect the calories we burn. For that, we need to focus on physical activity.

In the last chapter, we debunked the idea that exercise is a use-ful tool for losing weight. Faced with increasing daily physical activ-ity, the body adjusts, saving energy elsewhere to keep daily energy expenditure in check. Any lasting increase in daily expenditure is matched by increased intake, nullifying the potential for weight loss. But while exercise doesn't do much to change the number of calories we burn each day, it does change the way those calories are spent, and that can mean the difference between health and disease. To stay healthy like the Hadza, we need to move like hunter-gatherers. To see why, let's visit our ape cousins, deep in the African rain forest.

CHAPTER 7

Run for Your Life!

As my plane sailed through the night sky 35,000 feet above the Sahara Desert, I looked down through my little plastic window into the immense blackness below and wondered what I'd find when we landed. It was my first trip to Africa, and I was heading to Uganda to study chimpanzee climbing. I was traveling alone in the pre-cell-phone era, my only security blanket a printed sheet of paper—a handful of helpful tips compiled and passed down by other grad students on how to negotiate the trip from the airport in Entebbe to the capital in Kampala by taxi, then onward by bus to Kibale National Park in the heart of the country. I went through the checklists and gear I was carrying once more in my mind, and silently rehearsed the conversation I'd have with the crush of taxi drivers at the airport to negotiate the fare to Kampala. *Relax*, I reminded myself. *You're prepared.*

And for the most part, I was. I was a total noob to rain forest fieldwork, but I'd been prepping for weeks. Rubber boots, long-sleeve shirts and pants, rain gear. Two huge duffel bags full of equipment, most of it from my advisor, who (like all good advisors) used his grad students as mules to transport it to the field. I had gotten the full battery of vaccines and was taking my malaria prophylactics religiously. I got to my hotel in Kampala and then to

Kibale without being kidnapped. From the tip sheet, I'd learned how to greet folks in Rutoro, the local language (*"Oliota!"* for a single person, *"Mulimuta!"* for groups; the response is always *"Kurungi!"*). I was even ready for the bugs. The mosquitoes and other buzzing annoyances weren't as bad as I'd feared. I popped the occasional mango fly larva out of my skin like pimples, thankful they hadn't found my nether regions. The first time I was swarmed by biting army ants, I ripped off my pants and plucked them from my thighs like an old pro. I even managed to yank a tick from the depths of my nose, *way* up there practically between my eyes, with a little patience and a long pair of metal Revlon tweezers I borrowed from a helpful (and horrified) fellow researcher.

But I wasn't prepared for the smell of chimpanzees.

On my first day in the forest with the Kibale Chimpanzee Project research crew, we crested a small knob overlooking an open area and stopped, silent. Just ahead, maybe thirty yards away, a party of chimps sauntered up to an enormous, sprawling fig tree, their bodies a vibrant black against the muted greens and browns of the forest. One by one they scampered up into the canopy and began to eat, lounging in the massive branches and gobbling handfuls of figs like Greek gods. It was my first time ever seeing apes in the wild, and the vision is seared into my memory.

Like all researchers with the Kibale Chimpanzee Project, I knew the rules. We were to observe the chimps quietly and give them their space. We were in *their* world and needed to respect that. And for the first few days all went according to plan. We'd wake up before dawn, find the chimps, and follow them for as long as we could manage (often until dusk), always keeping a safe distance, twenty yards *minimum*. It was thrilling, but it still felt a bit like a trip to the zoo. The chimps kept far enough away that I was able to maintain my intellectual distance. *They* were animals and *I* was a serious researcher, studiously observing them with academic detachment.

Then, somewhere near the end of my first week, a party of chimpanzees surprised us as we followed them, doubling back and filing past us on the ground just a few feet away, close enough to smell. It was a pungent, woody musk that spoke of a life in damp forest but was still unsettlingly human. That visceral recognition seemed to wake me out of a fog. Suddenly it didn't feel like I was observing animals anymore. These creatures were something more.

Peter Singer, a moral philosopher at Princeton University, has argued quite powerfully that the boundary we draw around our species is arbitrary, that sentient animals are morally equivalent to humans. Growing up in rural western Pennsylvania, observing animals in forests, pastures, and occasionally through the scope of a hunting rifle, I understood that our species is just one thin twig among millions in the tree of life, but I'd never felt any confusion between human and other. The notion that humans aren't distinct, that the line between us and them is arbitrary and meaningless, would have seemed absurd to me, the abstract navel-gazing of effete dweebs who had never spent a day in the woods. Now, standing there in the middle of a Ugandan rain forest, I wasn't sure what I was looking at. The division in my mind between human and animal was still there, but the chimps had crossed over to our side of the fence. I mumbled something to a veteran researcher in our crew. She gave me a knowing look and turned to follow the chimps.

Of course, that uncanny kinship is the reason we find apes so fascinating. We can't help but see ourselves in them. It's their inescapable humanness that prompted a young Jane Goodall to break with tradition, giving the chimps of Gombe National Park names like Fifi and Gremlin rather than the inert serial number IDs that previous generations of bird and mammal ecologists had given to their subjects. Ever since Goodall, Dian Fossey, and Biruté Galdikas began their pioneering work with wild apes in the 1960s, we've learned just how similar our closest evolutionary relatives are to us in body and behavior (see Figure 4.1). Chimpanzees, bonobos, gorillas, and orangutans have complex social lives and long-lasting friendships. They hunt and use a broad variety of tools, wrestle and play, fight and complain, and seem to grieve when loved ones die. Apes even have something like culture, learning a variety of social norms and foraging tricks from their community.

We share a number of bad habits with our ape cousins as well. As I learned that summer in Kibale, chimpanzees are lazy. True, they are incredibly powerful, able to scale giant trees effortlessly, and the males occasionally thrash one another and display ferociously. But for every dash through the forest or bare-toothed screaming explosion from the alpha male, we'd spend hours watching the chimps just hanging out. Chimpanzees and the other great apes get nine or ten hours of sleep each night and spend another ten hours each day resting, grooming, or eating. They walk less each day than the typical American, and don't climb as much as you might think. My data from that summer in Kibale showed that chimpanzees climb about 330 feet per day, the energy equivalent of about one mile of walking. It's the same story for the other apes: they are an impressively indolent bunch.

For us, a life of apelike idleness is a recipe for disaster. Sedentary humans are far more likely to develop cardiometabolic disease, including heart disease and diabetes. Yet, despite their laziness, apes don't get sick. Diabetes is exceptionally rare among apes, even in zoos. They have naturally high cholesterol levels, but their arteries don't clog. The primary cause of death in captive apes is cardiomyopathy, a pathology of the heart muscle, the causes of which aren't entirely known. But they seem to be immune to the kind of heart disease that fells humans. Apes don't develop hardened vessels or have heart attacks from blocked coronary arteries. They stay lean, too. As my work with Steve Ross, Mary Brown, and others showed (Chapter 1), chimpanzees and bonobos in zoos carry less than 10 percent body fat.

The fact that our closest evolutionary cousins don't need to be active to stay healthy tells us that exercise isn't like water or oxygen, some required element that all animals need to survive. Our need to exercise is peculiar. It sets us apart. As our hominin ancestors evolved into hunter-gatherers, the body adapted to the incredible physical demands it entails. No part was left untouched. Muscles, heart, brain, guts—everything was affected. As we discussed in Chapter 4, this transformation fundamentally changed the pace at which our cells work, accelerating our metabolic rates to meet the energetic demands of our high-octane strategy. Those ancient adaptations have consequences for us today: our bodies are built to move. In our modern, industrialized world, free of the daily demands of foraging for our food, we need to exercise for our bodies to function properly. It's a legacy of our hunter-gatherer past.

Our hunter-gatherer past provides an evolutionary context for exercise, the answer to *why* exercise is so vital, but it doesn't tell us anything about *how* exercise works to keep us healthy. We know from our work with the Hadza and all the other research discussed in Chapter 5 that the standard line—that exercise helps us burn more calories—is wrong. Sadly, a lot of people, when they find out that exercise doesn't have a big effect on daily energy expenditure or a durable impact on weight, assume that exercise isn't important. That's precisely the *wrong* message to take home! Data from hundreds of studies and hundreds of thousands of subjects over the past several decades are clear: our bodies work better when we exercise. But if exercise isn't increasing the number of calories we burn each day, what exactly is it doing to keep us healthy?

In this chapter, we'll delve into the effects that exercise has on our body. Specifically, we'll look at the impact of exercise on our metabolism. As we'll see, the metabolic response to exercise—the myriad trade-offs and adaptations that keep daily energy expenditure in check—are a big reason that exercise is so beneficial. Rather than an excuse to avoid exercise, constrained daily energy expenditure is one of the main reasons regular physical activity is so important. Exercise doesn't change the number of calories you burn each day, but it does change how you spend them—and *that* makes all the difference.

Exercise Gets Everywhere

The benefits of exercise aren't limited to its effects on energetics. It makes you strong and fit, for one thing, which is a great way to keep the Reaper at bay. One fun example: men who can do more than ten pushups in one go reduce their risk of a heart attack by more than 60 percent compared to men who can't. (Go on, put the book down and check how you're doing. I'll wait.) Aerobic fitness is associated with better cardiometabolic health—and longer, healthier lives as well. The benefits of staying strong are particularly important as we age. One standard measure of fitness for older folks is a 6-minute walk test, wherein a person walks as far as they can in (you guessed it) six minutes. Older adults who can cover at least 1,200 feet in that time have half the risk of dying in the next decade compared to those who can't make 950.

Vigorous activity, defined as anything demanding 6 METS or more (Chapter 3), has positive effects all over the body. These are activities like jogging, playing soccer or basketball, backpacking, or bicycling that really get your heart rate up. Vigorous exercise gets the blood rushing through your arteries, triggering the release of nitric oxide, which keeps them open and elastic. Pliable vessels keep blood pressure low and are less likely to clog or burst, the catastrophes that cause heart attacks and strokes. Moderate activity (3 to 6 METS, things like a brisk walk, an easy bike ride, or gardening) is great, too. It helps with the trafficking of glucose out of the blood and into cells, and it is known to improve mood, stress, and can even help treat depression. Regular exercise also keeps you sharp mentally, slowing the rate of cognitive decline with age. Running and other aerobic exercise increases blood flow to the brain and causes the release of neurotrophins, molecules that promote the growth and health of brain cells. Dave Raichlen and colleagues have argued that walking and running improve cognitive function by challenging the brain to coordinate a rush of visual and other sensory information to navigate and maintain speed and balance.

Exercise doesn't stop there. As Dan Lieberman, my PhD advisor at Harvard, details in his book *Exercised*, physical activity affects every system in the body, from immune response to reproduction. The signaling mechanisms underlying its reach are still being worked out, but the range is staggering. In addition to directly engaging the nervous system and circulatory systems, both of which extend throughout the body, exercising muscles release hundreds of molecules into the bloodstream. We are only beginning to understand all the myriad ways that exercise affects us. No part of our body is untouched.

A Different Way of Thinking About Exercise Energetics

The fundamental insight from our work with the Hadza and other physically active populations is that our bodies work on a fixed energy budget. This is the constrained model of daily energy expenditure (Chapter 5). Like other animals, our evolved metabolic systems work to keep the total energy burned each day the same, even as demands shift and change. Sure, we'll experience day-to-day fluctuations in energy expenditure, burning more calories if we exercise and fewer if we don't. But our bodies adapt to our normal routines, our habitual workload. As you increase the amount of energy burned on physical activity, the energy available for other tasks is diminished (Figure 7.1).

Constrained daily energy expenditure changes the way we think about the role of exercise in our daily energy budget. With a fixed energy budget, everything is a trade-off. Instead of adding to the calories you burn each day, exercise will tend to reduce the energy spent on other activities. You can't spend the same calorie twice.

While the importance of trade-offs has been understood since Darwin, they've been largely ignored in public health. Instead, as we discussed in Chapter 3 and 4, clinicians and researchers in public health have adhered to the armchair engineer's view of metabolism, that exercise simply increases daily expenditure and doesn't affect the energy available for other tasks. Only recently, with the growth of doubly labeled water studies of daily expenditure across a wide variety of lifestyles, has the constrained model come to the fore. As a result, we're only beginning to understand the importance of metabolic trade-offs in exercise and health.

We've already seen in the last two chapters just how shrewd our evolved metabolic engines can be. Faced with calorie restriction, our hypothalamus reduces our metabolic rate and cranks up our drive to eat. When excess calories come pouring in, metabolic rates go up, burning off much of the excess intake. Think for a moment about what that means for your organs and all of their various tasks: when energy is scarce, some nonessential metabolic processes are suppressed; when times are good, some nonessential metabolic processes are promoted. The effect of daily physical activity on other metabolic expenditure is illustrated in Figure 7.1.

It should come as no surprise that humans and other animals, as the inheritors of half a billion years of vertebrate evolution, are very clever about which tasks are sacrificed when things get tough and which ones are protected. My favorite example comes from the mouse study out of John Speakman's lab that I mentioned in Chapter 5. His team subjected adult male mice to different degrees of calorie restriction and measured how their bodies responded as their energy deficit became more and more dire. Metabolic rates and body mass plummeted as expected, but the effects were unevenly distributed across the body. Most organs, like the heart, lungs, and liver, shrank (and burned less energy) as the mice lost weight. Brains were protected, maintaining their size. The stomach and intestines actually *grew*, in a costly effort to squeeze every last calorie from their food. The best comparison, though, is between the spleen and testes. The spleen, a major organ in the immune system, melted away immediately, shrinking more than other organs. Testes, on the other hand, were protected, changing very little until the energy deficit was truly desperate. I love the study because it lays bare the evolved metabolic strategy of mice: Life is short. Make babies. The immune system is optional.

In a long-lived species like us, the evolved metabolic strategy is different. Sam Urlacher's work with Shuar kids has shown that children fighting an infection increase the energy spent on immune defense while reducing their growth. Apparently, when times get tough, humans play the long game, allocating energy to maintenance and survival.

When exercise starts to take up a large chunk of the constrained daily energy budget, we see the same sort of prioritization at work. Other functions are squeezed out. Activities that aren't essential—luxuries to be indulged only when energy is plentiful—are shut down first. Essential activities are protected until the bitter end. As a result, exercise has wide-ranging effects on how our metabolism

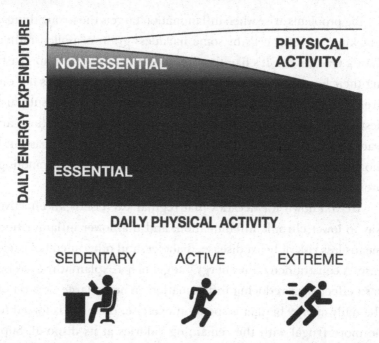

Figure 7.1. Daily energy expenditure is constrained and doesn't increase with daily physical activity in a simple linear manner (see Chapter 5). Instead, as daily physical activity increases with a more active lifestyle, the energy spent on physical activity grows (white portion), squeezing out energy spent on nonessential tasks. Under extreme workloads, physical activity can even cut into essential tasks, causing problems like overtraining syndrome.

is managed and where our calories are spent, which has enormous effects on our health.

Inflammation

When your body is under attack from bacteria, viruses, or parasites like the tick that lived deep inside my nose for five days in Kibale, the body's first line of defense is inflammation. Immune system cells are sent to the site of infection, a ton of signaling molecules called cytokines are released into the bloodstream, and the tissue swells. The inflammation response is energetically costly but essential. It's the emergency response team, and you need it to deal with invaders.

Big problems arise when inflammation targets the wrong things, attacking our own cells or some harmless grain of pollen rather than a true threat. It's like the fire department showing up, blasting their hoses and breaking down doors, at a house that's not on fire. With chronic inflammation, they never leave. The results are destructive. Depending on the tissues involved, inflammation can lead to everything from allergies to arthritis to arterial disease and more. Inflammation can also affect the hypothalamus, promoting overeating and other dysregulation.

We've known for decades that regular exercise is an effective way to lower chronic inflammation, and that lower inflammation means less risk of heart disease, diabetes, and other metabolic disease. A constrained daily energy budget helps explain why exercise is so effective at reducing inflammation. When a large portion of the daily energy budget is spent on exercise, the body is forced to be more frugal with the remaining calories at its disposal. Suppressing the inflammation response, limiting it to target real threats rather than sounding the alarm constantly, reduces the energy spent on unnecessary immune system activity.

Stress Reactivity

You need a healthy stress response to deal with the real emergencies that life inevitably throws at you. For our hunter-gatherer ancestors, a surge of adrenaline and cortisol—the hormonal cocktail at the heart of the fight-or-flight response—was essential to escape the occasional leopard. These days, it might be the fuel you need to outrun a mugger or dodge a taxi. But as is true with inflammation, when stress response is triggered incorrectly or never shuts off, the result is chronic stress, which is devastating to our health.

Exercise is well known to reduce stress and improve mood, in part by reducing the magnitude of the stress response. A nice example of this comes from a Swiss study that used public speaking to induce a stress response in two groups of men: endurance athletes and sedentary non-exercisers. The groups were similar in age, height and weight, and general anxiety levels, but their reactions to stress were remarkably different. Both groups showed elevated heart rate and cortisol levels, but the athletes' response was smaller and dissipated more quickly. Their bodies invested less energy in the stress response, just as the constrained daily energy model would predict.

Another great example of exercise's healthy, suppressive effects on stress response comes from a study of college-age women with moderate depression. These women enrolled in a four-month trial, with eight weeks of regular jogging and eight weeks without structured exercise. As we'd expect from our evolutionary perspective on metabolism, exercise had no effect on weight (their bodies adjusted to the increased workload perfectly), but it did reduce their stress response. When they were exercising regularly, their bodies produced 30 percent less adrenaline and cortisol each day. Their depression improved, too, demonstrating yet again the expansive reach of exercise on our bodies.

Reproduction

Pop quiz: Who has higher testosterone levels, a Hadza man in the prime of his life or a soft schlub from Boston? Turns out it's not even close. Testosterone levels among Hadza men are about half those of average U.S. men. It's not just the men, and it's not just the Hadza. Around the world, men and women in physically active, small-scale societies like the Hadza, Tsimane, and Shuar have much lower circulating reproductive hormone levels (testosterone, estrogen, and progesterone) than their counterparts in the sedentary industrialized world.

We can be confident that the low reproductive hormone levels in small-scale societies is due to their active lifestyles because they mirror the effects of exercise on hormones in experimental studies. College-age women enrolled in exercise studies routinely show lower levels of estrogen and progesterone, and they're more likely to have disruptions to their menstrual cycles. The suppressive effects of exercise on the reproductive system are hard to explain with the traditional armchair engineer's view of energy expenditure, but it makes all the sense in the world from a constrained energy expenditure perspective. With more energy spent on physical activity, less is available for reproduction.

Studies examining reproductive hormone responses to exercise also reveal just how long the process of adjustment can be, as our bodies adapt to different levels of physical activity. Anthony Hackney, an exercise physiologist at the University of North Carolina Chapel Hill, just down the road from me, has been investigating physiological responses to endurance training in men for decades. Comparing testosterone levels in endurance runners to age-matched sedentary men, he found about a 10 percent drop in testosterone, on average, among men who had been training for one year, a 15 percent or so drop for those training for two years, and about a 30 percent drop for those training five years or more, suggesting that it can take years for the body to fully adjust to different levels of exercise. These studies also provide a bridge between exercise physiology in the industrialized world and human ecology with groups like the Hadza. That 30 percent reduction in testosterone among longtime runners is roughly similar to what we see among men in small-scale traditional societies, who have had their entire lives to adjust to their high levels of physical activity.

Suppressing the reproductive system might sound like a bad thing, but in general it's quite the opposite. Exercise is one of the most effective ways to decrease the risk of cancers of the reproductive system (like breast and prostate cancer), in part because it keeps reproductive hormone levels in check. In fact, reproductive hormone levels in the sedentary industrialized world are likely much higher than they were in our hunter-gatherer past, judging from the levels seen in the Hadza and other physically active, traditional populations.

There is a cost to exercise-induced reproductive suppression, at least in terms of potential family size. In populations like the Hadza, where birth control is nonexistent and people usually want large families, mothers typically have babies every three to four years. In the United States, most mothers who want to can have babies every one to two years, even if they're breastfeeding. The lower activity levels and easier access to high-calorie foods experienced by women in the U.S. means their bodies can put more energy into reproduction and can recover from the last pregnancy sooner than Hadza moms can, something we'll discuss again in Chapter 9. The wider birth spacing for Hadza moms is probably closer to the "normal," evolved physiology for humans.

Taken to the extreme, exercise *can* begin to cut into normal reproductive system function. At unhealthy workloads, ovulatory cycles can stop completely, libido can evaporate, and sperm count can plummet. And that's just the beginning of your problems.

The Dark Side

Remember the early '90s, when the sport of cycling was rocked by doping scandals? Of course you don't, because I'm talking about the *1890s*. Using drugs is a human pastime that predates the wheel, so perhaps it's no surprise that doping was present at the birth of competitive cycling. The modern bicycle was invented in 1885, and in less than a decade, drug use in competition was widespread and generally accepted. People became understandably concerned when riders started dying in the 1890s. Apparently, the preferred performance cocktail at the time—a mix of cocaine, caffeine, strychnine, and heroin—had some nasty side effects.

Still, riders kept at it through the early and middle part of the twentieth century, using stimulants and painkillers to push themselves through grueling multiday races like the Tour de France, which premiered in 1903. After the development and widespread use of amphetamines to turbocharge soldiers on both sides of World War II, athletes started adding those into the mix as well. It wasn't until 1967 that the International Olympic Committee decided enough was enough and banned the use of stimulants and narcotics. The effect was immediate: cyclists and other athletes stopped admitting that they doped.

The 1960s also saw an expansion of the cyclist's pharmaceutical palette. They started doping with testosterone and testosterone mimics, powerful hormones that promote muscle growth and aggression. Those were banned by the IOC as well, in 1975, but their use remains widespread. A 2006 investigation by the World Anti-Doping Agency found that testosterone and its synthetic relatives accounted for 45 percent of all doping infractions that year. Later that summer, American cyclist Floyd Landis won the Tour de France, only to be stripped of the victory for failing a drug test. The culprit? Testosterone.

From a purely utilitarian perspective—putting aside the health risks of taking rat poison and narcotics, and the moral failure of cheating—one can understand why athletes might be tempted to take stimulants and painkillers to fuel a race and ignore screaming muscles. But *testosterone*? Why would cyclists risk their health and careers to take a hormone that their body makes on its own? Sure, testosterone helps grow muscle, which could be helpful during training, months before racing season. It also stokes competitive aggression, which could be good during the race if you weren't in a competitive mood. But why would a professional athlete in the final stages of his sport's biggest competition want to grow *more* muscle or need a chemical spark to push himself?

The answer lies in part with the suppressive effects that exercise has on the body. At the workloads that most of us—even the ambitious exercisers—are likely to experience, the suppressive effects are good for us. They help keep inflammation, stress response, and reproductive hormones at healthy levels. But at extreme workloads, exercise cuts deeper. As we'll discuss in the next chapter, Tour de France cyclists like Landis burn over 6,000 kcal each day on cycling, and the race lasts nearly a month. They are pushing their bodies to the brink. The consequence is stark: their bodies shut down other functions, cutting into the essential tasks that keep us healthy (Figure 7.1).

This is the dark side of constrained daily energy expenditure, and it helps explain a well-known but poorly understood phenomenon in athletics: overtraining syndrome. We've known for decades that too much exercise can be bad for your health. At the workloads that elite athletes often take on during training, their bodies break down. They get sick more often and take longer to recover because their immune system is weakened. Injuries take longer to heal. The cortisol bump that helps them wake up in the mornings is muted and they feel fatigued all the time. The reproductive system goes into hibernation. Libido drops. Women have irregular periods or stop cycling altogether. Men's sperm counts decline. Testosterone, the hormone that helps maintain muscle and keep their competitive edge, crashes—unless, of course, they can artificially elevate it with a few discreet injections.

Tellingly, giving overtrained athletes more food doesn't solve the problem (unless there's an underlying eating disorder—sadly, not uncommon among elite athletes). For example, a 2014 study by Karolina Lagowska and colleagues provided food supplements to thirty-one women endurance athletes (rowers, swimmers, and triathletes) who had irregular ovarian cycles and other symptoms of overtraining. After three months of being plied with extra calories, the women saw their daily energy expenditure increase by a modest amount: they were eating *and* burning about 10 percent more calories each day, the metabolic effect we'd expect given the body's usual response to overeating. The women's weight and body fat didn't change—they weren't storing the extra energy, they were using it. Some of those extra calories went to the reproductive system, increasing luteinizing hormone (which stimulates the ovary) by a modest amount. But it wasn't enough to make a meaningful impact on ovarian function. Daily energy expenditure was still too constrained to take in enough calories to make a difference, and their prodigious exercise regimens were still taking up too much of the energy budget for the reproductive system to function normally.

Interestingly, researchers like Lagowska hit upon the constraints in daily energy expenditure decades ago, from a different angle. They discovered that subtracting the energy burned during exercise from total daily energy expenditure produced a very useful estimate, energy availability, the calories available for non-exercise tasks like immune function and reproduction. As workload increases and an athlete's energy availability drops below 30 kcal per day for every kilogram of fat-free mass (an ungainly calculation for the recreational athlete, but one must account for body size), the risk of overtraining syndrome climbs. The intuitive treatment is to provide more calories, to try and increase daily energy expenditure. Constrained energy expenditure helps explain why that doesn't work very well. With daily energy expenditure fixed, the only way to increase energy availability is to decrease training workload.

Rather than some mysterious aberration or a lack of food, overtraining syndrome is just the logical extension of the same energetic trade-offs that make moderate exercise so good for us. As is true with sex, water, bluegrass music, beer, and all other wonderful things, there *is* such a thing as too much exercise. So how much exercise is enough, and how much leads to trouble?

Of Apes and Athletes

Finding the sweet spot for daily physical activity should be easy enough. There's loads of real estate between the chimps idling away the hours in Kibale and the chemically enhanced maniacs racing the Tour de France. Our hunter-gatherer past is, as usual, a good place to start.

Hunting and gathering is hard work, but it's not the Tour de France. Our research with the Hadza shows that men and women rack up about five hours of physical activity each day. A third of that—around one to two hours—is what physiologists call "moderate and vigorous" activity like fast walking or digging tubers, the kind of exertion that really gets your heart rate up. The rest is "light" activity, like strolling around camp or picking berries. Daily workloads for groups like the Tsimane and Shuar are similar. Living hunter-gatherers and other small-scale societies are culturally diverse, of course, but it's reasonable to take five hours of physical activity, with one or two hours in the "moderate" or "vigorous" range, as a reasonable guideline for the amount of physical activity our hunter-gatherer ancestors typically got each day. If we want to think of this in terms of steps per day, we'd be well north of 10,000. Hadza men and women average around 16,000 steps per day.

Compare that to the training regimes of elite athletes. Pro cyclists train about five hours each day, mostly at "vigorous" (6+ METS) levels of exertion. Olympic swimmers regularly log five to six hours of swimming each day during training. That's about three times more exercise than our bodies are evolved to handle, judging by Hadza standards. No wonder professional endurance athletes are tempted to experiment with hormones and other drugs that mask the metabolic consequences of their superhuman training programs.

On the other end of the spectrum, chimpanzees in the wild

rack up less than two hours of physical activity each day, and most of it is light. They average around 5,000 steps per day. That's remarkably similar to the typical U.S. adult, who gets about two hours of light activity (5,000 steps each day), and less than twenty minutes of moderate and vigorous activity. A lazy apelike existence is great for chimps—their bodies have been tuned to it over millions of years. But the human body has evolved to expect more—about three times more, if we use the Hadza and other foragers as a guide. Despite all the fascinating similarities that bind us to our ape relatives, our metabolic engines are fundamentally different. When we act like apes, we get sick.

As a first pass, then, we might aim to be on our feet for around five hours a day, with an hour or so of structured exercise or other activity where we get our heart rates up. That amount of physical activity would land us halfway between our ape cousins and overtrained Olympians, and in the good company of our hunter-gatherer friends. With a little luck, we'll grow old with strong hearts, fresh legs, and clear minds. Healthy as a Hadza.

That Hadza-approved level of physical activity jibes well with the clinical and epidemiological data. In cultures around the world, daily physical activity is one of the strongest predictors of whether you live well or die young. One large study followed nearly 5,000 U.S. adults for five to eight years to test whether daily activity affected their risk of dying during that period. People who got an hour or more of moderate and vigorous activity each day were 80 percent less likely to die than the most sedentary participants. A similar study of 150,000 Australian adults found that an hour of vigorous exercise each day helped counteract the negative health effects of sitting at a desk job all day. In Denmark, men and women in the famed Copenhagen City Heart Study cut their risk of dying in half if they averaged at least thirty minutes of exercise a day.

My favorite example of finding the sweet spot for daily physical activity comes from a study of postal workers in Glasgow. As you might guess, these men and women walk a lot each day carrying the mail. Mail carriers in the study who clocked 15,000 steps a day (about two hours of walking) were virtually free of heart problems and other metabolic disease. And this is in *Scotland,* land of the deep-fried Mars bar, with one of the lowest life expectancies in Western Europe. You don't have to move to the African savanna or cosplay as a hunter-gatherer to get the health benefits of an active lifestyle.

For those of us who spend our days banging away on a keyboard, delivering dank memes instead of the post, a Hadza-sized dose of daily activity can seem out of reach. The U.S. Centers for Disease Control recommend a modest 150 minutes of moderate and vigorous activity per *week*, and still only 10 percent of Americans meet that goal. Don't despair. Just try to get moving. Hunt around until you find an activity that you love. Take the stairs. Bike to work. It doesn't have to be exercise—any physical activity helps regulate your energy expenditure, reducing the calories spent on inflammation and other unhealthy activity.

While we're at it, we can learn from the Hadza and other hunter-gatherers about the best ways to rest as well. The difference is in quality, not quantity. Even without electric lights or the garden of televised delights that tempt us in the West, Hadza, Tsimane, and other traditional populations sleep about as much as adults in industrialized populations, averaging around seven to eight hours per night. But they keep a regular schedule dictated by the sun. Too many of us in the industrialized world have shifting schedules, and the misalignment between our body's internal clock and our sleep schedules can reduce daily energy expenditure and increase our risk of cardiometabolic disease. Hadza adults also accumulate the same amount of resting time as Westerners do during the day, hanging out around camp or resting on a foray. But in the industrialized world, we spend far too much of our lives in comfy chairs and sofas that leave our muscles limp. Hadza men and women use more active resting postures, like squatting, that engage the core and leg muscles. That low level of muscle activity helps reduce circulating levels of glucose, cholesterol, and triglycerides.

So how much exercise is best? *More* is the simple answer. The vast majority of us are far too chimpanzee-like in our daily activity, burning too many calories on nonessential (and potentially harmful) tasks like inflammation instead of exercise. Unless you're already pushing your physical limits on a regular basis, you really can't go wrong spending more time in motion, and your body will thank you. We should be cognizant of our inactive behavior as well, avoiding long periods of sitting in chairs and aiming to keep a regular sleep routine. And if you're one of the few who already spend hours exercising each day, look out for the warning signs of overtraining, like constant fatigue or colds that won't go away. If you find yourself in a French hotel room injecting synthetic testosterone into your ass, that's a definite sign to back it off a bit.

But Weight, There's Less

With all these metabolic benefits of exercise, is there really no effect on weight? Well, the short answer is still *no*. Decades of research are very clear. As we discussed in Chapter 5, exercise isn't effective for weight loss, and being more physically active is poor protection against the real problem in unhealthy weight gain: overeating. But there are two important caveats, curious wrinkles in the way exercise affects our bodies that deserve attention.

The first is that a complete absence of physical activity—sitting on the sofa or at a desk all day, every day—seems to mess up our body's ability to regulate its metabolic tasks, *including* the regulation of eating. Exercise gets everywhere, sending hormones and other molecules all over the body. Without those cues and communication, the system doesn't work right. Similar to what happens with a billionaire recluse who lives for months in the dark without human contact, things get weird. Basic tasks of cellular hygiene, like breaking down lipids in the blood or trafficking glucose into cells, start to fall apart.

Some of the best, early evidence for the dangers of inactivity come from an unlikely place, the Ludlow Jute factory in Chengail, India. In 1956, physiologist Jean Mayer of Harvard teamed up with a dietician and medical officer at the massive factory (at the time, it had more than 7,000 employees on site) to study the effects of daily activity on body weight. They ranked 213 workers by the physical demands of their job, from Stallholders who sat in a stall all day, six days a week, to Carriers, who ferried 190-pound bales of jute around the factory. In general, the amount of daily physical activity had no effect on weight: pencil-pushing clerks weighed the same as hardworking coalmen (Figure 7.2). But the extremely sedentary men were another story. Stallholders, who Mayer describes as having an "extraordinarily inert mode of life," were fifty pounds heavier than the other men. Supervisors, the second most sedentary group, were thirty pounds heavier. The usual checks and balances that match energy intake to expenditure weren't working.

The mechanisms that lead to overeating in "extraordinarily inert" people are still being worked out. It's not as simple as sedentary people having lower daily energy expenditures. If it were, we'd see that daily activity and weight were related for all the men, not just the most sedentary. The lack of correspondence between activity and weight is a widespread phenomenon. A recent study by Lara Dugas, Amy Luke, and colleagues followed nearly two thousand men and women from the United States and four other countries for two years, and showed that daily physical activity, measured by accelerometer, had no effect on weight gain. For the vast majority of people, physical activity and the energy it burns each day has no effect on weight.

A more compelling explanation is that physical activity changes the way the brain regulates hunger and metabolism. Regular exercise seems to help the brain match appetite to caloric needs. Inflammation might play a role here as well. Overconsumption of energy-rich fatty foods can cause inflammation in the hypothalamus, leading to poor regulation of hunger and satiety signals and weight gain, at least in rat studies. It's speculative, but perhaps chronic inflammation brought on by inactivity has similar ill effects in the brain.

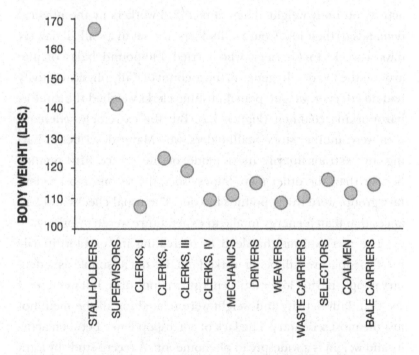

Figure 7.2. Average body weights for men in Mayer's 1956 Ludlow Jute factory study. Men were grouped and ranked by the physical demands of their occupation, from sedentary Stallholders to "very hardworking" Bale Carriers. Daily physical activity was unrelated to weight, except in the most sedentary men.

Whatever the mechanism, it's clear that spending hours each day being inactive is disastrous for your health. As we can see with the jute factory study, extreme inactivity can lead to dysregulated eating and unhealthy weight gain. Time spent sitting each day, either at your desk or watching TV, is a strong predictor of heart disease, diabetes, cancer, and a range of other serious problems. More than five million deaths around the world each year are attributable to sedentary lifestyles. Modernization is pulling us indoors, out of the sun, and into the warm embrace of a computer screen—and the apelike lethargy is killing us.

The second caveat in the relationship between activity and weight is that exercise can also be useful for managing weight once you're able to lose it. Exercise is a poor tool for *achieving* weight loss, but it does seem to help people *maintain* weight loss. A great example of this comes from a study of obese policemen in Boston (not the same men in the testosterone study mentioned above). The men were assigned to one of two weight-loss programs for two months: diet only or diet plus exercise. There was no difference between the groups in the amount of weight lost, just as we'd expect. But once the active weight-loss intervention was over, men who exercised were much more successful in keeping the weight off (Figure 7.3). This was true for both men who exercised during the first two months and those who started in the "diet only" condition. The opposite was true as well: men who didn't exercise after the weight-loss intervention gained all their weight back.

Some of the best evidence for the role of exercise in maintaining weight loss comes from the National Weight Control Registry, an online group of over ten thousand men and women who have lost at least thirty pounds and kept it off for at least a year. These folks defy the cynical view that meaningful, sustainable weight

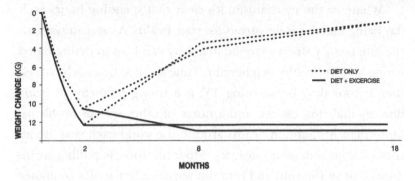

Figure 7.3. Weight loss and gain for men in the Boston policemen study. Adding exercise to a reduced calorie diet didn't improve weight loss during the two-month active weight-loss phase. However, men who exercised afterward kept the weight off. Those who didn't exercise in the in the months following the weight-loss phase gained all the weight back.

loss is impossible. The average Registry member has lost over sixty pounds and kept it off for more than four years. They are truly exceptional.

Much of what we know about Registry members comes from surveys, which is worth keeping in mind. People are notoriously unreliable when it comes to discussing their diet, exercise, or body weight. Still, the common threads among these weight-loss success stories are interesting. Nearly all of them (98 percent) report changing their diet to lose weight, which makes sense given how diet can affect the reward and satiety systems in our brain and impact how much we eat (Chapter 6). They report being more physically active, too, and the most common exercise added is walking.

More revealing are the empirical studies done with Registry members, from researchers collecting hard data on their metabolism and lifestyle. A 2018 study compared daily physical activity of Registry members (measured using accelerometers) to two other groups: obese adults who weighed the same as the Registry members did before their weight loss, and normal-weight adults who were never obese and weighed the same as Registry members do today. Just as we might expect from the Boston police study results, Registry members spent nearly an hour more each day engaged in light physical activity (like casual walking) and about forty minutes more in moderate and vigorous physical activity than the obese group. Exercise seemed to help Registry members keep weight off.

Tellingly, the Registry members also racked up more physical activity each day than the normal-weight adults who had never been obese. In other words, the Registry members worked harder than never-obese adults did to maintain the same body weight. A follow-up study that measured daily energy expenditures helps to explain why. Despite their smaller body size and lower BMRs, Registry members had the same daily energy expenditures as obese adults. Their bodies—or more specifically, the weight management systems in their brains—were stuck at their old, pre-weight-loss daily energy expenditures, targeting the same number of calories they burned before their weight loss, when they were a lot bigger. To stay in energy balance and keep the weight off, Registry members had to find a way to burn all those calories. Exercise provided the answer.

The daily energy expenditures of National Weight Control Registry members sheds light on the inner workings of our evolved metabolic engines. For one thing, they suggest that the daily energy intake that our hypothalamus targets doesn't change much after diet-induced weight loss, even after we've maintained a lower weight for years, and even when the starvation response has passed and BMR has returned to normal. Perhaps some deep, distant echo of the starvation response drives the hypothalamus to retain its old target for food intake. Another possibility is that the constraints on daily energy expenditure affect the regulation of energy intake as well, and that the body resists any changes to the calories it brings in. Either way, it's a problem. As we discussed in Chapter 3, weight loss lowers our daily energy expenditure. If our hypothalamic hunger and satiety systems continue to target our pre-weight-loss intake, we'll be pushed to eat more calories than we burn. As a result, we'll slowly gain the weight back, until our body weight and daily energy expenditure are right back where they were before we lost weight. Sound familiar?

Exercise is one way to maintain weight loss in a constrained energy expenditure world, allowing people who've lost weight to retain their old, pre-weight-loss daily intakes and expenditures without regaining weight. As we discussed above, exercise also seems to help the brain do a better job matching eating and expenditure. It's likely that exercise does both for successful weight-loss maintainers, pushing daily energy expenditure back toward pre-weight-loss levels and helping to regulate food intake.

Pushing the Limits

A few years ago, at a conference on metabolism, I found myself at the hotel bar late in the evening, talking to a colleague who has spent his career investigating energy expenditure and obesity. I had given a talk earlier in the day, laying out the evidence that daily energy expenditure is constrained. The details are a little foggy, but the conversation went something like this.

"You might be right," he said, "that exercise doesn't do much to increase daily energy expenditure or lose weight. But you have to be careful. Once people find out that exercise won't help them lose weight, they'll stop doing it. Avoiding death isn't a big enough incentive. The only reliable motivation to exercise is vanity."

It was an unfiltered take on the inherent weakness of the human species from a frustrated scientist who knew the score. I suspect he was right. When it comes to our inner desires, our lazy ape relatives are more of a mirror than we'd care to admit. Deep in our subconscious, we still yearn to lie around all day, eating and grooming. The industrialized human zoos we've built ourselves make it all too easy. *Of course* we'd like to avoid heart disease. But first we'd like to check our phones. Maybe get a snack. Relax a little. If exercise isn't going to make me look hot, it can wait.

The danger, though, in selling exercise as a way to lose weight is that it doesn't work. Eventually, people notice the results don't match the sales pitch. Some will keep with it anyway, hooked by the many other benefits of exercise—improved mood, clearer minds, stronger body—and willing to overlook the bait and switch. But there would be more happy customers if those of us in public health were honest about what we're selling. Exercise won't keep you thin, but it will keep you alive.

Exercise does much more than rev our metabolic engines. It's the rhythm section of our vast internal orchestra, keeping our 37 trillion cells on the same beat. Constrained daily energy expenditure doesn't diminish the importance of physical activity. To the contrary. The fact that daily energy expenditure is constrained helps explain why exercise has such pervasive effects throughout the body. My lab and others are busy with the painstaking work of unraveling the impact of exercise on our other systems. It's an exciting time to explore. There is undoubtedly much more to exercise's impact on metabolism and the rest of our body waiting to be discovered.

Still, the evidence for constrained daily energy expenditure raises other questions. How can we reconcile the idea that energy expenditure is limited with the jaw-dropping workout regimens we see in elite athletes, mountaineers, and Arctic explorers? As we'll see in the last two chapters, the metabolic machinery that powers an Ironman triathlete, a Tour de France cyclist, or an Arctic trekker is the same that fuels a pregnant mother. And yet those feats, impressive as they are, do not tell the whole story of our ravenous appetite for energy. As our species has evolved, our energy demands have grown beyond what our own bodies can provide. The calories that each of us command today shape the modern world—and threaten our long-term survival.

CHAPTER 8

Energetics at the Extreme: The Limits of Human Endurance

Bryce Carlson looks like a normal person. In his late thirties, with a lanky build and a big grin, he's clearly in good shape, but he wouldn't look out of place at the office holiday party—the kind of guy who wakes up chipper at some awful hour every day to exercise before coming into work, and casually mentions the marathon he's training for at lunch. Definitely a contender in the annual corporate 5K, but not a superhuman world record holder.

Looks can be deceiving.

On the morning of June 20, 2018, in Quidi Vidi Harbour on the coast of Newfoundland, Bryce grinned his big happy grin and waved goodbye to a small group of locals and journalists. He looked at his watch—8:00 A.M.—grabbed the handles of two long carbon-fiber oars and *pulled*, feeling the weight of his boat, *Lucille*, in his shoulders and back. *Lucille* wasn't your typical rowboat, more like a spacecraft with oars, with a smooth white ovoid hull and tiny cabin perched on the bow. And it wasn't your typical day on the water. As Bryce pulled away from shore, his back to the sea, he was attempting to make history. He was setting out to cross the North Atlantic, hoping to row over two thousand miles, solo and unsupported, to the Isles of Scilly just off England's southern coast.

Even with GPS and other modern tech on board, it was a dicey proposition. Of the fourteen people who had set out on this mad adventure before, only eight had completed the crossing. Two had drowned in the dark, frigid waters of the North Atlantic, their bodies lost at sea. But never mind that, Bryce was dreaming big. He didn't just plan to survive the crossing, he hoped to crush it. He wanted to claim the world record for the fastest human-powered trip across the North Atlantic. He and *Lucille* had fifty-three days to get to England.

Things could have gone better. Early in the journey the main desalinization unit used to supply fresh water broke. He capsized a dozen times, and salt water seeped into the onboard electronics and fried the navigation system. But Bryce endured. On an overcast Saturday evening in early August, Bryce pulled into St. Mary's Harbour on the Isles of Scilly and stepped off *Lucille* to a hero's welcome. Hundreds had gathered to catch a glimpse of the new world record holder. Bryce had made the crossing in 38 days, 6 hours, and 49 minutes, blasting the old record out of the water.

The trip had taken its toll. Bryce ate between 4,000 and 5,000 kilocalories each day during the journey, but he expended much more than that. He emerged from the Atlantic fifteen pounds lighter than when he'd started, burning off about 625 kcal of fat and muscle each day despite his huge energy intake. Add the energy consumed from his own body to the energy in his diet, and Bryce was burning well over 5,000 kilocalories per day during the row.

Bryce was all alone on the ocean, but his metabolism was in good company. Other endurance athletes register similarly high daily expenditures. Tour de France cyclists burn 8,500 kilocalories per day during the race. Triathletes can burn that much energy in a twelve-hour Ironman. Michael Phelps, human-dolphin chimera and winner of twenty-three gold medals in Olympic swimming, report-edly ate 12,000 kcal each day during training. Feats like these seem to challenge the idea that daily energy expenditure is constrained, our bodies adjusting to our exercise workload to keep daily expen-ditures in the normal range of 2,500 to 3,000 kcal per day. In this chapter, we'll explore this puzzle and map the limits of human en-ergy expenditure. As we'll see, the same metabolic machinery that constrains our expenditures during daily life also sets the limits on our most extreme ambitions. You don't have to be superhuman to push the boundaries of human endurance. Just ask your mom.

A Matter of Time

How fast can you run? It's a simple question without a simple an-swer. Your maximum speed depends on the reason you're running and the depth of your motivation. Escaping a lion? Playing some beer league softball? It also depends on how *long* you'll be running. You can sprint for a few seconds, but you'll need to dial it back if you're running a mile. Our top speed lies along a continuum from short, fast sprints to longer, slower jogs. Most of us have known this about our bodies since those early schoolyard afternoons play-ing tag.

The effect of time on endurance is so intuitive and instinctual that we don't tend to give it much thought. But the physiology of fa-tigue is anything but obvious. Sports scientists and physiologists still argue about the mechanisms in our body that set the limits (for ringside seats to this scientific brawl, check out Alex Hutchinson's excellent book, *Endure*). One thing is certain: hitting your limit is not simply a case of running out of fuel. Instead, your brain appears to be integrating signals from all over the body—including the met-abolic by-products of working muscles, body temperature, your per-ception of difficulty, and the expected amount of work left to do—and using that information to regulate how hard we can push ourselves. When you collapse from exhaustion, it's your brain that shuts you down. Not that you have any access to those decisions. Just as we see with the hypothalamus and its control of appetite and metabolism, the neural systems that shape endurance and fatigue do their work deep within the brain, beneath our consciousness.

Neural control of fatigue and endurance was a controversial concept in the 1990s, but it gained acceptance as the evidence grew. First, it became clear from lab studies and lived experience that a person who feels completely exhausted still has plenty of fuel on board. Even when we feel like we've reached our absolute limits, there's still plenty of ATP in our tired muscles and glucose and fatty acids circulating in our blood. We routinely watch elite runners fall to the ground at the end of a long race, totally spent, only to pick themselves up a minute later and jog a victory lap around the stadium, smiling. And second, neural control of fatigue helped explain the strange effects of mood and perception on performance. World-class marathoners pushing their limits for two hours are still able, somehow, to run even faster at the end for the finishing kick—desperation and determination can unlock hidden athletic potential. Conversely, lab studies show that mental fatigue reduces endurance. Athletes and coaches around the world know the importance of being in the right frame of mind if you want to win.

The central role of the brain in fatigue also helps to explain the relationship between energy expenditure and endurance (Figure 8.1). These effects are easiest to see with running, but the same physiology applies to swimming, cycling, and other sports. As we discussed in Chapter 3, when you run faster, you burn calories faster. The effect is linear, meaning that running 10 percent faster requires you to burn energy 10 percent faster. That's not so different from what we'd find with a car engine: a 10 percent increase in the speed generally means you burn gasoline at a 10 percent faster rate (or drain the battery 10 percent faster, if you drive an electric). But there are some important differences between your metabolic engine and the engine in your car. In your car, speed doesn't have much effect on how far you can drive on a full tank or a full battery, it just determines how quickly you run out of fuel. With running, speed has a huge effect on how much energy you burn before you reach your limit. The faster you run, the less energy you burn in total before hitting the wall. Race for a mile, and you'll collapse after burning 100 kcal. Race a marathon, and you'll collapse, just as exhausted, having burned 2,600. Our bodies don't just stop when we run out of fuel (even though it can feel that way). Intensity matters.

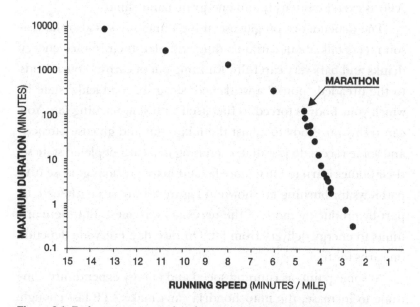

Figure 8.1. Endurance, measured as the maximum amount of time you can maintain a given workload, is closely related to power output. Here, world record race times are plotted against running speed for events ranging from 800 meters to over 600 miles in length. Marathons are run near the VO_2 max speed. At faster speeds, endurance drops precipitously as the body is forced to rely on anaerobic metabolism for an ever greater proportion of power.

One reason that speed affects fatigue is the change in the type of fuel your body burns during exercise. When we're resting and during low-intensity activity (reading this book or strolling around the park), our bodies burn fat as their primary fuel. That makes good sense as a biological strategy: you've got virtually unlimited energy stored as fat, and, although it takes longer to process and burn fat to make ATP, at low levels of energy expenditure, we don't require anything faster. As exercise intensity picks up, more glucose is added to the mix of fuel. Some of this additional glucose is supplied from circulating blood sugar; some of it is pulled from glycogen stores in the muscle. Compared to fat, glucose is easier and faster to burn (even if it's being converted from glycogen). This improved speed of availability helps keep the muscles supplied with ATP as exercise intensity and energy demand climb.

The dependence on glucose at high intensities is also the reason racers talk about carbo-loading and plan their in-race energy drinks and bars very carefully. Running out of carbs to burn leads to the dreaded "bonk," a weakened, sluggish, zombielike state in which your body is forced to fuel itself with slow-burning fats. You can train your body to adjust the mix of fat and glucose burned, and some racers do just that, exercising in a carb-depleted state so their bodies learn to burn more fat and spare precious glucose (the pathways for burning fat shown in Figure 2.1 are strengthened, in part by producing more of the necessary enzymes). But there are limits to energy delivery from fat. On race day, everyone depends on carbs for fuel.

At some point, as running speed and energy expenditure continue to increase, the mitochondria can't make ATP fast enough to meet demand, even with a steady supply of glucose. If we're measuring oxygen consumption in the lab when you hit this point, we'll see oxygen consumption plateau and remain steady even as your speed and energy demand continue to climb. You won't last much longer. This break point is your VO_2 max, the limit of your aerobic capacity. The supply chain that carries oxygen and glucose to your cells, then converts them to ATP via the mitochondria, has reached its limit. It simply can't supply energy any faster.

With your aerobic (oxygen-based) production of ATP maxed out, the muscles are forced to rely on anaerobic metabolism (Chapter 2). As anaerobic metabolism grows, CO_2 production continues to climb even as oxygen consumption remains stuck. Your blood pH becomes more acidic. Glucose in your cells is broken down into pyruvate, the molecule that will jump into the mitochondria, transform into acetyl CoA, and feed the Krebs cycle, ultimately paying off in tons of ATP (Figure 2.1). But there's a traffic jam getting into the mitochondria, and the excess pyruvate is diverted and converted to lactate and then to lactic acid. Your muscles start to burn. *How much longer can you hold on?* Your brain has the final say. A dark, shapeless voice, familiar to any runner, starts to moan from deep inside your head, imploring you to *stop.* Its volume and intensity grows until it swallows you whole. Eventually you give in. You simply can't push any longer. You slow down or collapse in a gasping heap.

Energy expenditure and the VO_2 max limit are only one piece of the puzzle that sets your endurance limit, but they're a crucial part. The brain is listening closely as the body switches from pure aerobic metabolism to a more troublesome mix of aerobic and anaerobic. As elite runners reach their VO_2 max speed, endurance plummets (Figure 8.1). A world-class marathoner can maintain a pace of 4:42 minutes per mile—*just* at the edge of hitting his VO_2 max—for a little over two hours. Increase his speed by just 5 percent, up to a 4:28 mile, and the amount of time he can maintain that pace is cut in half. He's crossed the VO_2 max threshold, and the reliance on anaerobic metabolism to help fuel his muscles signals the brain to pull the plug before any damage is done. Any faster, and his endurance—the maximum amount of time he can run before collapsing—will continue to fall precipitously as his body relies more and more on anaerobic metabolism.

Our metabolic machinery shapes the internal unseen landscape of every endurance race. Marathons are exciting because the entire race is run along the edge of a cliff, right up against the VO_2 max threshold (Figure 8.1), each racer monitoring their own body and trying to read their opponents', looking for the right time to give them a shove. The VO_2 max threshold makes shorter races into a sort of blood sport, each competitor trying to find the right mix of oxygen and pain to fuel faster and faster races without blowing up before the finish.

Still, the usual battery of track and field events are all fairly short. Even a marathon is over in less than three hours if you're fast. What about the *really* long events? The unglamorous, never-ending suffer-fests? The kind where you and a team of dogs pull sledges across Antarctica for three months, the sledge carrying all your food falls in a bottomless crevasse, and you resort to eating your dogs one by one in a desperate endless bid to get home? Extreme events like that are understandably rare, but a growing number of studies have tracked the energy expenditures of people like Bryce, who are out there pushing the boundaries of human performance. What they've taught us about endurance has changed the way we understand our metabolic limits.

Endurance over Days, Weeks, and Months

Impressive as it was, the North Atlantic row wasn't Bryce Carlson's longest expedition. Before he crossed an ocean, he crossed a continent.

On the morning of January 16, 2015, a brave and cheerful crew of runners gathered at Huntington Beach, California, with their shoes in the sand and the Pacific Ocean at their backs. Bryce was there, of course, along with about a dozen other men and women eager to get going. One of them, a man named Newton from Vermont, was celebrating his seventy-third birthday, but the runners hadn't gathered to blow out candles. They were about to set out on an audacious transcontinental run: the Race Across the USA.

At 8:00 A.M., they started off, gamboling at an easy pace through the urban sprawl of Southern California, heading east into the sun. By midafternoon, the runners had completed a marathon, the day's objective. They rested up at a temporary camp near the finish line, went to bed, and woke up the next day and did it again. And again. And again . . . Bryce and the other Race Across the USA runners, including Newton, ran a marathon a day, six days a week (and sometimes seven), for 140 days. They covered over three thousand miles, wending their way through the deserts of the American Southwest, across the hills and plains of Texas, through the green forests of the Carolinas, and north to Washington, D.C., finishing at the White House.

Lucky for us, Darren and Sandy Van Soye, the husband and wife team who organized the Race Across the USA, invited a gang of scientists along for the race (Darren was also one of the runners). Bryce, then a professor at Purdue University and one of the core team of runners, had the vision to organize a research component for the race, and the Van Soyes agreed to have him lead it. At an anthropology conference the year before the race, Bryce approached me out of the blue and asked if I wanted to measure the runners' energy expenditures. It was the first time I'd ever met Bryce or heard anything about the Race Across the USA, and I was sure he was delusional. A five-month, 3,000-mile footrace across the whole of North America? The entire thing sounded absurd. I immediately agreed to be involved.

With my collaborators, Cara Ocobock (a former PhD student from my lab) and Lara Dugas (whom we met in Chapter 5), we hatched a plan. We'd measure the runners' daily energy expenditures and BMRs before the race, and then twice during the run—at the beginning and the end. We figured those measurements would give us two critical pieces of information. First, with two measurements taken during the race, we'd have a solid measurement of the calories burned each day under extreme exercise workloads—a rare and valuable piece of data. Second, we could compare daily energy expenditures at the beginning and end of the race to test for energy compensation. Would the runners' bodies adapt to such an extreme workload, reducing energy expenditure to compensate for the huge increase in activity expenditure?

Six of the core runners agreed to participate in our metabolic study. Caitlin Thurber, a grad student in my lab, led the field effort to measure daily energy expenditures (using doubly labeled water). She traveled to California for the start of the race and then, five months later, to Virginia for the final week. She even tracked down two runners who split from the race midway through to follow a faster schedule (proving once again that ambition and sanity are relative). Lara Dugas collected careful BMR measurements of the runners at the beginning and end of the race as well, though she wasn't able to get the two rogue racers. One of the six runners in our sample quit the race a few weeks in due to injury.

As Caitlin churned through the doubly labeled water analyses that summer, an exciting set of results emerged. In the first week of the race, the runners burned exactly what we'd predict if we added the cost of a marathon (about 2,600 kcal) to their prerace daily expenditures. That's just what we expected. One week isn't enough time for the body to adjust to the new workload—a marathon per day—and so the cost of that activity was simply added to the body's usual, prerace energy budget. Bryce and the other runners were averaging an incredible 6,200 kcal per day.

But by the end of the race, 140 days later, their bodies had changed. Even with the same crazy marathon-a-day workload, runners were burning 4,900 kcal per day—still impressive, but a 20 percent decrease from the first week of the race. Some of that decrease could be attributed to the smaller hills out east and having lost a bit of weight over the course of the event, but at least 600 kcal per day seemed to have just vanished from their daily energy budget. This was energy compensation, their constrained metabolism at work: faced with an enormous exercise workload, the runners' bodies were reducing energy expenditure on other tasks to try to keep daily energy expenditures in check. The enormous cost of a daily marathon was more than the energy compensation could fully absorb—their daily expenditures during the final weeks of the race were still well above their prerace values—but their bodies were trying.

Another interesting detail emerged when we looked at Lara Dugas's BMR measurements: unlike the runners' daily energy expenditures, their BMRs didn't change at all between the beginning and the end of the race (if anything, they were a smidge higher). Energy compensation didn't show up in the BMR component of daily energy expenditure. Instead, the component of daily expenditure that shrank was what we usually call activity energy expenditure, or AEE, the portion of daily energy expenditure that's left after you subtract BMR and the costs of digestion. It's strange to think that AEE would shrink when the workload (a marathon each day) stayed the same, but in fact we see energy compensation showing up in the AEE component pretty regularly. How is it that activity expenditure decreases when exercise increases?

One possibility is that people reduce their non-exercise behavior—what the researcher James Levine called non-exercise activity thermogenesis, or NEAT—to reduce AEE when their exercise workloads increase. The idea here is that the body might unconsciously reduce small, overlooked behaviors that burn calories, like fidgeting or standing, in response to increased exercise demands. It's an interesting idea and could certainly contribute to energy compensation, but the evidence is mixed. As Ed Melanson and others have shown, most studies measuring the NEAT response to exercise have found little or no effect. Besides, it's hard to imagine the Race Across the USA runners were saving 600 kcal per day by fidgeting less.

The other possible explanation is that AEE is capturing more than just physical activity. Our bodies have a strong circadian rhythm: resting metabolic rate (the collective metabolism of our organs at work) follows a daily roller-coaster trajectory, up and down, rising to its peak in the late afternoon and hitting its valley in the early morning. We measure BMR during the valley, in the early morning. When we calculate AEE by subtracting BMR and digestion costs from daily energy expenditure, we implicitly ignore the daily rise in resting energy expenditure and instead lump all those non-activity calories into AEE. I strongly suspect that the energy compensation we often see coming out of AEE reflects decreasing amplitude of the circadian fluctuation in resting energy expenditure. Increasing exercise workload doesn't necessarily make the valleys of resting expenditure lower, but it squashes the peaks. The resulting decrease in AEE *looks* like the energy compensation is coming from changes in activity, but in fact it's due to decreased energy expenditure on everything else—for example, the healthy suppression of immune activity, reproductive hormones, and stress reactivity we discussed in the last chapter. This is a hot area of research, and my lab and others are working to test these ideas.

It's Alimentary, My Dear Watson

Curious to know how the daily energy expenditures of the Race Across the USA runners stacked up against other long-haul efforts, I dug into the scientific literature to find whatever I could on metabolism during extreme events: the Kona Ironman triathlon, Western States 100-mile ultramarathon, the Tour de France, Antarctic trekking, military expeditions, the whole lot. I tracked down credible estimates of daily expenditure of world records for ultralong distances, from the maximum distance run in 24 hours to the 46-day record for the 2,200-mile Appalachian Trail. I searched for endurance events that lasted longer than the Race Across the USA but was coming up empty-handed. The longest lasting, highest energy expenditure activity I could find was pregnancy: nine months long, with daily expenditures of 3,000 kcal per day or more in the third trimester.

When we look at these records of human endurance, one thing was obvious: daily expenditures were higher for shorter events like the triathlon, and lower for longer events like the Tour de France. Still, it was hard to compare among all the studies, in large part because the subjects of each one differed so much in body size, which we know affects metabolic rates (Chapter 3). To account for size, I did what metabolism researchers often do: I divided daily energy expenditure by BMR. That ratio, called metabolic scope, removes the effect of body size because size affects both daily expenditure and BMR in a similar manner. You can think of metabolic scope as a size-corrected daily energy expenditure.

When I plotted metabolic scope against duration, the result was startling and beautiful. Staring back at me from my laptop was an elegant crisp line, a graceful arc sweeping down from the high expenditures of the shortest events and out to the lower expenditures of the longest (Figure 8.2). I realized I was looking at a map.

Those points, that line, marked the boundaries of human endurance. Quickly, I added all the other high endurance studies I could find, from military endeavors to athletes in training. Every one of them fell dutifully within the bounds of human capability. Not one of them jumped the border. And pregnancy? It fell right along the boundary, marking the far end of our metabolic capacity. Expecting mothers were pushing the same metabolic limits as Tour de France cyclists. Pregnancy is the ultimate ultramarathon.

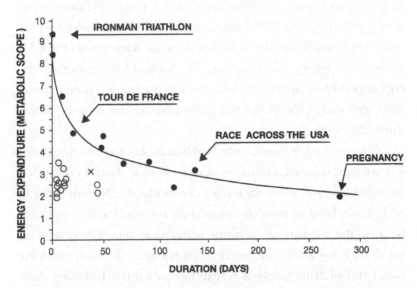

Figure 8.2. Endurance limit (shown as metabolic scope, or multiples of BMR) for events lasting days, weeks, or months. Solid black circles are from events at the limit of human endurance (some are labeled). Open gray circles are from studies of other long-duration, high-intensity endeavors, from mountaineering to Olympic training. Estimated expenditure for Bryce Carlson's North Atlantic row is marked ×.

We can be confident that the metabolic ceiling in Figure 8.2 is a real limit, because no one has ever punched through it. Elite cyclists, triathletes, and others who have ventured to the edge of our metabolic world train their whole lives to get as close to those limits as possible. Their competitors do the same, and so the races come down to the slimmest of margins, just seconds separating the top competitors after hours or even weeks of racing. If they could somehow break through the metabolic ceiling—if, for example, a cyclist could maintain the metabolic scope of a 100-mile ultramarathoner for the full four-week Tour de France—they'd win by hours, finishing each stage miles ahead of the pack. But they don't, because they can't. They can't exceed the limits of the human body; they can only push themselves to the brink and hope their competitors blink first.

Bryce Carlson is the only human I know of who has visited the metabolic boundary twice in widely different sports. He and the core Race Across the USA team hit the limit as they ran across the continent, and he nearly hit it again when he rowed *Lucille* across the North Atlantic.

Endurance Takes Guts

Shortly after we put the Race Across the USA measurements and all the other high-endurance studies together, I presented our discovery of human metabolic limits at an energetics conference in Switzerland. John Speakman, a pioneer in metabolic physiology, was complimentary but largely unimpressed. He had done a number of studies hunting down the physiological mechanisms that constrain maximum energy expenditures in mammals. John's work pointed toward thermoregulation as the critical issue: if metabolic rates get too high, the body overheats. In one memorable study, he shaved mouse mothers with nursing pups to show they could burn more calories and produce more milk when they were able to lose body heat faster. I may have mapped the boundary of human endurance, but John wanted to know the physiological mechanism that shaped it.

I hadn't given the mechanism much thought, but a thermoregulatory limit seemed unlikely. After all, in our diverse sample of studies, we had people racing triathlons in Hawaii, cycling through sweltering summers in Europe, and trekking across frigid Antarctica. They all fit the same limits of endurance. If overheating was the primary obstacle, then the Antarctic trekkers—like Speakman's shaved mice—should have been able to exceed the normal human limits of endurance.

John and I worked through the data and hit upon a stronger explanation. When we plotted weight loss against energy expenditure for the endurance athletes in our dataset, a clear pattern emerged. Daily weight loss increased in proportion to daily expenditure. These athletes weren't trying to lose weight—on the contrary, they were stuffing their faces with all the high-calorie performance foods they could manage to eat. But try as they might, they weren't able to get calories in fast enough to meet demands, and as expenditures climbed higher, the energy deficit grew.

Then another piece of the puzzle clicked into place. When we put the daily energy expenditure measurements together with the data on weight loss, we found that every athlete (and pregnant mother) in our dataset was taking in the same amount of energy per day. Across the board, from the Antarctic trekkers to elite distance runners, their bodies were absorbing about two and a half times their BMR (just as we did with energy expenditure, we calculated energy intake as multiples of BMR to account for differences in body size). All of the energy expenditure above the two and a half times BMR intake limit was coming out of their fat stores, which is why athletes above that level of expenditure were losing weight.

To test whether the body really can't absorb more energy, we included forced overeating studies in the analysis. In these studies, people eat far more calories than they burn each day. Here again, when we calculated the total number of calories absorbed into the body, everyone in the dataset was hovering around 2.5 times BMR. To put this in terms of calories: no matter the event or circumstances, the maximum amount of energy the body can absorb is around 4,000 to 5,000 kcal per day. Beyond that, and you'll be in negative energy balance, burning more fat and glycogen than you can replenish each day and slowly melting away.

Of course, you can maintain a negative energy balance for a few days or even a few months—that's what the steep part of the human endurance boundary reflects. But you can't keep it up forever. For truly limitless endurance you need to be able to maintain body weight, and to do that you have to keep your daily energy expenditure at around two and a half times BMR (around 4,000 to 5,000 kcal) or below. Your body simply can't digest and absorb calories any faster. For events that last days, weeks, or longer, it isn't our muscles that hold us back, it's our guts.

We don't yet know how the body interprets weight loss during multiday and multiweek events and translates that signal into fatigue and a loss of endurance. It's practically certain that the brain coordinates this response, just as it does in marathons and shorter races. After all, Tour de France cyclists don't stop because they're *hungry*, they stop because they're *exhausted*—a sensation manufactured entirely in the brain.

We do think, though, that the weight-loss signal plays a critical role. As we discussed in Chapter 5, the brain tracks changes in weight very precisely and responds accordingly. Consequently, the rate of weight loss would seem to be a critical signal for the brain as it regulates endurance and effort. And conversely, finding some way to enhance the body's ability to absorb calories could be an effective way to increase endurance in multiday and multiweek events. Tour de France cyclists—or their team doctors, in any case—would seem to agree. In the 1980s and '90s, some cyclists began injecting intravenous doses of lipids and glucose at night, between race stages. Delivering these nutrients directly into the bloodstream bypasses the digestive machinery, circumventing the usual limits on energy absorption. Maybe that's why cyclists in the Tour de France (who, we should be clear, were measured during a race in the 1980s) lost less weight than we'd expect. Compared to other athletes in our dataset, the Tour de France cyclists were outliers, losing less than three pounds over the course of the race. Fats and sugars aren't illegal in endurance sports (you have to eat *something*), but a nightly IV drip is frowned upon. A crackdown on intravenous energy delivery in the 1990s seems to have quashed the practice, but like other illicit performance enhancers, it may have just moved deeper underground.

Athletes Everywhere

Our metabolic limits aren't important only when we are trekking across Antarctica or cheating in the Tour de France. Constraints on energy absorption shape our daily lives. For mothers, the limits on energy absorption may prevent pregnancies from lasting too long. Throughout gestation, for the fetus to grow, mom has to take in more energy than she burns. This is the fundamental rule of pregnancy: mom has to gain weight. But as her weight increases, so does her daily energy expenditure. At nine months, the familiar duration of a typical pregnancy, mom is being pushed to the brink. If the baby gets much larger, mom won't be able to bring in enough calories to sustain them both. We think the signals of metabolic stress released as moms approach their metabolic limits help trigger the birth process.

Modern changes in diet and lifestyle might be affecting this metabolic trigger in ways that put moms and babies in greater danger. Birth has always been a tricky affair for our species, with big babies born right at the size limits of the bony birth canal. If the neonate is even a tiny bit too big, serious and often life-threatening complications arise. And how do babies get too big? They get too much energy from mom, either by annexing a greater share of the nutrients in mom's bloodstream or by overstaying their welcome. In populations like the Hadza, where pregnant mothers stay physically active through the third trimester and foods are unprocessed and slower to digest, less energy will be available for the fetus to commandeer. Their babies are unlikely to get too big before mom's metabolic limits trigger birth. We don't have great numbers on the rates of birth complications for the Hadza or other small-scale societies, but they appear to be quite low. In the United States and other sedentary, industrialized populations, mothers are awash in easy calories, and the fetus doesn't need to compete with the energy demands of physical activity. Perhaps this leads to babies being born a bit later and a bit larger—not by much, but enough to cause trouble. It's notable that the rates of delivery by cesarean section have skyrocketed over the past half century, along with modern changes in diet and physical activity.

Our digestive limits also put a cap on daily energy expenditure during normal daily life. Over the long haul, as months stretch into years and years into lifetimes, we simply can't burn more energy than we can bring in. We have to live within our metabolic means. No one can maintain a daily energy expenditure too far above two times their BMR. And guess what? No one does. Around the globe, when we look at daily energy expenditures during normal daily life for the hundreds of populations who have been measured, from Holland to the Hadza, everyone lives their lives well under the 2.5 times BMR limit. In physically active populations like the Hadza, the body adjusts to keep daily expenditures at a sustainable level.

We have just rediscovered the constrained model for daily energy expenditure, like Magellan sailing west, arriving where we left off in Chapter 5, but traveling from a different direction.

What's So Special About Michael Phelps?

Our study mapping the limits of human endurance also provided some cognitive relief on an issue I had been wrestling with for years. Ever since we published the first energy expenditure work with the Hadza showing that human energy expenditure is constrained, I would inevitably get the same question in conversations and public talks. It's such a regular occurrence that I gave it a name: The Michael Phelps Enigma. "How can it be," my skeptical colleagues would ask, "that Michael Phelps can eat 12,000 kcal a day if human energy expenditure is constrained?" It was a fair question, and I didn't have an easy answer. Michael Phelps haunted my dreams.

It says something about the human psyche that the eating habits of elite athletes are a key part of their mythology and the idolizing of their fans. Profiles of professional athletes often make a point of detailing their diets. Of all the incredible feats that Phelps has accomplished—the world records, the twenty-three Olympic gold medals, the countless trips to the podium—the number that sticks in people's heads is the amount of food he crammed in. Perhaps it's so powerful because food is so personal: *12,000 kilocalories per day?!* What stronger evidence do you need that these superheroes are fundamentally different from you and me?

Solving the Michael Phelps Enigma requires that we first get a handle on his actual food intake. No one has ever actually measured daily food intake by Phelps or his Olympic teammates (at least, no one has ever published those measurements). Instead, the 12,000 kcal per day figure floating around in the collective consciousness seems to have been a bluff from Phelps or the people in his orbit, a bit of Olympic exaggeration. He has since said that his daily energy intake during training was closer to 7,000 to 8,000 kcal per day. Even that number is a gross estimate based on recollections of his training days, and there's reason to question it. Self-reported energy intake is unreliable, even in the most rigorous studies, and other swimmers report much more mundane diets. Katie Ledecky, another star Olympic swimmer, reports a diet that's well under 4,000 kcal per day. But let's take 7,000 kcal per day as a first-pass estimate for Phelps.

Like most elite swimmers, Michael Phelps is a large guy, well above average for height (six-four) and weight (194 pounds) in his competition days. Plugging those numbers into our BMR equations from Chapter 3, we'd expect him to have a BMR of around 1,900 kcal per day. There's a fair amount of uncertainty around that prediction, though. People can easily deviate from their expected BMR by 200 kcal per day or more. Someone like Phelps, with a lower body-fat percentage than the average adult (and thus more energy-burning lean mass), would be expected to have above average BMR. For the sake of argument, let's estimate his BMR at 2,100 kcal per day.

Next, let's think about what it means to eat 7,000 kcal per day. Your digestive tract doesn't extract every last calorie from the food you eat (if it did, you'd hardly ever poop). Instead, human digestive efficiency—the ratio of energy absorbed over energy eaten—is about 95 percent. Your mileage will vary depending on your diet and the particulars of your digestive anatomy and physiology. If Phelps ate 7,000 kcal per day, he'd be absorbing about 6,650 kcal for his body to burn. The remainder would be lost in the bathroom.

At 6,650 kcal per day, Phelps would be absorbing a little over three times his BMR. That would put him in the very upper range of energy absorption in our human endurance dataset. We found that elite athletes were absorbing two and a half times BMR on average, but (like everything in the biology of metabolism) there was a bit of variation around that average value. A few athletes in our sample had estimated rates of energy absorption just above three times BMR. Eating 7,000 kcal per day, Phelps would be stretching the limits of the rule of 2.5 times BMR, but not breaking it. Elite, but not superhuman.

Every year, tens of thousands of kids in the United States and around the world churn their way through swim practices and meets, many with big dreams of becoming the next Michael Phelps or Katie Ledecky. What separates the tiny fraction of swimmers who become truly elite from the thousands upon thousands who will never make it? No doubt you need opportunity, good coaching, strong support, and a rare mental determination to win. But maybe there's more to it. Maybe you also need a digestive tract that's *really* good at absorbing calories, so that you can fuel the endless hours in the pool without your body shutting down. Maybe Phelps, Ledecky, and the other ultra-elite athletes in our modern Olympic pantheon are distinguished as much by their remarkable guts as their ferocious strength.

Evolved to Break the Rules

We humans like our origin stories simple. One cause, one effect, one lesson. Vishnu built the world and Shiva will destroy it. We can cook our food because Prometheus stole fire. Grandma has to die because Eve ate the apple. John and Paul built the Beatles and Yoko tore them apart. It's turtles all the way down.

We gravitate toward simple evolutionary stories, too. But natural selection rarely targets one trait in isolation, and most traits have multiple effects that all contribute to evolutionary success or failure. The obvious utility of a trait today might not be the reason it arose. We think of feathers as adaptations for flight, but they began in the earliest avian ancestors as insulation. Darwin thought that human ancestors began walking on two legs so that they could use their hands to wield weapons—not a bad guess (since we do that today) but clearly wrong, in the light of the archaeological record. I've seen colleagues argue endlessly whether natural selection favored bigger brains in hominins because it improved their foraging prowess or because it increased their social savvy (surely it was both, and more). Language has so many benefits and uses that in 1866, the French Academy famously banned any discussion of its origins, since there was no way to distinguish the myriad explanations. But frustrating as it might be, we have to embrace the complexity of evolution and the interdependence of our features and abilities if we want to develop a deep and real understanding of our evolutionary past. Grappling with evidence and weighing competing ideas is what distinguishes science from mythology.

Our metabolic machinery provides a perfect demonstration of our body's physiological interconnections. The same machinery that limits our athletic endurance also shapes gestation and pregnancy and constrains daily energy expenditure. Tellingly, *all* of these aspects of our metabolism are enhanced compared to our ape cousins. We have better endurance, larger babies, and higher daily energy expenditures than chimpanzees, bonobos, or any other great ape. Natural selection pushed our metabolic capacity skyward, increasing expenditures across the board. A rising tide lifts all boats.

So which trait was The One Big Thing that led natural selection to increase our metabolic capacity? Improved endurance to forage and run down prey? The capacity to have bigger babies, more often? Greater daily energy expenditures to fuel larger brains and more daily physical activity? Like most arguments about The One Big Thing that explains human evolution, the premise is faulty. It's most likely that all of these advantages (and possibly others) strengthened natural selection for enhanced metabolic capacity in our hominin ancestors. Each is an integral part of what makes us human today.

One thing is certain: we have moved the metabolic boundaries upward and outward compared to those of our ape relatives. As we discussed in Chapter 4, hunting and gathering changed the way we acquire energy from the world around us and use it for growth, reproduction, and survival. We evolved a larger energy footprint. Like language, tool use, and walking on two legs, a greater metabolic capacity has affected nearly every aspect of our lives.

But our evolutionary drive for increased energy expenditure didn't end with a revved-up metabolism. We have broken the rules in a more fundamental way. Over the past two million years, we have figured out how to harness energy outside our own bodies to use toward our own ends. It's an unprecedented innovation in the history of life. The future of our species will depend on how well we manage our ever-increasing hunger for energy. Maybe the Hadza have some insight to share.

CHAPTER 9

The Past, Present, and Uncertain Future of *Homo energeticus*

How long would it take to walk to your house?" asked Onawasi as we sat around the men's area in a camp called Setako, down in the hot dry flats at the foot of the Tli'ika Hills.

It was a reasonable question. With no alternative means of transportation, Hadza men and women walk everywhere. No place is too far away. They aren't fazed by the prospect of a two-day walk to the village to trade honey for some new clothes or a cooking pot, or even longer hikes to visit friends in far-off camps. If that sounds hard to wrap your head around, you're not alone. The average American hops in a car for any trip longer than a mile.

In a seminomadic community like the Hadza, where people move among camps fluidly, you adapt early to spending your days on foot. I remember talking to a couple of boys, maybe ten years old, about a wild escape from boarding school. Their parents had saved enough shillings to put them in classes for a month or so—a big investment for a Hadza family—but the boys, like children everywhere, weren't crazy about school. Other kids might have stuck it out, if only because leaving wasn't much of an option: the school was several days' walk from home, through a wild savanna full of big cats, deadly snakes, and other dangers. But these were Hadza kids. A few days' walk didn't scare them. The three of them sneaked out of the dorms before dawn one morning and headed home. They couldn't have been more than eight years old at the time, sleeping on the ground at night and walking miles each day under the hot sun, through unfamiliar terrain, with nothing to eat. It's not every day that I talk to kids who were braver at eight years old than I am as an adult, but this, apparently, was one of those times.

As they told the story, I searched their eyes for some flicker of fear from the trek or maybe a sense of pride in the adventure, but all I found was that usual implacable Hadza nonchalance. I don't think they understood why I was so interested in the story. They didn't like school, so they walked home. What was the big deal about that?

Onawasi's question was more about distance than time. The Hadza know that researchers and others like to measure distances in miles or kilometers, but that's not the measurement system they grew up with. The number of days it takes to walk somewhere is probably the most meaningful measure of distance to far-flung places for a Hadza man or woman. He knew my home was far away, but how far, exactly? Onawasi wanted to get a handle on that, maybe mull over the journey in his mind for fun. He wasn't planning to walk to my house, but then again it might not be out of the question. His kids were grown, and he had no earthly obligations. He could set out tomorrow with his bow in his hand and the sun in his face, free as a honey badger. It isn't like he'd have to call off of work or worry about his mortgage.

Except, of course, it was completely unreasonable to consider walking to my house—it was over eight thousand miles away, across two continents and an ocean. Even if he could somehow walk across the Atlantic, a Hadza man covering his typical ten miles (sixteen kilometers) per day would take two and a half years to get there. That much walking would burn 400,000 kcal.

Onawasi deserved a serious answer, so I started in. It would be a long trip, *years* long. And he wouldn't be able to walk the whole way. There was an ocean in between. He couldn't walk *around* the ocean—it was too big. He'd need to get on a boat . . .

That's when Onawasi lost interest. Walking for a couple of years was one thing, but Hadza guys don't do boats.

I left that conversation with Onawasi smiling to myself about the absurdity of his question. Years later, I see it differently. Traveling eight thousand miles in two and a half years isn't ridiculous—that's normal speed for a human. What was absurd is that I had made that journey in less than a day. I had traveled nearly one thousand times faster than a human is built to go, *through the air,* and ended up in a Hadza camp so quickly that my body was jet-lagged. My trip cost at least ten times more energy than walking would have, burning over five million kilocalories worth of jet fuel per passenger. The energy my body would typically burn over five years was consumed in a day. But I hadn't broken a sweat. I had hardly even noticed. *That* was absurd.

Life takes energy. Every physiological task, every metabolic chore, burns calories. The way we take those calories in and burn them off shapes every aspect of our existence, from the pace of our lives to our health and fitness. We've explored this metabolic landscape throughout the course of this book, dissecting everything from mitochondria to marathons. But we have remained within ourselves, examining only the energy our bodies consume.

The modern energy economy, the massive global market of renewable and fossil fuels, feels divorced from our internal metabolic energy budget. We don't even use the same language. Our bodies run on calories, while our homes run on kilowatt-hours and our transportation burns gallons of gasoline or barrels of oil. But the distinction between our internal metabolic engine and the external engines that run our world is largely an invention of language, a verbal sleight of hand we've played on ourselves. A calorie is a calorie, whether it's in the food we eat, the sunlight we trap in a solar panel, or the fossilized plants we burn in our cars. Our two engines, internal and external, are deeply interdependent and intertwined in ways we rarely appreciate. We've been burning energy externally, harnessing it for our purposes, ever since our hunter-gatherer ancestors got hold of fire, hundreds of thousands of years ago. As we shaped fire, it shaped us. Just as our metabolism today reflects its evolutionary roots, our modern energy economy, and our dependence on it, is an extension of our hunter-gatherer past.

Today, as we speed headlong into a strange and wonderful future, we find ourselves drifting uncomfortably close to the cliff's edge, with no guardrails. We have more control over our energetic environment than ever before, with breathtaking new technologies that energize our world and fuel our bodies. We can feed billions with food to spare, zip around the planet and touch the moon, and move mountains and rivers at will. Yet, the mismanagement of our energy environment has also led to existential crises: obesity and climate change. Our ability to navigate these dual energy crises will determine our species' collective future.

Throughout this book, we've discussed the new science of human metabolism, focusing on how our bodies actually work from an evolutionary perspective. We've gazed inward and back through time. Let's wrap things up by focusing outward and looking ahead. Humans have developed incredible godlike powers for controlling our energetic environments, both internal and external. In less than a century, some of the wildest science fiction has become a daily reality. But with great power comes incredible responsibility and the potential to royally screw things up. Our track record isn't particularly encouraging. How can we use our powers to keep ourselves healthy and avoid burning out as a species?

From Focusing Your Energy to Playing with Fire

We had been walking and hunting most of the morning, up and down the rocky, brushy shoulder of the Tli'ika escarpment, when Danfort started doing something I hadn't seen before. As he breezed past low acacia trees, he started snapping off thumb-sized dead branches without slowing down, and inspecting the centers of their broken ends. He did this a few times, tossing each branch on the ground as he went. They clearly weren't what he was looking for. But what *was* he looking for? I couldn't figure it out. I made a note of this strange behavior and planned to ask him the next time we stopped for a break.

The break came sooner than I anticipated. A branch finally met his criteria, and he immediately found a patch of shade to sit down and get to work. Before I could ask what he'd been up to, it became obvious. He was building a fire. It had rained a bit the night before, and the sticks on the ground were damp. But he'd found a branch that was dry inside, and was ready to go. He split a finger-length section of the branch down the middle and gouged a small divot into the exposed dry surface. Then he pulled the metal head out of an arrow and carefully placed the blank wooden end into the divot. Clamping the broken stick against the ground with the toe of his sandal, he clapped his hands together with the arrow shaft between them and began to spin it, back and forth, forcing it downward in the dry wood below.

Within minutes a thin tendril of smoke began to dance lightly upward, curling around the arrow shaft as it spun furiously. Soon he had an ember, a live bit of glowing dust resting atop the exposed face of the broken stick. I sat a few feet away, marveling at the speed and competence with which he'd started the fire. Still, though, I couldn't quite understand why he was going to all the trouble. He'd been hunting all morning and had a bit of luck, taking shots at a klipspringer and a hyrax, but he hadn't hit anything. There was nothing to cook, and it certainly wasn't cold. *Why did he need a fire?*

Danfort placed a cupped hand over the embryonic flame and began to dig into his shorts pocket. Deftly, with one hand, he extracted a stubby, half-smoked, hand-rolled cigarette. He gripped the butt between his lips and bent gingerly over the glowing ember. A couple of puffs and he was lit. Danfort sat up, took a drag, and gave me a smile. The point of the fire was clear: the universal satisfaction of a smoke break.

Technology has been a defining element of the human strategy since the origins of our genus and the early days of hunting and gathering. In 1964, Louis Leakey and his team at Olduvai Gorge announced their discovery of fossil remains from an extinct hominin with a brain roughly half the size of humans today—just a smidge larger than apes'. But Leakey looked past the small brain. He was drawn to the simple stone tools associated with the fossils, crude choppers and flakes for dismantling game or cutting up plants. Ever the provocateur, Leakey named the species *Homo habilis*, placing this small-headed creature in the human genus. His argument was clear: anything clever enough to use tools, particularly in the service of hunting and gathering, had crossed the threshold. They were more human than ape.

Leakey's sober, tweed-clad contemporaries pushed back against his bold claims, arguing he'd stretched the limits of our genus too far. Discoveries over the subsequent decades have muddied the picture even more: using tools doesn't mark a clean break between animal and human, as Leakey proposed. The oldest stone tools predate *habilis*, and we know now that apes regularly use simple tools (but not flaked stones) in the wild. Still, Leakey's broader point has grown into something as close to consensus as you'll find in paleoanthropology. A dependence on stone tools marks a sea change in the way our hominin ancestors made a living. We're the only predators on the planet who rely on technology to kill and consume our prey. Those stone blades made hunting and gathering— the quintessential human lifestyle—possible.

Simple tools, from the stone choppers at Olduvai to the knives in your kitchen, are useful because they allow us to concentrate our energy. You have the strength to cut a steak with your bare hands, but only if you can focus your power along the edge of a blade. Without that tool, you're stuck trying in vain to tear it apart with nubby fingertips and dull teeth. The same goes for other simple hand tools, from shovels to crowbars to a bow and arrow. They don't make us stronger or provide any extra energy—they are powered entirely by our bodies. Instead, they allow us to use our energy in smarter ways.

Simple tools are so useful they've never faded away. Instead, over the past two million years, we have been refining the classics (there's an infomercial for a new and improved knife seemingly every day) and inventing new ones. Your house is full of them, from all the handheld gadgetry in your kitchen to the gardening tools in the garage. For the first two million years or so, the hunter-gatherer tool kit was limited to digging sticks and stone flakes and hammers. Around seventy thousand years ago, people starting figuring out nifty ways to store up muscle energy and concentrate it to send a spear or arrow flying. The Hadza bow is a direct descendant of this innovation, and a nice example of its effectiveness. When Hadza men draw their bows, the force with which they pull the bowstring often exceeds their own body weight—the equivalent of doing a one-arm pull-up. That energy is stored in the strain of the bow staff and is released in an instant when the arrow is fired. The arrow leaves the bow at over 100 mph, with enough energy to blow right through the rib cage of an unsuspecting warthog.

But as clever and important as these simple tools are, their impact pales in comparison to the control of fire. Fire was the great technological leap forward. Stone tools, a bow and arrow, and other simple tools allow you to manipulate the way you store, focus, and release your body's own energy. With fire, our hominin ancestors had access to a completely new engine. Unlike their internal metabolic engines, our hunter-gatherer ancestors could burn these fires as hot as they liked, for as long as they wanted. They could walk away and let them grow cold, then restart them again later. Most important, they could harness the power of fire in service of essential evolutionary tasks: growth, maintenance, and reproduction. It was a first in the two-billion-year history of life: external energy expenditure to augment your own metabolism.

Exactly when hominins got control of fire remains hotly contested. Some argue it began early in our genus, with *Homo erectus*, over a million years ago. The more conservative estimate, based on clear evidence of cooking hearths and burned animal bones, puts the date at around 400,000 years ago. Regardless of the exact timing, it seems fire initially had three uses: cooking food, staying warm, and keeping potential predators away.

The use of fire for warmth meant our ancestors didn't have to shiver through the night. As we discussed in Chapter 3, even mild cold can elevate our metabolic rates by 25 percent, or around 16 kcal per hour. Sleeping cold for eight hours could cost a stone-age hunter-gatherer over 100 kcal. With fire to keep warm, those calories could be spent on other important physiological tasks, like growth, reproduction, and repair. Our ancestors might have also slept more soundly knowing that big cats and other species instinctively shied away from fire.

Fire's impact on our diet and digestion was even more profound. As Richard Wrangham lays out in great detail in his excellent book *Catching Fire*, cooking completely changed our diets and in turn changed our bodies. Wood fires release about 1,600 kcal per pound of fuel. In a simple campfire, most of that energy is lost to the air. The energy that is captured as heat in the food changes its structure and chemistry. Meat becomes easier to chew. Proteins are denatured, making them easier to digest. Starches that are otherwise indigestible are transformed, their carbohydrates accessible in our guts. The effects are largest with root vegetables, which are full of resistant starches that our guts can't digest: we get double the calories from a cooked potato as we do if we eat one raw. In short, fire supercharged the hominin diet, increasing the amount of energy per bite and decreasing the energy spent on digestion.

Over time, our hunter-gatherer ancestors evolved to rely on fire to prepare our food. Digestive capabilities were reduced, the energy for a big gut and intensive digestion diverted to other tasks. Some of this extra energy seems to have been allocated to reproduction, just as we'd expect from natural selection. As we discussed in Chapter 5, humans have bigger babies, more often, than any of our ape relatives. The energy boost from cooking may have also contributed to the evolution of larger, more energetically expensive brains.

The catch was that hominins became physiologically dependent on cooking. Every culture ever recorded, from the tropics to the Arctic, cooks their food. And while it would be unethical to test whether cooking is truly necessary by depriving people of cooked food, there are enough folks in the Raw Foodist movement to provide a natural experiment. Raw Foodists eschew cooking for a variety of philosophical reasons or misguided ideas about the "life force" in food. The largest study of their health and physiology comes from a group of over three hundred men and women following raw food diets (with varying degrees of strictness) in Germany. People eating uncooked diets have a hard time maintaining healthy weight, with many below a BMI of 18.5, the threshold for being considered malnourished. Women on raw food diets often stopped ovulating, and the degree of ovarian disruption was directly correlated with the proportion of uncooked food in the diet. Men's reproductive function was sometimes compromised as well, with some reporting a loss of libido. Without cooked food, humans' ability to survive and reproduce—the two nonnegotiable measures of evolutionary fitness—are seriously diminished.

Tellingly, these men and women had access to calorie-rich, low-fiber, domesticated foods. They had cold-pressed vegetable oils and other energy-concentrating innovations of modern food preparation. It wasn't enough. Even with these modern advantages, the human body doesn't run very well on a raw food diet. There's no way our fire-adapted hunter-gatherer ancestors, with only wild foods to eat, could have subsisted entirely on a raw food diet.

With our dependence on fire built into our bodies, our internal and external engines were irrevocably conjoined. Our own metabolism was no longer enough. We became reliant on a second, external energy source, fire, to power our lives. We became a pyrobiological species: *Homo energeticus.*

Of course, fire brought more than just an extra source of calories. Fires could be used to change the landscape, burning swaths of forest or scrub to push game and promote new plant growth. Flame also unlocked a universe of chemistry and new materials. Paleolithic hunter-gatherers learned to use fire to harden the tips of wooden spears, a practice Hadza women still use today to prepare their digging sticks. Our ancestors discovered that fire-treated rocks often made better stone tools. Neanderthals and modern humans learned to use kilns to made bitumen, a strong adhesive derived from birch sap, to glue stone axe heads and other blades onto wooden handles. As early as thirty thousand years ago, humans were building fires hot enough to fire pottery. Around seven thousand years ago, early farming cultures were figuring out how to smelt ore to make copper and other metals. By three thousand years ago, they had figured out how to make iron and glass. The floodgates were open. One hundred generations later, their descendants would be walking around with smartphones in their pockets and sending rocket-powered robots to distant planets.

The Technology Tsunami

Our command and consumption of external energy has grown exponentially over the past ten thousand years. We've moved beyond fire, harnessing energy from every conceivable source. But even as the technologies have changed and developed, we've applied them to the same ancient objectives. As our control of external energy sources has grown, so has our physiological dependence on them.

The biggest change in our energy economy, after the introduction of fire, was the domestication of plants and animals. Starting around twelve thousand years ago, several populations around the world began to converge on a game-changing insight. Rather than trekking into the wild to try and find plants and animals to eat, they could bring their food home and grow it there. In the time-compressed archaeological record, where a thousand years might be captured in a half-inch layer of sediment, the switch to agriculture seems to have happened in an instant. In reality, it's not hard to imagine how it would have developed gradually. I've seen Hadza men experimenting with growing bushes of desert roses, the plants they use to make arrow poison, in the soils near camp. They often curate the bees' nests they exploit, filling the holes they make in the tree with rocks so the bees will return and rebuild the hive. Feral dogs will sometimes loiter around a camp, pilfering scraps and occasionally getting conscripted into service for hunting small game. In a world full of hunter-gatherer societies twelve thousand years ago, trials like these were probably happening all over the globe.

The successful experiments gave early agriculturalists control over the metabolic engines of plants and animals. Human selection usurped the role of natural selection. In the wild, a plant that invested too heavily in its fruit or grew too quickly might be at a disadvantage, having allocated too little energy to the hardy stems and roots that keep them upright in a storm or the fibers, thorns, and toxic chemicals that keep herbivores at bay. But in a horticulturalist's garden, those fruit-heavy plants were prized and replanted, their reproductive success much greater than that of their stingy neighbors. Over time, we manipulated the metabolisms of our domesticated plants to divert their energy into the starches and sugars that fuel our bodies. Today, the fruits and vegetables we find in the market look like grotesque energy-packed carnival freaks compared to their wild ancestors.

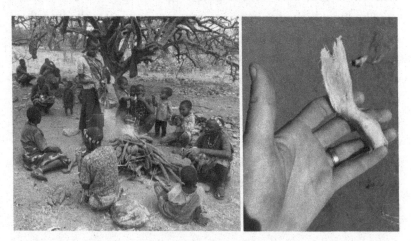

Figure 9.1. Hadza women roasting *makalitako* tubers. Wild tubers are woody and fibrous compared to their domesticated relatives. You chew on them and suck out the starch, then spit out the fibrous quid.

We played the same trick with our domestic animals. By protecting them from natural predators and picking the winners and losers in reproduction, we favored those that allocated more energy into growth and milk production. Under our management, these species evolved into soft, dumb, reliable sources of fat and protein. They provided a metabolic engine for converting grasses and other forage that was inedible to us into milk, blood, and meat for our consumption.

Horses and other large species provided a new kind of engine as well—a source of mechanical work to augment or replace our own physical abilities. As James Watt, inventor of the steam engine, deduced through experiments at the dawn of the Industrial Revolution, a horse can comfortably produce around 640 kcal of work per hour (the definition of *horsepower*) and sustain that output for ten hours, day after day. That number is even more impressive than it might seem. Muscles are, at best, only about 25 percent efficient at converting metabolic fuel into mechanical work. To produce 6,400 kcal of work in a ten-hour day, a horse burns over 25,000 kcal of energy—and that's *in addition* to the energy spent on BMR, digestion, and its other physiological needs.

The advent of draft animals must have been an incredible jolt to the economy and psyche of early farmers. A human with a horse had superhuman powers. She could do the work of ten men and command Herculean strength. On horseback, she could easily cover thirty miles in a day, twice that if needed, without breaking a sweat. That's more than three times the daily range of a hunter-gatherer on foot. Suddenly, what once seemed distant was close enough to touch.

Like the control of fire, the domestication of plants and animals increased the energy content of our food and reduced the energy needed to acquire it. Early farmers experienced an energy windfall. With less energy needed for physical activity and digestion, their internal engines could plow energy into other tasks. As we'd expect from any evolved organism, those extra calories went to reproduction. In early farming cultures around the world, fertility rates accelerated as mothers and babies benefited from the extra calories that domestication provided. In the centuries that followed the adoption of agriculture, family sizes grew by an additional two children per mother. We can see these effects in hunter-gatherer and mixed foraging-farming populations today. A typical Hadza woman will have six children over the course of her lifetime, while a Tsimane woman, with the caloric benefits of some traditional farming, will have nine.

As populations grew, early farmers encountered strange new problems that their hunter-gatherer forebears never had to deal with, like overcrowding and the difficulties of public sanitation. Communicable diseases that would have fizzled out quickly in sparse hunter-gatherer encampments became full-blown plagues, tearing through early farming towns and cities. As the Covid-19 pandemic has made all too clear, we're still grappling with these age-old challenges today.

But larger populations also spurred innovation. Larger populations meant more people living, working, and thinking together. Putting more heads together has a synergistic effect on the development of new ideas, a phenomenon that Joe Henrich, a human evolutionary biologist at Harvard, calls the collective brain. Greater capacity to produce food also meant that people could diversify. Some were free to spend their adult lives on tasks other than food production, a luxury that no hunter-gatherer would recognize. Whole new crafts and trades were born. Over three thousand years ago, cultures in the Mediterranean, South Pacific, and elsewhere had figured out how to harness the power of the wind to sail. Watermills appeared over two thousand years ago, as people learned to harness the energy of a flowing river to grind grain, lift water into irrigation systems, and perform a wide range of other work. Windmills joined them a few centuries later. Each invention and refinement expanded our external engines and the energy we could command.

The latest chapter in the history of our external energy economy, the one we're still living in today, began in the 1700s with the use of coal to heat the steam engines and factories of the Industrial Revolution. Fossil fuels represent the collective metabolisms of uncountable plants and animals in the distant past, toiling away over millions of years. When we burn them, we're releasing the energy stored in those ancient organisms. Coal has been mined and burned for millennia, but the advances in mining techniques and a burgeoning industrial sector sent coal use soaring in eighteenth-century Europe. Oil and natural gas production followed, moving from marginal sources of fuel to mainstays of global energy use following the development of commercial drilling in the mid-1800s. Today, these fossil fuels combine to provide over 35,000 kcal of energy every day for every person on Earth, 80 percent of our species' external energy expenditure.

In the industrialized world, the quantum leap in energy consumption through the exploitation of fossil fuels has completely changed the way we produce our food. In 1840, the early days of the Industrial Revolution in the United States, farmers made up 69 percent of the American workforce, or 22 percent of the total U.S. population. Each farmer produced enough to feed himself or herself and four others. As energy from fossil fuels poured into food production over subsequent decades, in the form of motorized machinery, petroleum-based fertilizers, and advanced transportation and refrigeration, the amount of food a farmer could produce soared. Today, farmers and ranchers make up only 1.3 percent of the U.S. workforce, just 0.8 percent of the total U.S. population. Food processing, transportation, and retail employ another approximately 1 percent of working adults. Together, people working in agriculture and food processing produce enough food to feed themselves and thirty-five others.

Our modern food system requires an immense amount of energy. Food production in the United States consumes roughly 500 trillion kilocalories each year. A third is burned as gasoline or diesel in farm machinery and transportation. Another third is the fossil fuel used to make fertilizers and pesticides. Electricity to run farms, storehouses, and supermarkets takes up most of the rest.

Those trillions of kilocalories channeled into food production have profound effects on both the energy cost and energy content of our diet. To see how, let's first consider the energy and time cost that goes into transforming a plant or animal into a meal. In hunter-gatherer societies like the Hadza, producing food requires a person to walk, combing the landscape to locate their target. Then they've got to harvest, through some combination of shooting and tracking their prey, digging up tubers, picking berries, or chopping into trees for honey. Next they've got to carry it home, but they're still not done. Animals need to be butchered and cooked (and firewood gathered), tubers need to be roasted and peeled, baobab kernels need to be crushed to extract the nutmeat inside. Finally, only after all that effort, do they have a meal. All that effort directly affects the rate of food production. Hadza adults acquire roughly 1,000 to 1,500 kcal per hour of foraging.

Traditional farming practices make things a bit easier. Fields and flocks are near your house, so you spend less time and energy walking to get to your food. Crops can be harvested in bulk, providing advantages of scale. If the plants and animals are domesticated, they likely pack a bit more energy per ounce. As a result, for the Tsimane and other foraging-farming societies, the rate of energy production is around 1,500 to 2,000 kcal per hour.

In a modern industrialized society, few people work in food production, and those that do usually contribute to just one aspect of the job (the people who grow wheat aren't the same people who transform it into breakfast cereal). That makes it hard to calculate the rate of food production for one person, but there's an alternative approach. Industrialized economies use money to exchange work for various goods and services. In a free labor market, an hour's worth of work in one trade, such as manufacturing, should earn roughly enough wages to pay for an hour's production in another, like food production. Rather than measure food production directly, we can ask, "How much food can a blue-collar worker buy with an hour's wages?"

In the United States in 1900, with industrialization already in stride, an hour of physical labor in a manufacturing job could buy you more than 3,000 kcal of flour, eggs, bacon, and other staples (Figure 9.2). As the flow of fossil fuel energy increased, so did our purchasing power. Today, an hour's wage could buy an American laborer roughly 20,000 kcal of those same staples. The basic elements of food production aren't much different than they are in a Hadza camp or Tsimane village, but the human time and energy required has been greatly reduced through the reliance on external energy expenditure. The time and energy needed to grow, harvest, transport, and process our food is provided by fossil-fuel-powered machinery that does it all at incredible scale and efficiency. Large numbers of poorly paid (often exploited) farmworkers add their energy as well, working alongside behemoth fossil-fuel-powered machines to pick, process, and package our food. All of that cheap energy is embodied in the food that ends up in your supermarket. It allows you to acquire more calories with three hours' work than a Hadza man or woman produces in a week.

Industrialized processing has also increased our food's energy density, the calories packed into each bite. All of the modern processing techniques, like extracting oils and sugars, manufacturing syrups and sweeteners, and threshing and milling grains to extract the starchy center of each kernel, require an incredible amount of energy. In the preindustrial world, all that effort acted as a brake on food processing, keeping processed foods rare and expensive. Sugar was a luxury item. Today, cheap energy from fossil fuels makes processing profitable. The foods with the most calories per gram are also the cheapest to produce and consume. Sweeteners like beet sugar and high-fructose corn syrup have become the single largest component of the American diet, comprising 20 percent of the calories we consume. Oils are the next largest component, accounting for 13 percent of our calories. In fact, processing has flipped the usual relationship between cost and energy content on its head. The result is a highly processed, supercharged diet. The energy density of an industrialized diet is 20 percent higher than the Hadza diet, and it requires little or no physical effort to acquire. Our hunter-gatherer ancestors would be stunned.

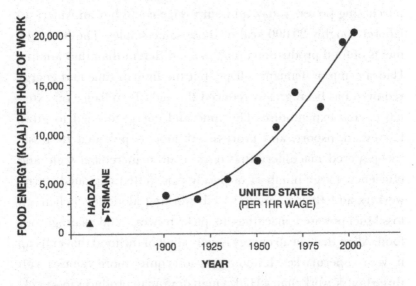

Figure 9.2. Men and women in industrialized populations can acquire far more food energy for an hour of work than is possible for hunter-gatherers or subsistence farmers.

The combination of easily digested calories and reduced cost of food brought about by the Industrial Revolution might have led to a fertility boom. Luckily, that didn't happen. But all those extra calories have affected *potential* fertility. The combination of energy-rich, processed diets (including baby formula) and sedentary lifestyles reduce the energy burden of reproduction, shortening the amount of time it takes for a mother's body to recover between pregnancies. For American mothers in their teens and twenties with more than one child, time between births is often two years or less, on par with—or even a bit faster than—the interbirth intervals we see among the Tsimane. At those rates, an American mother could easily have ten or more kids during her childbearing years.

But instead of taking off with the Industrial Revolution, fertility rates around the world declined as societies modernized, a phenomenon known as the demographic transition. Women began having fewer kids and investing more time and resources in each one. The precise mix of cultural and biological factors behind this change in reproductive strategy aren't yet clear. Many note that the decline in fertility rate follows an increase in life expectancy, suggesting families are responding (consciously or not) to the greater likelihood that their kids will survive to adulthood. Others argue cultural changes, including women's access to education and family planning, are what changes the tide. Whatever the cause, we should be grateful. The demographic transition has slowed global population growth, buying us time to save the planet.

Unintended Consequences

The enormous energy cost of food production puts industrialized human populations in strange and ominous territory. It is a basic rule of life that no species can persist if it spends more energy foraging than it acquires in food. Mammals in the wild typically get around 40 calories of food for every calorie they spend foraging. Humans in hunter-gatherer societies like the Hadza or mixed foraging-farming societies like the Tsimane fare a bit worse, with each calorie of work spent on food production yielding around 10 calories of food. Our modern food production system violates the fundamental laws of ecology. When we include the fossil fuel energy consumed in food production, we burn 8 calories for every calorie of food we produce. That's not a great recipe for avoiding extinction.

It gets worse. The energy consumed in food production is just one part of our energy economy. Each year in the United States, we consume a staggering 25 *quadrillion* kilocalories. With a population of approximately 330 million, annual U.S. energy expenditure works out to 77 million kilocalories per person. That's 210,000 kcal per day, equivalent to the daily energy expenditure of a nine-ton mammal (African elephants weigh only seven tons). Each American consumes more energy than do seventy hunter-gatherers.

In a few countries, per capita energy consumption is even higher. Countries sitting on massive supplies of oil, like Saudi Arabia, or blessed with lots of alternative energy sources, like Iceland, tend to consume energy freely. But most of the world lacks the easy access to external energy that those of us in industrialized countries take for granted. Globally, our species consumes 141 quadrillion kilocalories each year, an average of 47,000 kcal per person per day, nearly sixteen times the energy expenditure of our internal metabolic engine. There are 7.7 billion people on the planet, but we're burning energy like there's 120 billion of us.

If all of this sounds somewhat unsustainable and slightly terrifying, you're wrong: it's completely unsustainable and totally terrifying. Current best estimates suggest we've got around fifty years' worth of oil and natural gas left, and perhaps 110 years' worth of coal. Those horizons will likely expand a bit as the technologies to find and extract these fuels improve, but all that will do is lengthen the fall. The impact is coming, either this century or the next. With fossil fuels spent, nearly 80 percent of the energy we burn externally will be gone. People living through the end of fossil fuels could be the first generation since our Paleolithic ancestors controlled fire to have a smaller external energy economy than their parents. Without some other energy source to replace fossil fuels, local and global systems of food production and transportation will collapse. It will be *The Hunger Games* without the gadgets, *Mad Max* without the motors.

The only thing more terrifying than running out of fossil fuel is the catastrophe we'll unleash if we burn it all. Human-caused climate change is well under way, with the Earth 0.8°C (1.4°F) warmer than it was in the late 1800s, when fossil fuel use began to take off. The current generation of climate models, which have done an incredibly accurate job predicting our increasingly warm and wild weather, predict an additional 8°C warming globally in the next century or two if we burn the remainder of known fossil fuel reserves. The last time the planet was that hot was 55 million years ago, during the Paleocene-Eocene Thermal Maximum. The oceans got so warm that nearly everything in the deep ocean went extinct. Sea levels were at least a hundred meters (328 feet) higher than today. If we even approach that degree of sea level rise with human-caused climate change, we're in trouble. Roughly 10 percent of the world's population, including two-thirds of the largest cities, are less than ten meters above sea level, and half of us live less than a hundred meters above sea level. Burning all of our fossil fuel reserves would reshape our planet, drowning our major cities and wiping out entire countries.

• • •

Avoiding the worst of the many dystopian climate change scenarios will require us to kick our fossil fuel habit, the sooner the better. Some of these changes are easy and should have been done a long time ago. More efficient cars and buildings, less waste in our packaging and products, better public transportation, and smarter farming and manufacturing will all reduce our energy usage. Despite resistance to regulating fuel efficiency and investments in mass transit, there are some hopeful glimmers that we're getting a bit smarter in how we use energy. In the developed world, energy consumption per capita has been steadily, if slowly, declining since the 1970s. Energy consumption per capita in the United Kingdom is down nearly 30 percent since 2000. In the United States, it's down 30 percent since the peak in the late 1970s, and down 15 percent since 2000.

But better efficiency alone won't save us. Our species, *Homo energeticus*, demands an enormous amount of energy. Culturally and biologically, we have evolved to rely on our massive external energy supply to power every aspect of our daily lives. A preindustrial energy economy just isn't tenable anymore, not if we want to maintain some semblance of modern life. As we've already seen, in the United States alone it takes 500 trillion kilocalories of external energy expenditure each year for a vanishingly small number of farmers and food producers to nourish hundreds of millions of people, most of them hundreds of miles away in dense urban centers. We spend *ten times* that amount of energy to heat, cool, and illuminate our modern homes and apartment buildings. Without the climate control that energy provides, the Sunbelt would still be sparsely inhabited desert. The United States consumes over 7 quadrillion kilocalories of external energy each year on the transportation that connects us to our families, our stuff, and our jobs.

Hadza men, with only their feet to carry them, walk about eight miles per day. Work commutes in the United States and Europe average nearly eight miles *each way*, and we can fly anywhere on the planet tomorrow for the price of plane ticket. That same Hadza man might carry thirty pounds of food home on a good day, at an energy cost of 10 kcal per mile. A diesel freight train can carry thirty pounds of goods anywhere on the continent for about 1 kcal per mile. Food, shelter, movement—we are wholly reliant on our modern external energy supply for life in our industrialized world.

It's easy to see where we need to go, even if it's hard to get there. If we want to continue on as *Homo energeticus*, we've got no choice but to find some way to power our external engines without burning fossil fuels. Climate scientists agree that we need to get to zero carbon emissions globally by 2050 to have a reasonable chance of avoiding catastrophe. So far, our species has figured out four ways to generate power at meaningful scale that don't emit greenhouse gases: hydropower, wind turbines, solar power, and nuclear fission. Hydropower is essentially maxed out. We've run out of big rivers to dam, and it causes massive ecological damage in any case. That leaves solar and wind, which currently combine to provide 2 percent of global energy, and nuclear, which generates 5 percent. We'll need to greatly expand these capacities in some combination to take the place of fossil fuels. It's a big hill to climb, but there are several plausible strategies to get us there. And there are hopeful examples to guide our way. France generates over 70 percent of its electricity, and 45 percent of its total energy demand, from nuclear and renewables (mostly nuclear). Expanding nuclear energy production as either an interim or long-term strategy might seem scary, but it's worth noting that fossil fuels kill thousands more people per unit of power generation than nuclear power. Whatever solutions we settle on for this long journey, the important thing is to get started and keep moving.

What we cannot do is assume that success is inevitable. The end of fossil fuels is coming soon, one way or the other. It will take concerted effort and political bravery to forge a new and sustainable external energy system. I worry that our species' recent history of unbridled progress and technological breakthrough makes us too complacent and blinds us to the lessons of deep time. As we see at sites like Dmanisi (Chapter 4), extinction is the norm. Our planet is a challenging and unpredictable place to live. Species and societies are repeatedly tested, and usually fail. If we don't figure out a sustainable way to maintain our species' external energy supply, we'll fail, too. The Earth will swallow us up and move on, uncaring, our bones and ruins frozen in the dirt. There's plenty of room in the ground.

Building a Better Zoo

Even as we rush to preserve our species' lifeline of external energy, we must wrestle with the damage that it's doing to our bodies. Our industrialized energy economy makes modern life possible, but it also makes us sick. We've been engineering our world with an eye toward growth and comfort. We need to do a better job shaping our environments to protect our internal metabolic engines.

Without decisive action to change our food environment, we'll never turn the tide in the global obesity pandemic. As we discussed in Chapters 5 and 6, weight gain is fundamentally a problem of energy imbalance, of eating more food calories than you burn. The lesson that the Hadza and others teach us is we can't do much to change the calories we burn. Daily energy expenditure is constrained, stuck within a narrow range that your body works hard to maintain. Obesity, then, is primarily a problem of overconsumption. And to fix that, we need to fix our food.

We should all take responsibility for our diets, but overeating isn't simply a failure of willpower or discipline. It's much more insidious than that. Our brains regulate intake subconsciously, using ancient, evolved systems to manage metabolic rate, hunger, and satiety. The energy we pour into producing and processing our food transforms it from a source of nourishment to something more akin to a drug. The highly processed, flavor-engineered foods that dominate our supermarket shelves and commercials easily overwhelm our brain's capacity to regulate energy balance. As Kevin Hall's work has shown (Chapter 6), diets dominated by processed foods lead to overeating and weight gain.

Cheap processed high-calorie foods are a direct consequence of industrialized food production and our reliance on easy external energy (Figure 9.2). It's a stunning achievement, really. We've managed to turn one of the fundamental principles of ecology on its head. In nature, energy-rich foods like honey, prey, or fruit are always less abundant and harder to get than low-calorie foods like leaves. In a modern supermarket, it's just the opposite. Highly processed items like oils, sweeteners, and junk food pack more calories per ounce *and* cost less per calorie. A double chocolate Dunkin' donut holds 350 kilocalories and costs 83 cents, when you buy a dozen. That's 25 cents for every 100 kcal. At a dollar a pound, red delicious apples costs 37 cents per 100 kcal, 60 percent more than the donut. The apple is obviously better for you, and we know from Susan Holt's work on satiety (Chapter 6) that apples are more than twice as satiating as donuts, but come on. Donuts are designed to be obscenely delicious. If you've got a dollar in your pocket and you're feeling hungry, do you buy a donut or a pound of apples?

If we engineered these freakish foods into our lives, we should be able to engineer them out. No one (at least not me) wants to live in a world without donuts. But we have to make the cost of food more reflective of its impact on our health. One approach is to increase the cost of unhealthy foods. Taxes on soda and other sugar-sweetened beverages are often unpopular, but they seem to work, reducing the amount people consume. Extending those taxes to other highly processed foods might lower their intake as well, and in any case would provide a source of revenue for governments grappling with the ever-expanding health costs of our ever-expanding waistlines.

We also need to make healthy unprocessed foods cheaper and easier to find. In 2015, more than 39 million Americans with low incomes lived in food deserts, defined as areas where grocery stores are more than a half-mile walk if you're urban or a ten-mile drive if you're rural. Even if these folks can get to a supermarket, they face the perverse pricing of our industrialized food system: processed foods are usually much cheaper per kilocalorie than fresh fruit and vegetables, meat and fish, and other unprocessed foods. Unsurprisingly, obesity and cardiometabolic disease disproportionately impact poor communities. We already manipulate the food and energy markets through billions of dollars in subsidies each year. If we were smarter about it, we would use those funds to ensure that healthy foods were cheaper and more plentiful. Since health trajectories are shaped during childhood, we should make school nutrition a priority, restricting access to junk food and increasing the proportion of whole foods on the menu.

And we don't need to wait for regulations or societal shifts to make helpful changes in our personal food environments. As Stephan Guyenet and others have argued, doing little things to keep tempting, high-calorie foods away from you could have a big impact. You can't mindlessly plow through a soda and a box of cookies if you don't have any in your house. The bowl of candies on your desk at the office doesn't need to be there, and isn't helping anyone. Keeping processed, energy-rich foods out of arm's reach makes them harder to get, and can make you more mindful and discerning about when and how you decide to indulge.

Modernization has also made us sedentary. Our evolution as hunter-gatherers left us with bodies that are built for action (Chapters 4 and 7). Like sharks, we need to keep moving to survive. But all the external energy we pour into food production and transportation has made physical effort optional in our industrialized environments. Over the past century, the percentage of the U.S. workforce employed in white-collar jobs, like lawyers, doctors, and administrators, has tripled, from roughly 25 percent in 1910 to 75 percent in 2000. Today, more than 13 percent of all jobs in the U.S. are classified as "sedentary," and another 24 percent require only "light work." Those percentages are higher among white-collar professions. In the not-so-distant past, our hunter-gatherer ancestors regularly racked up 15,000 steps or more over the course of a day. Now, for the first time in the evolution of our lineage, the average man or woman can make a living without ever leaving their chair.

Externally powered transportation and mechanization make modern life work. No one is going to walk the sixteen miles round trip to work each day or climb thirty flights of stairs to get to the office. Still, we need to engineer more physical activity into our daily lives. Exercise is great, and we need more of that, too. But we need to move beyond an exercise mind-set, where our physical activity is structured into a few discrete hours each week. Sitting for hours on end is deadly, even if we spend our nights and weekends at the gym. We need walkable cities and towns, and real investment in human-powered movement. Cities like Copenhagen are leading the way on this, designing bicycle friendly urban areas that favor people over cars. Bike share systems have enormous potential to help, too, increasing daily physical activity and reducing disease.

Industrialization and modernization carry other costs as well, costs that are harder to quantify. Like the Hadza, our hunter-gatherer ancestors spent their lives enmeshed in a rich social fabric of family and friends. They spent their days outdoors, under the sun. With everyone in the same line of work and no durable wealth to concentrate over generations, social and economic inequality would have been low. The Hadza are proudly egalitarian, and they answer to no one but themselves.

With farming, and then again with industrialization, came major revisions to the social contract. Class differences and hierarchies emerged as wealth was consolidated in land and then in capital. This worked well for the upper class, of course, but was a disaster for those stuck at the bottom, who were used as slaves or otherwise exploited for their labor. The rest were caught somewhere in the middle, eager to climb the socioeconomic ladder but also desperate not to be caught in the gears below.

The stresses that result from this socioeconomic arrangement, from fears about money to the aching feeling that we're being left behind to the daily assaults on our dignity, are new for our species. We don't seem to handle them well. Living at the unhappy end of the socioeconomic spectrum makes us sick and shortens our lives. People living in poverty suffer from higher rates of obesity, diabetes, heart disease, and other cardiometabolic illness than the wealthy, and the effect is larger than anything we'd expect from diet and exercise differences alone. Likewise, people of color and other marginalized communities have worse health and shorter lives. If we're serious about changing our environments to improve our metabolic health, then we need to address socioeconomic disparities, not just diet and exercise.

Unfortunately, industrialization has also diminished some of the tools that might help counteract the effects of stress. Daily physical activity is lower, for one thing. We are also less socially connected. Families are smaller and more dispersed. Loneliness has become so prevalent that it's now a recognized medical condition. Modernization also brought us indoors. Time outside can relieve stress and promote physical activity, and it seems to improve cardiometabolic health more than physical activity alone. Hadza spend essentially all of their waking lives outdoors. The typical American spends 87 percent of his life in buildings and another 6 percent of his life in cars. As we work to bring the healthy elements of our hunter-gatherer past back into our modern lives, we need to think broadly, holistically. There's more to it than just the tubers.

Back in Camp

I wanted them to be fires.

I sat on a sweep of warm flat rock outside of Mkelenge, a Hadza camp perched on an escarpment in the Tli'ika Hills, and looked out through a clearing in the acacia over the wide valley floor below. I was in a reflective mood. It was my first trip back to Hadzaland in a couple of years, and ten years since the first days of the Hadza energetics project. Moments before, the orange sun had splashed its last against the cliffs on the far side of the wide valley and sank beneath the western horizon. As the world lost its color and started to go dark, I saw something in the flat distance below that I had never witnessed before in a Hadza camp: lights.

I counted five of them, scattered like misplaced stars, spread far apart in the distance a few miles off. They probably weren't Hadza. The sweeping expanse below was more popular with the Datoga pastoralists who grazed their cattle and goats on the dry scrub. My brain registered them initially as cooking fires, but the color was wrong. Fires are orangey-red, these were unmistakably electric white. And why would Datoga families be cooking outside their houses?

The obvious conclusion sank in. Electricity was seeping into Hadzaland.

I tried to be *hamna shida* about it. Maybe even happy. Lights are helpful, and god knows I depend on them in my own daily life (I had a flashlight in my pocket and two more in my tent). Who was I to judge? A light in a Datoga home would be a huge help to the women and kids doing evening chores. And these were small solar panel systems, not a power line running through the heart of Hadza territory. At least the energy was clean.

I reminded myself that the Hadza have been dealing with the encroachment of the industrialized world for decades, ceding land but trying to make the best of a difficult situation. They've happily adopted some modern technology. You'll find the occasional flashlight or radio in camp, though batteries are hard to come by. Cell phones have grown more common, and in every camp you'll find someone who knows the right hill to climb in search of a signal, even if they don't have a cell phone themselves. They're happy to take advantage of the sacks of corn the Tanzanian government occasionally doles out as food assistance. Through it all, Hadza culture has remained incredibly resilient and intact. They've accepted the modern world on their terms, piece by piece.

Still, I couldn't shake some darker feeling, a sense of loss. The industrialized world was slowly, implacably, forcing its way into Hadzaland. Not today of course, probably not next year, maybe not even next decade. But the glacier was advancing, the untold weight of civilization forcing it through the valley in front of me, tearing at the fabric beneath it. Hadza had lived in these hills, hunting and gathering for hundreds, maybe thousands of generations. How many more until it was all gone? How long until the Hadza were forced to join the industrialized world and relegated, like countless native cultures before them, to the bottom rung of the socioeconomic ladder? Would the young men and women in camp today live out their golden years in dirty cinder-block houses, dreaming of their lives in the bush and watching their grandchildren struggle with obesity, heart disease, and the other burdens of the modern world? After all they've taught us about how to live well, was this how the industrialized world would repay them?

What I saw during my time at Mkelenge gave me hope. Hadza men and women were hunting and gathering as they always had, following the old traditions. The women, old and young alike, spent their mornings out foraging for *makalitako* and *ewka* tubers and bringing them home to roast on a communal fire (Figure 9.1). They'd make tangy baobab fruit smoothies and pound the kernels to extract the meaty centers. Men spent their days out hunting or back in camp working on arrows and bows. It was a special time of year, late dry season, when the baobab trees were flowering. Heavy white fragrant flowers danced in the branches and littered the ground, attracting herbivores. The men would leave camp before sunrise to hunt from blinds near flowering baobabs. Game was plentiful, and the camp dined on impala, bush duiker, and dikdik.

There was reason for hope for the future as well. The camp was full of playful kids, running around and speaking Hadza. Boys would head out of camp carrying a light bow and their dad's axe, looking for honey and game. Girls were foraging with their moms and aunts, learning how to assess the quality of tubers by tamping the ground near the vine. Friends and family spent their days together, sharing food, laughing and talking. Neighbors from other camps near and far would pass through to visit, rest, and maybe snag a snack. The community was strong.

I left Mkelenge feeling optimistic, and not just about the Hadza but about the rest of us, too. There's still plenty to learn about our bodies and our metabolic health, but we understand enough to get started, taking better care of ourselves and raising a generation of healthier kids. It starts with an understanding of where we come from, a willingness to learn from cultures like the Hadza who hold on to old traditions, and the creativity to bring those lessons into our own lives in a sustainable way. We are the smartest, most creative species on the planet, with godlike technological powers at our disposal. Surely, we can learn to treat our bodies, our neighbors, and our planet with care.

ACKNOWLEDGMENTS

The material in this book came together over more than a decade with the help and input of countless family, friends, and collaborators. First and foremost I thank my wife, Janice, and children, Alex and Clara, for their support and good humor while I was off doing field-work, stuck in the lab measuring urine samples, or cloistered in the basement pounding out this book. Thanks, guys. Love you.

I'm likewise grateful to my family (Mom, Dad, George, Heide, Holly, and Emily) for raising me to think critically and enjoy a good argument. Jeff Kurland, Alan Walker, Bob Burkolder, and others at Penn State provided guidance and opportunities during those forma-tive undergrad years that shaped my trajectory as a scientist and ultimately made this book possible.

The Hadza community has been incredibly generous and welcom-ing to my colleagues and me, graciously welcoming us into their camps and putting up with our endless questions and requests. Stories and conversations in this book from my research with the Hadza (and else-where) all come from real experiences, and are rendered as accurately as my memory and occasional journal entries will allow. I thank the Hadza for their hospitality and friendship, and I hope the accounts of their life in this book paint an accurate portrait of their remarkable culture. To learn more about the Hadza community, please visit HadzaFund.org.

None of my work with the Hadza would have been possible with-out my close friends and collaborators, Brian Wood and David Raich-len. My work in Tanzania over the years has also been facilitated and enriched by a long list of friends, including Mariamu Anyawire, Heri-eth Cleophas, Jake Harris, Christian Kiffner, Fides Kirei, Lieve Lynen,

Nathaniel Makoni, Audax Mabulla, Ibrahim Mabulla, Carla Mallol, Frank Marlowe, Ruth Mathias, Elena Mauriki, Bunga Paolo, Daudi Peterson, and Christopher and Nani Schmelling.

Science is a team sport, and I've had the great fortune of learning from and working with many of the best researchers in human evolution and energetics. Stephan Guyenet, Kevin Hall, Daniel Lieberman, and John Speakman have shared critical insights over the years as well as feedback on an early draft of this book. The ideas and material here also benefited from conversations and collaborations with Leslie Aiello, Andrew Biewener, Rick Bribiescas, John Buse, Vincent Careau, Eric Charnov, Steve Churchill, Meg Crofoot, Maureen Devlin, Lara Dugas, Holly Dunsworth, Peter Ellison, Melissa Emery Thompson, Reid Ferring, Michael Gurven, Anthony Hackney, Lewis Halsey, Steve Heymsfield, Kim Hill, Richard Kahn, Hillard Kaplan, William Kraus, Christopher Kuzawa, Mitchell Irwin, Karen Isler, Amy Luke, Paul Mac-Lean, Felicia Madimenos, Andrew Marshall, Ed Melanson, Deborah Muoio, Martin Muller, Guy Plasqui, Susan Racette, Eric Ravussin, Leanne Redman, Jessica Rothman, Stephen Ross, Robert Shumaker, Joshua Snodgrass, Dale Schoeller, Lawrence Sugiyama, Benjamin Trumble, Claudia Valeggia, Carel Van Schaik, Erin Vogel, Kara Walker, Christine Wall, Klaas Westerterp, William Wong, Richard Wrangham, and Yosuke Yamada. I thank the U.S. National Science Foundation, the Wenner-Gren Foundation, and the Leakey Foundation for supporting my research.

I've also been fortunate to work closely with a great team of students, postdocs, and research assistants who made much of the research in this book possible and nearly all of it fun. I thank them for their collegiality, clever ideas, and hard work. A full list would be a book unto itself, but I'd be remiss not to mention Caitlin Thurber (who led the Race Across the USA study), Sam Urlacher (who led the Shuar studies featured in this book), Mary Brown, Eric Castillo, Martin Hora, Jörg Jäger, Elaine Kozma, Myra Laird, Cara Ocobock, Jenny

Paltan, Rebecca Rimbach, Khalifa Stafford, Zane Swanson, and Anna Warrener.

I'm indebted to Max Brockman, my agent, for his work to find this book a home. I thank Caroline Sutton, my keen-eyed and encouraging editor, along with Hannah Steigmeyer, Dorian Hastings, and the production team at Penguin Random House, for shepherding me through the long process of making this book. Kasia Konopka produced the graphs in this book. Victoria Ehrhardt, Holly Daniels, Emily Khan, Saleem Khan, and Janice Wang read a draft of this book and provided helpful feedback. Finally, I thank the community here at Duke University, particularly Brian Hare and Vanessa Woods, for their friendship and support while I wrote this book.

NOTES

Chapter I: The Invisible Hand

2 The Hadza are hunter-gatherers: For a thorough discussion of everything Hadza, see: Frank Marlowe, *The Hadza: Hunter-Gatherers of Tanzania* (Univ. of California Press, 2010).

6 37 trillion cells: E. Bianconi et al. (2013). "An estimation of the number of cells in the human body." *Ann. Hum. Biol.* 40 (6): 463–71, doi: 10.3109/03014460.2013.807878.

6 an ounce of the Sun: A 70-kg human burns approximately 2,800 kilocalories per day, or 40 kcal/kg per day. The Sun has a mass of 1.989×10^{30} and produces 7.942×10^{27} kcal per day, or a paltry 0.004 kcal/kg per day. See Vaclav Smil, *Energies: An Illustrated Guide to the Biosphere and Civilization* (MIT Press, 1999).

7 Nine-year-olds burn 2,000 calories: N. F. Butte (2000). "Fat intake of children in relation to energy requirements." *Am. J. Clin. Nutr.* 72 (suppl): 1246S–52S.

7 most doctors don't, either: R. Meerman and A. J. Brown (2014). "When somebody loses weight, where does the fat go?" *BMJ* 349: g7257.

7 U.S. federal government: Chris Cilliza, "Americans know literally nothing about the Constitution," CNN, last modified September 13, 2017, https://www.cnn.com/2017/09/13/politics/poll-constitution/index.html.

11 dead by twenty-five: Author's unpublished analyses, calculated from allometric regressions between body mass and age at maturity, maximum lifespan, and neonate size for placental mammals, using the AnAge database. R. Tacutu et al. (2018). "Human Ageing Genomic Resources: new and updated databases." *Nucl. Acids Res.* 46 (D1): D1083–90. doi: 10.1093/nar/gkx1042.

12 compared to other mammals: E. L. Charnov and D. Berrigan (1993). "Why do female primates have such long lifespans and so few babies? *or* Life in the slow lane." *Evol. Anthro.* 1 (6): 191–94.

12 killed early by a predator or other malefactor favor a slower pace of life: S. C. Stearns, M. Ackermann, M. Doebeli, and M. Kaiser (2000). "Experimental evolution of aging, growth, and reproduction in fruitflies." *PNAS* 97 (7): 3309–13; S. K. Auer, C. A. Dick, N. B. Metcalfe, and D. N. Reznick (2018). "Metabolic rate evolves rapidly and in parallel with the pace of life history." *Nat. Commun.* 9: 14.

13 stronger, pound for pound, than humans: M. C. O'Neill et al. (2017). "Chimpanzee super strength and human skeletal muscle evolution." *PNAS* 114

(28): 7343–48; K. Bozek et al. (2014). "Exceptional evolutionary divergence of human muscle and brain metabolomes parallels human cognitive and physical uniqueness." *PLoS Biol.* 12 (5): e1001871. doi: 10.1371/journal.pbio.1001871.

14 proponents of this hypothesis, like Brian McNab: Brian K. McNab (2008). "An analysis of the factors that influence the level and scaling of mammalian BMR." *Comp. Biochem. Phys. A—Mol. Integ. Phys.* 151: 5–28.

14 faster pace of life presumably requires a faster metabolic engine: T. J. Case (1978). "On the evolution and adaptive significance of postnatal growth rates in the terrestrial vertebrates." *Quar. Rev. Biol.* 53 (3): 243–82.

14 studies built upon these results, and a consensus developed: P. H. Harvey, M. D. Pagel, and J. A. Rees (1991). "Mammalian metabolism and life histories." *Am. Nat.* 137 (4): 556–66.

18 Orangutans burned fewer calories each day than humans: H. Pontzer et al. (2010). "Metabolic adaptation for low energy throughput in orangutans." *PNAS* 107 (32): 14048–52.

19 three-toed sloths and pandas: Y. Nie et al. (2015). "Exceptionally low daily energy expenditure in the bamboo-eating giant panda." *Science* 349 (6244): 171–74.

19 everything we knew about orangutan ecology and biology: Serge A. Wich, S. Suci Utami Atmoko, Tatang Mitra Setia, and Carel P. van Schaik, *Orangutans: Geographic Variation in Behavioral Ecology and Conservation* (Oxford Univ. Press, 2008).

21 Primates burn only *half* as many calories: H. Pontzer et al. (2014). "Primate energy expenditure and life history." *PNAS* 111 (4): 1433–37.

23 1995 paper by Leslie Aiello and Peter Wheeler: L. C. Aiello and P. Wheeler (1995). "The Expensive Tissue Hypothesis: the brain and the digestive system in human and primate evolution." *Curr. Anthropol.* 36: 199–221.

24 "nature is forced to economise on the other side": Charles Darwin, *On the Origin of Species* (John Murray, 1861), 147.

24 primates in Southeast Asia: Arthur Keith (1891). "Anatomical notes on Malay apes." *J. Straits Branch Roy. Asiatic Soc.* 23: 77–94.

24 the first doubly labeled water study in a wild primate: K. A. Nagy and K. Milton (1979). "Energy metabolism and food consumption by howler monkeys." *Ecology* 60: 475–80.

24 smaller brains than fruit-eating species: K. Milton (1993). "Diet and primate evolution." *Scientific American*, August, 86–93.

24 arguing that the cost of bigger brains: K. Isler and C. P. van Schaik (2009). "The Expensive Brain: A framework for explaining evolutionary changes in brain size." *J. Hum. Evol.* 57: 392–400.

25 had evolved distinct daily energy expenditures: H. Pontzer et al. (2016). "Metabolic acceleration and the evolution of human brain size and life history." *Nature* 533: 390–92.

Chapter 2: What Is Metabolism Anyway?

33 the combination of work done and heat gained: I'm simplifying slightly by lumping the formation energy of making molecules (which should also be included in an exhaustive accounting of energy) along with the mechanical work of moving things.

33 releases enough energy (730 kilocalories): J. Taylor and R. L. Hall (1947). "Determination of the heat of combustion of nitroglycerin and the thermochemical constants of nitrocellulose." *J. Phys. Chem.* 51 (2): 593–611.

34 by one degree Celsius (1.8 degrees Fahrenheit): The energy needed to raise a milliliter of water 1 degree Celsius depends slightly on the starting temperature of the water. The modern definition of a calorie is the energy equivalent of 4.184 joules. One joule is defined as the energy needed to lift 1 kilogram of mass upward by 1 meter (against gravity). Joules are named after the English scientist James Prescott Joule, who figured out the relationship between mechanical work and heat energy in the 1800s.

34 capitalize "Calories" when referring to kilocalories: J. L. Hargrove. (2006). "History of the Calorie in Nutrition." *J. Nutr.* 136: 2957–61.

34 to convert joules on their food labels to calories: There are actually 4.18 joules per calorie, but dividing by four will be accurate to about 5 percent, which is close enough for daily use. Also, be aware that kJ is kilojoules (1,000 joules) and MJ is megajoules (1,000,000 joules).

36 little machine that builds baby flies: I thank Dr. Kenneth Weiss, professor at Penn State, for blowing my mind with this perspective during my formative college years.

38 65-million-year history of relying on them: R. W. Sussman (1991). "Primate origins and the evolution of angiosperms." *Am. J. Primatol.* 23 (4): 209–23.

41 80 percent of the starches and sugars that you eat: R. Holmes (1971). "Carbohydrate digestion and absorption." *J. Clin. Path.* 24, Suppl. (Roy. Coll. Path.) (5): 10–13.

42 blood flow to our guts more than doubles: P. J. Matheson, M. A. Wilson, and R. N. Garrison (2000). "Regulation of intestinal blood flow." *Jour. Surg. Res.* 93: 182–96.

42 low glycemic index foods might be better for you: The evidence from carefully done studies on glycemic index are mixed. M. J. Franz (2003). "The glycemic index: Not the most effective nutrition therapy intervention." *Diabetes Care* 26: 2466–68.

42 compared to a piece of orange, which does: F. S. Atkinson, K. Foster-Powell, and J. C. Brand-Miller (2008). "International tables of glycemic index and glycemic load values: 2008." *Diabetes Care* 31 (12): 2281–83.

43 With trillions of bacteria: R. Sender, S. Fuchs, and R. Milo (2016). "Revised estimates for the number of human and bacteria cells in the body." *PLoS Biol.* 14 (8): e1002533.

43 the microbiome is like a four-pound superorganism: I. Rowland et al. (2018). "Gut microbiota functions: Metabolism of nutrients and other food components." *Eur. J. Nutr.* 57 (1): 1–24.

43 Carbs are energy: Sugars are also used to make some structures in the body. For example, the D in DNA is deoxyribose, which is a sugar molecule built from dietary carbohydrate.

45 Bile is a green juice produced by your liver: "Secretion of Bile and the Role of Bile Acids in Digestion," Colorado State University, accessed March 13, 2020, http://www.vivo.colostate.edu/hbooks/pathphys/digestion/liver/bile.html.

45 Bile acids (also called bile salts): M. J. Monte, J. J. Marin, A. Antelo, and J. Vazquez-Tato (2009). "Bile acids: Chemistry, physiology, and pathophysiology." *World J. Gastroenterol.* 15 (7): 804–16.

46 obesity is a major risk factor: S. L. Friedman, B. A. Neuschwander-Tetri, M. Rinella, and A. J. Sanyal (2018). "Mechanisms of NAFLD development and therapeutic strategies." *Nat. Med.* 24 (7): 908–22.

47 a typical alkaline battery: Wikipedia, accessed March 13, 2020, https://en .wikipedia.org/wiki/Energy_density.

48 sequence of amino acids to make a protein: I'm massively simplifying here, skipping over several steps from DNA to RNA to amino acid sequence. For a nice primer, see "Essentials of Genetics," Nature Education, https://www.nature.com /scitable/ebooks/essentials-of-genetics-8/contents/.

48 tissues and molecules break down over time: G. E. Shambaugh III (1977). "Urea biosynthesis I. The urea cycle and relationships to the citric acid cycle." *Am. J. Clin. Nutr.* 30 (12): 2083–87.

49 providing around 15 percent of our calories each day: C. E. Berryman, H. R. Lieberman, V. L. Fulgoni III, and S. M. Pasiakos (2018). "Protein intake trends and conformity with the Dietary Reference Intakes in the United States: Analysis of the National Health and Nutrition Examination Survey, 2001–2014." *Am. J. Clin. Nutr.* 108 (2): 405–13.

50 each molecule cycles from ADP to ATP and back: Lawrence Cole, *Biology of Life Biochemistry, Physiology and Philosophy* (Academic Press, 2016).

50 the story is essentially the same for fructose and galactose: J. M. Rippe and T. J. Angelopoulos (2013). "Sucrose, high-fructose corn syrup, and fructose, their metabolism and potential health effects: What do we really know?" *Adv. Nutr.* 4 (2): 236–45.

51 circular track called the Krebs cycle: Discovered by Hans A. Krebs and William A. Johnson in 1937, earning Krebs a Nobel Prize in medicine. Krebs and his student Kurt Henseleit discovered the urea cycle in 1932. Krebs was probably happy to have been known for energy production rather than pee production.

52 *not* the atoms themselves: If we converted the mass of those atoms to energy, we have to follow Einstein's famous formula, $E = mc^2$, and we'd need a nuclear reactor. A gram of glucose would yield 21 billion kilocalories, vaporizing everything in sight.

57 Dogs have evolved to prey on our emotions: Brian Hare and Vanessa Woods, *The Genius of Dogs: How Dogs Are Smarter Than You Think* (Dutton, 2013).

57 a new recipe for photosynthesis evolved: R. M. Soo et al. (2017). "On the origins of oxygenic photosynthesis and aerobic respiration in Cyanobacteria." *Science* 355 (6332): 1436–40.

58 struck by lightning, which are 1 in 700,000: "Flash Facts About Lightning," *National Geographic*, accessed March 13, 2020, https://news.nationalgeographic .com/news/2004/06/flash-facts-about-lightning/.

58 over a million bacteria in an ounce: K. Lührig et al. (2015). "Bacterial community analysis of drinking water biofilms in southern Sweden." *Microbes Environ.* 30 (1): 99–107.

58 about 330 million cubic miles of water: "How Much Water Is There on Earth?" USGS, https://water.usgs.gov/edu/earthhowmuch.html

60 championed by the visionary evolutionary biologist Lynn Margulis: Lynn Margulis, *Origin of Eukaryotic Cells* (Yale University Press, 1970).

Chapter 3: What Is This Going to Cost Me?

66 Phlogiston was thought to be the essential stuff: Wikipedia, accessed March 13, 2020, https://en.wikipedia.org/wiki/Phlogiston_theory.

66 the chemist Joseph Priestley: "Joseph Priestley and the Discovery of Oxygen," American Chemical Society, International Historic Chemical Landmarks, accessed March 13, 2020, http://www.acs.org/content/acs/en /education/whatischemistry/landmarks/josephpriestleyoxygen.html.

67 They placed a guinea pig in a small metal container: Esther Inglis-Arkell, "The Guinea Pig That Proved We Have an Internal Combustion Engine," Gizmodo, last modified June 23, 2013, https://io9.gizmodo.com/the-guinea-pig -that-proved-we-have-an-internal-combusti-534671441.

68 oxygen consumption and CO_2 production as the main measure: See pioneering work by Max Rubner, such as Max Rubner (1883). "Über den Einfluss der Korpergrosse auf Stoff- und Kraftwechsel." *Zeitschr. f. Biol.* 19: 535–62.

69 The Compendium of Physical Activity: B. E. Ainsworth et al. (2011). "Compendium of Physical Activities: A second update of codes and MET values." *Medicine and Science in Sports and Exercise* 43 (8): 1575–81.

75 a large meta-analysis by Jonas Rubenson and colleagues: Jonas Rubenson et al. (2007). "Reappraisal of the comparative cost of human locomotion using gait-specific allometric analyses." *J. Experi. Biol.* 210: 3513–24.

75 Hadza data fell right in line with this much larger sample: H. Pontzer et al. (2012). "Hunter-gatherer energetics and human obesity." *PLoS One* 7 (7): e40503.

75 Studies of elite swimmers by Paola Zamparo: P. Zamparo et al. (2005). "Energy cost of swimming of elite long-distance swimmers." *Eur. J. Appl. Physiol.* 94 (5–6): 697–704.

76 riding a bicycle is much cheaper: P. E. di Prampero (2000). "Cycling on Earth, in space, on the Moon." *Eur. J. Appl. Physiol.* 82 (5–6): 345–60.

76 the cost of ascent increases with body weight: Elaine E. Kozma (2020), *Climbing Performance and Ecology in Humans, Chimpanzees, and Gorillas* (PhD dissertation, City University of New York).

79 Walking at our most economical pace, about 2.5 mph: D. Abe, Y. Fukuoka, and M. Horiuchi (2015). "Economical speed and energetically optimal transition speed evaluated by gross and net oxygen cost of transport at different gradients." *PLoS One* 10: e0138154.

79 close to the energetically optimal speed: H. J. Ralston (1958). "Energy–speed relation and optimal speed during level walking." *Int. Z. Angew. Physiol. Einschl. Arbeitphysiol.* 17 (4): 277–83.

79 People in big, fast-paced cities: M. H. Bornstein and H. G. Bornstein (1976). "The pace of life." *Nature* 259: 557–59.

79 the inherent mechanics of a walking gait: Andrew Biewener and Shelia Patek, *Animal Locomotion*, 2nd ed. (Oxford Univ. Press, 2018).

80 the effect is typically small, around 1 to 4 percent: M. I. Lambert and T. L. Burgess (2010). "Effects of training, muscle damage and fatigue on running economy." *Internat. SportMed J.* 11(4): 363–79.

81 increases the calories burned by only 3 to 13 percent: C. J. Arellano and R. Kram (2014). "The metabolic cost of human running: Is swinging the arms worth it?" *J. Exp. Biol.* 217: 2456–61.

81 half of a Big Mac (270 kcal): "McDonald's Nutrition Calculator," McDonald's, accessed March 13, 2020, https://www.mcdonalds.com/us/en-us/about-our-food/nutrition-calculator.html.

81 calories in a chocolate glazed donut (340 kcal): "Nutrition." Dunkin' Donuts, accessed March 13, 2020, https://www.dunkindonuts.com/en/food-drinks/donuts/donuts.

83 BMR (in kcal per day) increases with body weight: Condensed from C. J. Henry (2005). "Basal metabolic rate studies in humans: Measurement and development of new equations." *Publ. Health Nutr.* 8: 1133–52.

84 about 85 kcal per day for a typical 150-pound adult with 30 percent body fat: For a review of organ costs see: ZiMian Wang et al. (2012). "Evaluation of specific metabolic rates of major organs and tissues: Comparison between nonobese and obese women." *Obesity* 20 (1): 95–100.

85 the low, low cost of about 2 calories per beat: M. Horiuchi et al. (2017). "Measuring the energy of ventilation and circulation during human walking using induced hypoxia." *Scientific Reports* 7 (1): 4938. doi: 10.1038/s41598-017-05068-8

85 converting lactate, glycerol (from fat), and amino acids (from proteins): J. E. Gerich, C. Meyer, H. J. Woerle, and M. Stumvoll (2001). "Renal gluconeogenesis: Its importance in human glucose homeostasis." *Diabetes Care* 24 (2): 382–91.

86 Like every other animal with a distinct mouth and butt: Many animals, like starfish, have only one hole, which serves for both bringing nutrients in and getting waste out. See A. Hejnol and M. Q. Martindale (2008). "Acoel development indicates the independent evolution of the bilaterian mouth and anus." *Nature* 456 (7220): 382–86. doi: 10.1038/nature07309.

86 A recent study in mice by Sarah Bahr, John Kirby, and colleagues: S. M. Bahr et al. (2015). "Risperidone-induced weight gain is mediated through shifts in the gut microbiome and suppression of energy expenditure." *EBioMedicine* 2 (11): 1725–34. doi: 10.1016/j.ebiom.2015.10.018.

87 providing nutrients and cleaning up waste: M. Bélanger, I. Allaman, and P. J. Magistretti (2011). "Brain energy metabolism: Focus on astrocyte-neuron metabolic cooperation." *Cell Metabolism* 14 (6): 724–38.

87 increased their metabolic rates by only around 4 kcal per hour: R. W. Backs and K. A. Seljos (1994). "Metabolic and cardiorespiratory measures of mental effort: The effects of level of difficulty in a working memory task." *Int. J. Psychophysiol.* 16 (1): 57–68; N. Troubat, M.-A. Fargeas-Gluck, M. Tulppo, and B. Dugué (2009). "The stress of chess players as a model to study the effects of psychological stimuli on physiological responses: An example of substrate oxidation and heart rate variability in man." *Eur. J. Appl. Physiol.* 105 (3): 343–49.

88 Work by Christopher Kuzawa and colleagues: C. W. Kuzawa et al. (2014). "Metabolic costs of human brain development." *Proc. Nat. Acad. Sciences* 111 (36): 13010–15. doi: 10.1073/pnas.1323099111.

89 thermoneutral zone is roughly between 75°F and 93°F: B. R. M. Kingma, A. J. H. Frijns, L. Schellen, and W. D. V. Lichtenbelt (2014). "Beyond the classic thermoneutral zone: Including thermal comfort." *Temperature* 1 (2): 142–49.

89 a couple of degrees colder than adults who aren't: R. J. Brychta et al. (2019). "Quantification of the capacity for cold-induced thermogenesis in young men with and without obesity." *J. Clin. Endocrin. Metab.* 104 (10): 4865–78. doi: 10.1210 /jc.2019-00728.

89 in the Arctic tend to have about 10 percent higher BMRs: W. R. Leonard et al. (2002). "Climatic influences on basal metabolic rates among circumpolar populations." *Am. J. Hum. Biol.* 14 (5): 609–20.

89 shivering can cause our resting metabolic rate to climb: F. Haman and D. P. Blondin (2017). "Shivering thermogenesis in humans: Origin, contribution and metabolic requirement." *Temperature* 4 (3): 217–26. doi: 10.1080/23328940.2017.1328999.

90 acute infections kill four out of ten children: M. Gurven and H. Kaplan (2007). "Longevity among hunter-gatherers: A cross-cultural examination." *Pop. and Devel. Rev.* 33 (2): 321–65.

90 college men who reported to a student health clinic found their BMRs: M. P. Muehlenbein, J. L. Hirschtick, J. Z. Bonner, and A. M. Swartz (2010). "Toward quantifying the usage costs of human immunity: Altered metabolic rates and hormone levels during acute immune activation in men." *Am. J. Hum. Biol.* 22: 546–56.

91 populations without the antiseptic advantages of modernization: M. D. Gurven et al. (2016). "High resting metabolic rate among Amazonian forager-horticulturalists experiencing high pathogen burden." *Am. J. Physical Anth.* 161 (3): 414–25. doi: 10.1002/ajpa.23040.

91 Shuar kids five to twelve years old have BMRs that are about 200 kcal: S. S. Urlacher et al. (2019). "Constraint and trade-offs regulate energy expenditure during childhood." *Science Advances* 5 (12): eaax1065. doi: 10.1126/sciadv.aax1065.

92 The cost of growth, then, is about 2,200 kcal per pound: J. C. Waterlow (1981). "The energy cost of growth. Joint FAO/WHO/UNU Expert Consultation on Energy and Protein Requirements." Rome, accessed March 14, 2020, http://www.fao.org/3/M2885E/M2885E00.htm.

93 total cost of a healthy nine-month pregnancy is about 80,000 kcal: N. F. Butte and J. C. King (2005). "Energy requirements during pregnancy and lactation." *Publ. Health Nutr.* 8: 1010–27.

94 directly tied to changes in the way these animals grow and reproduce: T. J. Case (1978). "On the evolution and adaptive significance of postnatal growth rates in the terrestrial vertebrates." *Quar. Rev. Biol.* 53 (3): 243–82.

94 burning ten times more calories per day than their reptilian ancestors: K. A. Nagy, I. A. Girard, and T. K. Brown (1999). "Energetics of free-ranging mammals, reptiles, and birds." *Ann. Rev. Nutr.* 19: 247–77.

94 Mammals grow five times faster than reptiles: Author's unpublished analyses, calculated from allometric regressions between adult body mass and growth rate (g/yr) and reproductive output (g/yr), using the AnAge database. R. Tacutu et al. (2018). "Human Ageing Genomic Resources: New and updated databases." *Nucleic Acids Research* 46 (D1): D1083–90.

95 Kleiber's law of metabolism, named for the pioneering Swiss nutritionist: Max Kleiber, *The Fire of Life: An Introduction to Animal Energetics* (Wiley, 1961). Samuel Brody and Francis Benedict also contributed to this discovery.

95 in the neighborhood of Kleiber's 0.75, ranging from 0.45 to 0.82: Author's unpublished analyses, calculated from allometric regressions between adult body mass and growth rate (g/yr) and reproductive output (g/yr), using the AnAge database. R. Tacutu et al. (2018). "Human Ageing Genomic Resources: New and updated databases." *Nucleic Acids Research* 46 (D1): D1083–90.

97 *On Longevity and the Shortness of Life* in 350 B.C.: Aristotle, *On Longevity and Shortness of Life. Written 350 B.C.E.* Translated by G. R. T. Ross, accessed March 16, 2020, http://classics.mit.edu/Aristotle/longev_short.html.

98 Rubner observed that the total energy expended per gram: Max Rubner, *Das Problem det Lebensdaur und seiner beziehunger zum Wachstum und Ernarnhung* (Oldenberg, 1908).

98 the American biologist Raymond Pearl: Raymond Pearl, *The Biology of Death* (J. B. Lippincott, 1922).

98 the free radical theory of aging: Denham Harman (1956). "Aging: A theory based on free radical and radiation chemistry." *J. Gerontol.* 11 (3): 298–300.

99 don't always show the expected effects on life span: Some studies find positive effects of antioxidant intake on mortality risk (e.g., L.-G. Zhao et al. [2017]. "Dietary antioxidant vitamins intake and mortality: A report from two cohort studies of Chinese adults in Shanghai." *J. Epidem.* 27 [3]: 89–97), while others find no effect at all (e.g., U. Stepaniak et al. [2016]. "Antioxidant vitamin intake and mortality in three Central and Eastern European urban populations: The HAPIEE study." *Eur. J. Nutr.* 55 [2]: 547–60).

99 researchers lamenting whether such links exist at all: For a skeptical view, see J. R. Speakman (2005). "Body size, energy metabolism, and lifespan." *J. Exp. Biol.* 208: 1717–30.

100 reducing how much they're allowed to eat leads to longer life spans: J. R. Speakman and S. E. Mitchell (2011). "Caloric restriction." *Mol. Aspects Med.* 32: 159–221.

100 Greenland sharks can live four hundred years: J. Nielsen et al. (2016). "Eye lens radiocarbon reveals centuries of longevity in the Greenland shark (*Somniosus microcephalus*)." *Science* 353 (6300): 702–04.

100 heart rates (beats per minute) match the cellular metabolic rates: C. R. White and M. R. Kearney (2014). "Metabolic scaling in animals: Methods, empirical results, and theoretical explanations." *Compr. Physiol.* 4 (1): 231–56. doi: 10.1002/cphy.c110049.

101 Frank Benedict and his colleague J. Arthur Harris had been amassing: J. A. Harris and F. G. Benedict (1918). "A biometric study of human basal metabolism." *PNAS* 4 (12): 370–73. doi: 10.1073/pnas.4.12.370.

102 PARs are essentially the same as MET values: MET values are always 1 kcal per kg per hour, which is the average person's BMR. PAR values are tailored to each individual's BMR or estimated BMR.

102 still used by the World Health Organization: FAO Food and Nutrition Technical Report Series 1, FAO/WHO/UNU (2001). "Human energy requirements." http://www.fao.org/docrep/007/y5686e/y5686e00.htm#Contents.

103 adults underreported actual food intake by 29 percent on average: L. Orcholski et al. (2015). "Under-reporting of dietary energy intake in five populations of the African diaspora." *Brit. J. Nutri.* 113 (3): 464–72. doi: 10.1017 /S000711451400405X.

104 you thought that the typical American eats a 2,000-kilocalorie diet: Marion Nestle and Malden Nesheim, *Why Calories Count: From Science to Politics* (Univ. of California Press, 2013).

104 Nathan Lifson, a physiologist at the University of Minnesota: A. Prentice (1987). "Human energy on tap." *New Scientist*, November: 40–44.

105 oxygen atoms in the body water pool have an alternative: N. Lifson, G. B. Gordon, M. B. Visscher, and A. O. Nier (1949). "The fate of utilized molecular oxygen and the source of the oxygen of respiratory carbon dioxide, studied with the aid of heavy oxygen." *J. Biol. Chem.* 180 (2): 803–11.

106 Lifson used those isotopes to track the flow oxygen and hydrogen: N. Lifson, G. B. Gordon, R. McClintock (1955). "Measurement of total carbon dioxide production by means of $D_2^{18}O$." *J. Appl. Physiol.* 7: 704–10.

106 isotope needed for a 150-pound human would cost more than $250,000: J. R. Speakman (1998). "The history and theory of the doubly labeled water technique." *Am. J. Clin. Nutr.* 68 (suppl): 932S–38S.

107 the first doubly labeled water study in humans in 1982: D. A. Schoeller and E. van Santen (1982). "Measurement of energy expenditure in humans by doubly labeled water." *J. Appl. Physiol.* 53: 955–59.

108 hundreds of doubly labeled water measurements of men, women, and children: L. Dugas et al. (2011). "Energy expenditure in adults living in developing compared with industrialized countries: A meta-analysis of doubly labeled water studies." *Am. J. Clin. Nutr.* 93: 427–441; N. F. Butte (2000). "Fat intake of children in relation to energy requirements." *Am. J. Clin. Nutr.* 72 (5 Suppl): 1246S–52S; H. Pontzer et al. (2012). "Hunter-gatherer energetics and human obesity." *PLoS One* 7 (7): e40503.

Chapter 4: How Humans Evolved to Be the Nicest, Fittest, and *Fattest* Apes

120 Georgians reported two new skulls along with solid dates: L. Gabunia et al. (2000). "Earliest Pleistocene hominid cranial remains from Dmanisi, Republic of Georgia: Taxonomy, geological setting, and age." *Science* 288 (5468): 1019–25.

122 uncovered yet *another* skull, the fourth from the area: D. Lordkipanidze et al. (2005). "The earliest toothless hominin skull." *Nature* 434: 717–18.

122 Wild plants and game are nearly all hard to chew: Like nearly all else in human evolution, the need for teeth, or for help in the absence of them, is hotly debated. Some have argued that this unlucky soul might have soldiered on without help, mashing his food with stone tools or just choking down big chunks. It's impossible to be certain. But it's difficult for me to see how he could have survived, particularly through the serious illness, without help—much more help than apes give one another.

123 early primates coevolved with flowering plants: R. W. Sussman (1991). "Primate origins and the evolution of angiosperms." *Am. J. Primatol.* 23 (4): 209–23.

125 hominin evolution lasted from seven to four million years ago: For a more thorough account of our species' evolution than the short overview here, see Glenn C. Conroy and Herman Pontzer, *Reconstructing Human Origins*, 3rd ed. (W. W. Norton, 2012).

125 the topic of another larger book: Conroy and Pontzer, *Reconstructing Human Origins*.

126 stone tools from a 3.3-million-year-old site in northern Kenya: S. Harmand et al. (2015). "3.3-million-year-old stone tools from Lomekwi 3, West Turkana, Kenya." *Nature* 521: 310–15.

127 Figure 4.1. The Human Family Tree: Adapted from Herman Pontzer (2017). "Economy and endurance in human evolution." *Curr. Biol.* 27 (12): R613–21. doi: 10.1016/j.cub.2017.05.031.

128 animal fossils from sites in Kenya and Ethiopia show signs of butchery: M. Domínguez-Rodrigo, T. R. Pickering, S. Semaw, and M. J. Rogers (2005). "Cutmarked bones from Pliocene archaeological sites at Gona, Afar, Ethiopia: Implications for the function of the world's oldest stone tools." *J. Hum. Evol.* 48 (2): 109–21.

130 "to attack their prey, or otherwise to obtain food": Charles Darwin, *The Descent of Man* (D. Appleton, 1871).

131 Orangutan mothers in the wild share food: A. V. Jaeggi, M. A. van Noordwijk, and C. P. van Schaik (2008). "Begging for information: Mother-offspring food sharing among wild Bornean orangutans." *Am. J. Primatol.* 70 (6): 533–41. doi: 10.1002/ajp.20525.

131 Gorillas have *never* been observed sharing food: A. V. Jaeggi and C. P. Van Schaik (2011). "The evolution of food sharing in primates." *Behav. Ecol. Sociobiol.* 65: 2125–40.

131 chimpanzees in the Sonso community in the Budongo Forest of Uganda: R. M. Wittig et al. (2014). "Food sharing is linked to urinary oxytocin levels and bonding in related and unrelated wild chimpanzees." *Proc. Biol. Sci.* 281 (1778): 20133096. doi: 10.1098/rspb.2013.3096.

131 adult bonobos (mostly females) share a particular fruit: S. Yamamoto (2015). "Non-reciprocal but peaceful fruit sharing in wild bonobos in Wamba." *Behaviour* 152: 335–57.

133 behaviors arise and the body adapts: A. Lister (2013). "Behavioural leads in evolution: Evidence from the fossil record." *Bio. J. Linnean Soc.* 112: 315–31.

135 channel their maternal efforts into sharing food with their daughters: K. Hawkes et al. (1998). "Grandmothering, menopause, and the evolution of human life histories." *PNAS* 95 (3): 1336–39. doi: 10.1073/pnas.95.3.1336.

135 fossil hominins with brains nearly 20 percent larger: S. C. Antón, R. Potts, and L. C. Aiello (2014). "Evolution of early *Homo*: An integrated biological perspective." *Science* 345 (6192): 1236828. doi: 10.1126/science.1236828.

137 early members of the genus *Homo* were adapted for endurance running: D. M. Bramble and D. E. Lieberman (2004). "Endurance running and the evolution of *Homo*." *Nature* 432: 345–52. doi: 10.1038/nature03052.

138 trade networks for highly prized raw materials stretch for miles: A. S. Brooks et al. (2018). "Long-distance stone transport and pigment use in the earliest Middle Stone Age." *Science* 360 (6384): 90–94.

139 harvesting shellfish on an annual schedule: A. Jerardino, R. A. Navarro, and M. Galimberti (2014). "Changing collecting strategies of the clam *Donax serra* Röding (Bivalvia: Donacidae) during the Pleistocene at Pinnacle Point, South Africa." *J. Hum. Evol.* 68: 58–67. doi: 10.1016/j.jhevol.2013.12.012.

139 murals on cave walls from Bordeaux to Borneo: M. Aubert et al. (2018). "Palaeolithic cave art in Borneo." *Nature* 564: 254–57.

139 VO$_2$ max, a common measure of peak aerobic power: H. Pontzer (2017). "Economy and endurance in human evolution." *Curr. Biol.* 27 (12): R613–21. doi: 10.1016/j.cub.2017.05.031.

140 **tool technology and hunting techniques were quite sophisticated:** H. Thieme (1997). "Lower Palaeolithic hunting spears from Germany." *Nature* 385: 807–10. doi: 10.1038/385807a0.

141 **until late in their teenage years:** H. Kaplan, K. Hill, J. Lancaster, and A. M. Hurtado (2000). "A theory of human life history evolution: Diet, intelligence, and longevity." *Evol. Anthro.* 9 (4): 156–85.

141 **interbirth intervals for chimpanzees, gorillas, and orangutans:** M. E. Thompson (2013). "Comparative reproductive energetics of human and nonhuman primates." *Ann. Rev. Anthropol.* 42: 287–304.

141 **world was already full of strange and wonderful humanlike species:** Nick Longrich, "Were other humans the first victims of the sixth mass extinction?" The Conversation, November 21, 2019, accessed March 16, 2020, https:// theconversation.com/were-other-humans-the-first-victims-of-the-sixth-mass -extinction-126638.

142 **bits of their DNA in our chromosomes today:** S. Sankararaman, S. Mallick, N. Patterson, and D. Reich (2016). "The combined landscape of Denisovan and Neanderthal ancestry in present-day humans." *Curr. Biol.* 26 (9): 1241–47. doi: 10.1016/j.cub.2016.03.037.

143 **Neanderthals had brains a bit larger than ours and were making cave art, :** D. L. Hoffmann et al. (2018). "U-Th dating of carbonate crusts reveals Neandertal origin of Iberian cave art." *Science* 359 (6378): 912–15. doi: 10.1126/ science.aap7778.

143 **playing music:** N. J. Conard, M. Malina, and S. C. Münzel (2009). "New flutes document the earliest musical tradition in southwestern Germany." *Nature* 460: 737–40.

143 **and burying their dead:** W. Rendu et al. (2014). "Neandertal burial at La Chapelle-aux-Saints." *PNAS* 111 (1): 81–86. doi: 10.1073/pnas.1316780110.

143 *Homo sapiens* **became hyper-social through a long process:** Brian Hare and Vanessa Woods, *Survival of the Friendliest* (Random House, 2020); Richard W. Wrangham, *The Goodness Paradox* (Pantheon, 2019).

147 **they kill more people globally each year than violence:** Risk Factors Collaborators (2016). "Global Burden of Disease 2015." *Lancet* 388 (10053): 1659–1724.

147 **by some accounts, human societies globally have become less violent:** Steven Pinker, *The Better Angels of Our Nature* (Penguin, 2012).

147 **Chimpanzees and bonobos put on less than 10 percent body fat:** H. Pontzer et al. (2016). "Metabolic acceleration and the evolution of human brain size and life history." *Nature* 533: 390–92.

148 **hunter-gatherers like the Hadza put on more fat than that:** H. Pontzer et al. (2012). "Hunter-gatherer energetics and human obesity." *PLoS One* 7 (7): e40503. doi: 10.1371/journal.pone.0040503.

154 life as a hunter-gatherer is tough: For descriptions and data regarding
Hadza life and daily activity, see Frank W. Marlowe, *The Hadza: Hunter-Gatherers of
Tanzania* (Univ. of California Press, 2010); D. A. Raichlen et al. (2017). "Physical
activity patterns and biomarkers of cardiovascular disease risk in hunter-
gatherers." *Am. J. Hum. Biol.* 29: e22919. doi: 10.1002/ajhb.22919.

156 hunter-gatherers lead lives that would make Westerners melt: H. Pontzer,
B. M. Wood, and D. A. Raichlen (2018). "Hunter-gatherers as models in public
health." *Obes. Rev.* 19 (Suppl 1): 24–35.

158 Hadza data sat right on top of the measurements: H. Pontzer et al. (2012).
"Hunter-gatherer energetics and human obesity." *PLoS One* 7: e40503.

162 daily energy expenditures among five- to twelve-year-old Shuar kids:
S. Urlacher et al. (2019). "Constraint and trade-offs regulate energy expenditure
during childhood." *Science Advances* 5 (12): eaax1065. doi: 10.1126/sciadv.aax1065.

162 daily energy expenditure in men and women among the Tsimane: M. D.
Gurven et al. (2016). "High resting metabolic rate among Amazonian forager-
horticulturalists experiencing high pathogen burden." *Am. J. Phys. Anth.* 161 (3):
414–25. doi: 10.1002/ajpa.23040.

**162 daily energy expenditures in African American women from Maywood and
rural Nigeria:** K. E. Ebersole et al. (2008). "Energy expenditure and adiposity in
Nigerian and African-American women." *Obesity* 16 (9): 2148–54. doi: 10.1038
/oby.2008.330.

163 same daily energy expenditures as pampered urbanites: L. R. Dugas et al.
(2011). "Energy expenditure in adults living in developing compared with
industrialized countries: A meta-analysis of doubly labeled water studies."
Am. J. Clin. Nutr. 93: 427–41.

**164 no difference between moderately active adults and those with the highest
levels:** H. Pontzer et al. (2016). "Constrained total energy expenditure and
metabolic adaptation to physical activity in adult humans." *Curr. Biol.* 26 (3):
410–17. doi: 10.1016/j.cub.2015.12.046.

164 a year-long program to train them to run: K. R. Westerterp et al. (1992).
"Long-term effect of physical activity on energy balance and body composition."
Brit. J. Nutr. 68: 21–30.

164 were running roughly 25 miles per week: The protocol was described as 60
minutes per session, 4 days a week, which would be about 25 miles per week at a
9:36 minutes/mile pace.

165 the rule among warm-blooded animals: H. Pontzer (2015). "Constrained
total energy expenditure and the evolutionary biology of energy balance." *Exer.
Sport. Sci. Rev.* 43: 110–16; T. J. O'Neal et al. (2017). "Increases in physical activity
result in diminishing increments in daily energy expenditure in mice." *Curr. Biol.*
27 (3): 423–30.

165 Same goes for kangaroos and pandas: H. Pontzer et al. (2014). "Primate energy expenditure and life history." *PNAS* 111 (4): 1433–37; Y. Nie et al. (2015). "Exceptionally low daily energy expenditure in the bamboo-eating giant panda." *Science* 349 (6244): 171–74.

166 daily energy expenditures and the PAL ratio have stayed the same: K. R. Westerterp and J. R. Speakman (2008). "Physical activity energy expenditure has not declined since the 1980s and matches energy expenditures of wild mammals." *Internat. J. Obesity* 32: 1256–63.

168 Midwest Exercise Trial 1 study conducted: J. E. Donnelly et al. (2003). "Effects of a 16-month randomized controlled exercise trial on body weight and composition in young, overweight men and women: The Midwest Exercise Trial." *Arch. Intern. Med.* 163 (11): 1343–50.

168 a more demanding workout regime in Midwest 2: S. D. Herrmann et al. (2015). "Energy intake, nonexercise physical activity, and weight loss in responders and nonresponders: The Midwest Exercise Trial 2." *Obesity* 23 (8):1539–49. doi: 10.1002/oby.21073.

169 two years, average amount of weight lost is less than five pounds: D. L. Swift et al. (2014). "The role of exercise and physical activity in weight loss and maintenance." *Prog. Cardiov. Dis.* 56 (4): 441–47. doi: 10.1016/j.pcad.2013 .09.012.

170 elevated daily expenditures in a small sample of Shuar men: L. Christopher et al. (2019). "High energy requirements and water throughput of adult Shuar forager-horticulturalists of Amazonian Ecuador." *Am. J. Hum. Biol.* 31: e23223. doi: 10.1002/ajhb.23223.

170 Obese people burn just as much energy each day: D. A. Schoeller (1999). "Recent advances from application of doubly labeled water to measurement of human energy expenditure." *J. Nutr.* 129: 1765–68.

170 children have shown the same result: S. R. Zinkel et al. (2016). "High energy expenditure is not protective against increased adiposity in children." *Pediatr. Obes.* 11 (6): 528–34. doi: 10.1111/ijpo.12099.

172 study metabolic changes among *The Biggest Loser* **contestants:** D. L. Johannsen et al. (2012). "Metabolic slowing with massive weight loss despite preservation of fat-free mass." *J. Clin. Endocrinol. Metab.* 97 (7): 2489–96. doi: 10.1210/jc.2012-1444.

173 their BMRs were *still* **lower than expected:** E. Fothergill et al. (2016). "Persistent metabolic adaptation 6 years after 'The Biggest Loser' competition." *Obesity* 24 (8): 1612–19. doi: 10.1002/oby.21538.

174 studies was conducted in 1917 by Francis Benedict: F. G. Benedict (1918). "Physiological effects of a prolonged reduction in diet on twenty-five men." *Proc. Am. Phil. Soc.* 57 (5): 479–90.

175 Ancel Keys and colleagues at the University of Minnesota: Ancel Keys, Josef Brozek, and Austin Henschel, *The Biology of Human Starvation*, vol. 1 (Univ. of Minnesota Press, 1950).

175 overshooting phenomenon isn't as well studied: A. G. Dulloo, J. Jacquet, and L. Girardier (1997). "Poststarvation hyperphagia and body fat overshooting in humans: A role for feedback signals from lean and fat tissues." *Am. J. Clin. Nutr.* 65 (3): 717–23.

178 metabolic manager isn't just a metaphor or a cartoon: For an excellent review of the neural control of hunger and satiety, read Stephan Guyenet, *The Hungry Brain: Outsmarting the Instincts That Make Us Overeat* (Flatiron Books, 2017).

180 thyroid hormone, the main control hormone for our metabolic rate: L. M. Redman and E. Ravussin (2009). "Endocrine alterations in response to calorie restriction in humans." *Mol. Cell. Endocrin.* 299 (1): 129–36. doi: 10.1016/j. mce.2008.10.014.

180 humans are quick to put reproduction on the back burner: For a thorough discussion of the role of energy availability in human reproduction, see Peter Ellison, *On Fertile Ground* (Harvard Univ. Press, 2003).

180 food restriction is sufficiently severe, will stop ovulating: N. I. Williams et al. (2010). "Estrogen and progesterone exposure is reduced in response to energy deficiency in women aged 25–40 years." *Hum. Repro.* 25 (9): 2328–39. doi: 10.1093/humrep/deq172.

180 mice faced with starvation maintain two organs: S. E. Mitchell et al. (2015). "The effects of graded levels of calorie restriction: I. Impact of short term calorie and protein restriction on body composition in the C57BL/6 mouse." *Oncotarget* 6: 15902–30.

181 body weights and BMIs hardly change: H. Pontzer, B. M. Wood, and D. A. Raichlen (2018). "Hunter-gatherers as models in public health." *Obes. Rev.* 19 (Suppl 1): 24–35.

182 our body tries to make use of some: R. L. Leibel, M. Rosenbaum, and J. Hirsch (1995). "Changes in energy expenditure resulting from altered body weight." *N. Engl. J. Med.* 332 (10): 621–28.

182 the average American adult gains about half a pound: S. Stenholm et al. (2015). "Patterns of weight gain in middle-aged and older US adults, 1992–2010." *Epidemiology* 26 (2): 165–68. doi: 10.1097/EDE.0000000000000228.

183 gain weight around the holidays: E. E. Helander, B. Wansink, and A. Chieh (2016). "Weight gain over the holidays in three countries." *N. Engl. J. Med.* 375 (12): 1200–02. doi: 10.1056/NEJMc1602012.

183 moths mistaking a porch light for the moon: R. Hertzberg, "Why insects like moths are so attracted to bright lights." *National Geographic*, October 5, 2018, accessed March 18, 2020, https://www.nationalgeographic.com/animals/2018/10 /moth-meme-lamps-insects-lights-attraction-news/.

186 the venerable Weight Watchers: "Dieters move away from calorie obsession," CBS, April 12, 2014, https://www.cbsnews.com/news/dieters-move-away-from -calorie-obsession/.

Chapter 6: The Real Hunger Games: Diet, Metabolism, and Human Evolution

189 European taxonomists named it *Indicator indicator*: It was originally named *Cuculus indicator* because honeyguides lay their eggs in other birds' nests, cuckolding the unwitting parents. See A. Spaarman, "An account of a journey into Africa from the Cape of Good-Hope, and a description of a new species of cuckow." *Phil. Trans. Roy. Soc. London* (Royal Society of London, 1777), 38–47.

189 honeyguide split from the other species: B. M. Wood et al. (2014). "Mutualism and manipulation in Hadza–honeyguide interactions." *Evol. Hum. Behav.* 35: 540–46.

193 the Dunning-Kruger effect: J. Kruger and D. Dunning (1999). "Unskilled and unaware of it: How difficulties in recognizing one's own incompetence lead to inflated self-assessments." *J. Pers. Soc. Psych.* 77 (6): 1121–34.

193 "ignorance more frequently begets confidence than does knowledge": Charles Darwin, *Descent of Man* (John Murray & Sons, 1871), 3.

193 competence in governing and expertise in world affairs: Could you tell this was a joke? If not, you might be a victim of the Dunning-Kruger effect.

194 talking points from PETA: "Is It Really Natural? The Truth About Humans and Eating Meat," PETA, January 23, 2018, accessed March 18, 2020, https://www.peta.org/living/food/really-natural-truth-humans-eating-meat/.

194 our hominin ancestors got their start: H. Pontzer (2012). "Overview of hominin evolution." *Nature Education Knowledge* 3 (10): 8, accessed March 18, 2020, https://www.nature.com/scitable/knowledge/library/overview-of-hominin-evolution-89010983/.

195 Insects may have been a regular part of the menu: L. R. Backwell and F. d'Errico (2001). "Evidence of termite foraging by Swartkrans early hominids." *PNAS* 98 (4): 1358–63. doi: 10.1073/pnas.021551598.

195 the exploitation of tubers: G. Laden and R. Wrangham (2005). "The rise of the hominids as an adaptive shift in fallback foods: Plant underground storage organs (USOs) and australopith origins." *J. Hum. Evol.* 49 (4): 482–98.

196 the telltale isotopic signatures of their bones: K. Jaouen et al. (2019). "Exceptionally high $\delta^{15}N$ values in collagen single amino acids confirm Neandertals as high-trophic level carnivores." *PNAS* 116 (11): 4928–33. doi: 10.1073/pnas.1814087116.

196 our digestive tracts are 40 percent smaller: L. C. Aiello and P. Wheeler (1995). "The expensive tissue hypothesis: The brain and the digestive system in human and primate evolution." *Curr. Anthropol.* 36: 199–221.

197 but they balanced all that meat with carb-rich grains: A. G. Henry, A. S. Brooks, and D. R. Piperno (2014). "Plant foods and the dietary ecology of Neanderthals and early modern humans." *J. Hum. Evol.* 69: 44–54; R. C. Power et al. (2018). "Dental calculus indicates widespread plant use within the stable Neanderthal dietary niche." *J. Hum. Evol.* 119: 27–41.

197 bread remnants dated to over 14,000 years ago: A. Arranz-Otaegui et al. (2018). "Archaeobotanical evidence reveals the origins of bread 14,400 years ago in northeastern Jordan." *PNAS* 115 (31): 7925–30. doi: 10.1073/pnas.1801071115.

198 the anthropologist George Murdock in his *Ethnographic Atlas*: G. P. Murdock, *Ethnographic Atlas* (Univ. Pittsburgh Press, 1967).

198 pillaging rodent burrows to steal their stores: S. Ståhlberg and I. Svanberg (2010). "Gathering food from rodent nests in Siberia." *J. Ethnobiol.* 30 (2): 184–202.

200 blood sugar and fat metabolism respond identically to honey: S. K. Raatz, L. K. Johnson, and M. J. Picklo (2015). "Consumption of honey, sucrose, and high-fructose corn syrup produces similar metabolic effects in glucose-tolerant and -intolerant individuals." *J. Nutr.* 145 (10): 2265–72. doi: 10.3945 /jn.115.218016.

200 they have exceptionally healthy hearts: H. Pontzer, B. M. Wood, and D. A. Raichlen (2018). "Hunter-gatherers as models in public health." *Obes. Rev.* 19 (Suppl 1): 24–35.

201 ancestral diet was only 5 percent carbs and 75 percent fat!: David Perlmutter, *Grain Brain: The Surprising Truth About Wheat, Carbs, and Sugar* (Little, Brown Spark, 2013), 35.

201 These analyses spawned a number of peer-reviewed scientific papers: L. Cordain et al. (2000). "Plant-animal subsistence ratios and macronutrient energy estimations in worldwide hunter-gatherer diets." *Am. J. Clin. Nutr.* 71: 682–92.

201 Cordain's influential book, *The Paleo Diet*: Loren Cordain, *The Paleo Diet* (John Wiley & Sons, 2002).

202 Phinney, a doctor, biochemist, and vocal advocate: S. D. Phinney (2004). "Ketogenic diets and physical performance." *Nutr. Metab.* (London) 1 (2). doi: 10.1186/1743-7075-1-2.

202 gets going only around 6,500 years ago in Africa: B. S. Arbuckle and E. L. Hammer (2018). "The rise of pastoralism in the ancient Near East." *J. Archaeol. Res.* 27: 391–449. doi: 10.1007/s10814-018-9124-8.

202 bison-hunting cultures of the Plains weren't established: D. G. Bamforth (2011). "Origin stories, archaeological evidence, and post-Clovis Paleoindian bison hunting on the Great Plains." *American Antiquity* 76 (1): 24–40.

202 Arctic cultures are even a bit younger: "Inuit Ancestor Archaeology: The Earliest Times." CHIN, 2000, accessed March 18, 2020, http://www .virtualmuseum.ca/edu/ViewLoitLo.do?method=preview&lang=EN&id=10101.

203 diets in populations like the Hadza, Tsimane, Shuar: H. Pontzer, B. M. Wood, and D. A. Raichlen (2018). "Hunter-gatherers as models in public health." *Obes. Rev.* 19 (Suppl 1): 24–35; L. Christopher et al. (2019). "High energy requirements and water throughput of adult Shuar forager-horticulturalists of Amazonian Ecuador." *Am. J. Hum. Biol.* 31: e23223. doi: 10.1002/ajhb.23223.

204 happened twice, independently, among early pastoralist groups: S. A. Tishkoff et al. (2007). "Convergent adaptation of human lactase persistence in Africa and Europe." *Nature Genetics* 39 (1): 31–40. doi: 10.1038/ng1946

204 humans have more copies of the gene that makes salivary amylase: G. H. Perry et al. (2007). "Diet and the evolution of human amylase gene copy number variation." *Nature Genetics* 39 (10): 1256–60. doi: 10.1038/ng2123.

205 decreasing levels of dietary folate: A. Sabbagh et al. (2011). "Arylamine N-acetyltransferase 2 (NAT2) genetic diversity and traditional subsistence: A worldwide population survey." *PloS One* 6 (4): e18507. doi: 10.1371/journal. pone.0018507.

205 changes in the fatty acid desaturase genes (FADS1 and 2): S. Mathieson and I. Mathieson (2018). "FADS1 and the timing of human adaptation to agriculture." *Mol. Biol. Evol.* 35 (12): 2957–70. doi: 10.1093/molbev/msy180.

205 high levels of arsenic in their groundwater: M. Apata, B. Arriaza, E. Llop, and M. Moraga (2017). "Human adaptation to arsenic in Andean populations of the Atacama Desert." *Am. J. Phys. Anthropol.* 163 (1): 192–99. doi: 10.1002/ ajpa.23193. Epub 2017 Feb 16.

205 FADS genes have changed in these groups as well: M. Fumagalli et al. (2015). "Greenlandic Inuit show genetic signatures of diet and climate adaptation." *Science* 349 (6254): 1343–47.

206 most people in these groups can't go into ketosis: F. J. Clemente et al. (2014). "A selective sweep on a deleterious mutation in CPT1A in Arctic populations." *Am. J. Hum. Gen.* 95 (5): 584–89. doi: 10.1016/j.ajhg.2014.09.016.

208 Dr. Oz is pushing "detox water": "Dr. Oz's detox water," *Women's World Magazine*, May 27, 2019.

209 "Negative calorie" foods that supposedly take more energy to digest: M. E. Clegg and C. Cooper (2012). "Exploring the myth: Does eating celery result in a negative energy balance?" *Proc. Nutr. Soc.* 71 (oce3): e217.

209 ice water won't change the amount of energy you burn: There's no evidence that the body burns extra energy to warm up ice water. Even if it did, the 240 ml in a glass of ice water (0°C) would only require 240 × 37 = 8,880 calories to warm up to body temp, or about 9 kcal.

209 caffeine in a cup of coffee: A. G. Dulloo et al. (1989). "Normal caffeine consumption: Influence on thermogenesis and daily energy expenditure in lean and postobese human volunteers." *Am. J. Clin. Nutr.* 49 (1): 44–50.

209 saturated fats and trans fats as important risk factors: L. Hooper, N. Martin, A. Abdelhamid, and G. D. Smith (2015). "Reduction in saturated fat intake for cardiovascular disease." *Cochrane Database Syst. Rev.* 6: CD011737. doi: 10.1002/14651858.CD011737; F. M. Sacks et al. (2017). "Dietary fats and cardiovascular disease: A presidential advisory from the American Heart Association." *Circulation* 136 (3): e1–e23. doi: 10.1161/CIR.0000000000000510.

210 cookbook promoting them, *The Benevolent Bean*: Margaret Keys and Ancel Keys, *The Benevolent Bean* (Doubleday, 1967).

211 insulin stimulates the conversion of excess glucose into fat: K. N. Frayn et al. (2003). "Integrative physiology of human adipose tissue." *Int. J. Obes. Relat. Metab. Disord.* 27: 875–88.

211 accumulation of fat is the cause of overeating: D. S. Ludwig and M. I. Friedman (2014). "Increasing adiposity: Consequence or cause of overeating?" *JAMA* 311: 2167–68.

212 Hall's team kept men who were overweight or obese: K. D. Hall et al. (2016). "Energy expenditure and body composition changes after an isocaloric ketogenic diet in overweight and obese men." *Am. J. Clin. Nutr.* 104 (2): 324–33. doi: 10.3945/ajcn.116.133561.

212 achieved either through cutting carbs or cutting fat: K. D. Hall et al. (2015). "Calorie for calorie, dietary fat restriction results in more body fat loss than carbohydrate restriction in people with obesity." *Cell Metabolism* 22 (3): 427–36. doi: 10.1016/j.cmet.2015.07.021.

213 no difference in daily energy expenditure: W. G. Abbott, B. V. Howard, G. Ruotolo, and E. Ravussin (1990). "Energy expenditure in humans: Effects of dietary fat and carbohydrate." *Am. J. Physiol.* 258 (2 Pt 1): E347–51.

213 DIETFITS study . . . randomly assigned 609 men and women: C. D. Gardner et al. (2018). "Effect of low-fat vs low-carbohydrate diet on 12-month weight loss in overweight adults and the association with genotype pattern or insulin secretion: The DIETFITS randomized clinical trial." *JAMA* 319 (7): 667–79. doi: 10.1001 /jama.2018.0245.

213 In the 1960s and '70s, when John Yudkin: John Yudkin, *Pure, White and Deadly: The Problem of Sugar* (Davis-Poynter, 1972).

213 Heart disease deaths, while still alarmingly high: H. K. Weir et al. (2016). "Heart disease and cancer deaths: Trends and projections in the United States, 1969–2020." *Prev. Chron. Dis.* 13: 160211.

213 the prevalence of overweight, obesity: C. D. Fryar, M. D. Carroll, and C. L. Ogden, "Prevalence of Overweight, Obesity, and Extreme Obesity Among Adults Aged 20 and Over: United States, 1960–1962 Through 2013–2014," Centers for Disease Control and Prevention, July 18, 2016, accessed March 18, 2020, https: //www.cdc.gov/nchs/data/hestat/obesity_adult_13_14/obesity_adult_13_14.htm.

213 diabetes have continued to climb: CDC's Division of Diabetes Translation, "Long-term Trends in Diabetes April 2017," April 2017, accessed March 18, 2020, https://www.cdc.gov/diabetes/statistics/slides/long_term_trends.pdf.

213 even as people eat less sugar: "Food Availability (Per Capita) Data System," USDA Economic Research Service, last updated January 9, 2020, accessed March 18, 2020, https://www.ers.usda.gov/data-products /food-availability-per-capita-data-system/.

214 In China, the percentage of calories from fats has risen: J. Zhao et al. (2018). "Secular trends in energy and macronutrient intakes and distribution among adult females (1991–2015): Results from the China Health and Nutrition Survey." *Nutrients* 10 (2): 115.

214 obesity and diabetes have steadily climbed: R. C. W. Ma (2018). "Epidemiology of diabetes and diabetic complications in China." *Diabetologia* 61: 1249–60. doi: 10.1007/s00125-018-4557-7.

214 obesity and metabolic disease have taken hold: T. Bhurosy and R. Jeewon (2014). "Overweight and obesity epidemic in developing countries: A problem with diet, physical activity, or socioeconomic status?" *Sci. World J.* 2014: 964236. doi: 10.1155/2014/964236.

214 Ludwig and colleagues examined metabolic rates: C. B. Ebbeling et al. (2018). "Effects of a low carbohydrate diet on energy expenditure during weight loss maintenance: Randomized trial." *BMJ* (Clinical research ed.) 363: k4583. doi: 10.1136/bmj.k4583.

214 reanalysis of their data by Kevin Hall: K. D. Hall (2019). "Mystery or method? Evaluating claims of increased energy expenditure during a ketogenic diet." *PloS One* 14 (12): e0225944. doi: 10.1371/journal.pone.0225944.

215 the ratio of carbs to fats has little or no effect: K. D. Hall and J. Guo (2017). "Obesity energetics: Body weight regulation and the effects of diet composition." *Gastroenterology* 152 (7): 1718–27.e3. doi: 10.1053/j.gastro.2017.01.052.

215 calories from sugar (including high fructose corn syrup): T. A. Khan, and J. L Sievenpiper (2016). "Controversies about sugars: Results from systematic reviews and meta-analyses on obesity, cardiometabolic disease and diabetes." *Eur. J. Nutr.* 55 (Suppl 2): 25–43. doi: 10.1007/s00394-016-1345-3.

216 leads to water loss and a rapid reduction in body weight: S. N. Kreitzman, A. Y. Coxon, and K. F. Szaz (1992). "Glycogen storage: Illusions of easy weight loss, excessive weight regain, and distortions in estimates of body composition." *Am. J. Clin. Nutr.* 56 (1 Suppl): 292S–93S. doi: 10.1093/ajcn/56.1.292S.

217 one of four popular diets for twelve months: M. L. Dansinger et al. (2005). "Comparison of the Atkins, Ornish, Weight Watchers, and Zone diets for weight loss and heart disease risk reduction: A randomized trial." *JAMA* 293 (1): 43–53. doi: 10.1001/jama.293.1.43.

217 Penn Jillette reportedly lost over a hundred pounds: Susan Rinkunas, "Eating Only One Food to Lose Weight Is a Terrible Idea," The Cut, August 16, 2009, accessed March 18, 2020, https://www.thecut.com/2016/08/mono-diet -potato-diet-penn-jillette.html.

217 followed a junk food diet for ten weeks: Madison Park, "Twinkie diet helps nutrition professor lose 27 pounds," CNN, November 8, 2010, http://www.cnn .com/2010/HEALTH/11/08/twinkie.diet.professor/index.html.

218 low-carb diets were used to treat diabetes: William Morgan, *Diabetes Mellitus: Its History, Chemistry, Anatomy, Pathology, Physiology, and Treatment* (The Homoeopathic Publishing Company, 1877).

218 eliminated their need for insulin and other diabetes medication: S. J. Athinarayanan et al. (2019). "Long-term effects of a novel continuous remote care intervention including nutritional ketosis for the management of type 2 diabetes: A 2-year non-randomized clinical trial." *Fron. Endocrinol.* 10: 348. doi: 10.3389/fendo.2019.00348.

218 weight loss can reverse type 2 diabetes: R. Taylor, A. Al-Mrabeh, and N. Sattar (2019). "Understanding the mechanisms of reversal of type 2 diabetes." *Lancet Diab. Endocrinol.* 7 (9): 726–36. doi: 10.1016/S2213-8587(19)30076-2.

219 intermittent fasting diets are no more successful: I. Cioffi et al. (2018). "Intermittent versus continuous energy restriction on weight loss and cardiometabolic outcomes: A systematic review and meta-analysis of randomized controlled trials." *J. Transl. Med.* 16: 371. doi: 10.1186/s12967-018-1748-4.

220 a thorough and engaging book, *The Hungry Brain*: Stephan Guyenet, *The Hungry Brain: Outsmarting the Instincts That Make Us Overeat* (Flatiron Books, 2017).

221 respond strongly to food, particularly fat and sugar: M. Alonso-Alonso et al. (2015). "Food reward system: Current perspectives and future research needs." *Nutr. Rev.* 73 (5): 296–307. doi: 10.1093/nutrit/nuv002.

222 Protein intake is monitored as well: M. Journel et al. (2012). "Brain responses to high-protein diets." *Advances in Nutrition* (Bethesda, Md.) 3 (3): 322–29. doi: 10.3945/an.112.002071.

222 which communicates with the hypothalamus: K. Timper and J. C. Brüning (2017). "Hypothalamic circuits regulating appetite and energy homeostasis: Pathways to obesity." *Disease Models & Mechanisms* 10 (6): 679–89. doi: 10.1242/dmm.026609.

223 they will inevitably overeat and get fat: A. Sclafani and D, Springer (1976). "Dietary obesity in adult rats: Similarities to hypothalamic and human obesity syndromes." *Physiol. Behav.* 17 (3): 461–71.

223 from monkeys to elephants, and, unsurprisingly, in humans: Monkeys: P. B. Higgins et al. (2010). "Eight week exposure to a high sugar high fat diet results in adiposity gain and alterations in metabolic biomarkers in baboons (*Papio hamadryas* sp.)." *Cardiovasc. Diabetol.* 9: 71. doi: 10.1186/1475-2840-9-71; **Elephants:** K. A. Morfeld, C. L. Meehan, J. N. Hogan, and J. L. Brown (2016). "Assessment of body condition in African (*Loxodonta africana*) and Asian (*Elephas maximus*) elephants in North American zoos and management practices associated with high body condition scores." *PLoS One* 11: e0155146. doi: 10.1371/journal. pone.0155146; **Humans:** R. Rising et al. (1992). "Food intake measured by an automated food-selection system: Relationship to energy expenditure." *Am. J. Clin. Nutr.* 55 (2): 343–49.

223 sugars and oils are the two leading sources of calories: S. A. Bowman et al., "Retail Food Commodity Intakes: Mean Amounts of Retail Commodities per Individual, 2007–08," USDA Agricultural Research Service and USDA Economic Research Service, 2013.

224 foods that always leave you wanting more: George Dvorsky, "How Flavor Chemists Make Your Food So Addictively Good," Gizmodo, November 8, 2012, accessed March 18, 2020, https://io9.gizmodo.com /how-flavor-chemists-make-your-food-so-addictively-good-5958880.

224 just how powerful processed foods can be: K. D. Hall et al. (2019). "Ultra-processed diets cause excess calorie intake and weight gain: An inpatient randomized controlled trial of ad libitum food intake." *Cell Metabol.* 30 (1): 67–77.e3.

225 explains the increase in the average weight: S. H. Holt, J. C. Miller, P. Petocz, and E. Farmakalidis (1995). "A satiety index of common foods." *Eur. J. Clin. Nutr.* 49 (9): 675–90.

225 they gain similar amounts of fat: C. Bouchard et al. (1990). "The response to long-term overfeeding in identical twins." *N. Engl. J. Med.* 322 (21): 1477–82.

225 Twins respond in similar ways to underfeeding: A. Tremblay et al. (1997). "Endurance training with constant energy intake in identical twins: Changes over time in energy expenditure and related hormones." *Metabolism* 46 (5): 499–503.

225 nine hundred gene variants associated with obesity: L. Yengo et al. and the GIANT Consortium (2018). "Meta-analysis of genome-wide association studies for height and body mass index in ~700000 individuals of European ancestry." *Hum. Mol. Gen.* 27 (20): 3641–49. doi: 10.1093/hmg/ddy271.

226 in 1995 tested thirty-eight different foods: S. H. Holt, J. C. Miller, P. Petocz, and E. Farmakalidis (1995). "A satiety index of common foods." *Eur. J. Clin. Nutr.* 49 (9): 675–90.

227 people eat more after a stressful experience: B. Hitze et al. (2010). "How the selfish brain organizes its supply and demand." *Frontiers in Neuroenergetics* 2: 7. doi: 10.3389/fnene.2010.00007.

227 gain an average of one to two pounds over the holidays: E. E. Helander, B. Wansink, and A. Chieh (2016). "Weight gain over the holidays in three countries." *N. Engl. J. Med.* 375 (12): 1200–2. doi: 10.1056/NEJMc1602012.

227 poverty and lack of opportunity are so strongly associated: K. A. Scott, S. J. Melhorn, and R. R. Sakai (2012). "Effects of chronic social stress on obesity." *Curr. Obes. Rep.* 1: 16–25.

229 Hadza eat about five times as much fiber each day: H. Pontzer, B. M. Wood, and D. A. Raichlen (2018). "Hunter-gatherers as models in public health." *Obes. Rev.* 19 (Suppl 1): 24–35.

229 which likely helps protect them against heart disease: L. Hooper, N. Martin, A. Abdelhamid, and G. D. Smith (2015). "Reduction in saturated fat intake for cardiovascular disease." *Cochrane Database Syst. Rev.* 6: CD011737. doi: 10.1002/14651858.CD011737.

Chapter 7: Run for Your Life!

235 great apes get nine or ten hours of sleep each night: C. L. Nunn and D. R. Samson (2018). "Sleep in a comparative context: Investigating how human sleep differs from sleep in other primates." *Am. J. Phys. Anthropol.* 166 (3): 601–12.

235 chimpanzees climb about 330 feet per day: H. Pontzer and R. W. Wrangham (2014). "Climbing and the daily energy cost of locomotion in wild chimpanzees: Implications for hominoid locomotor evolution." *J. Hum. Evol.* 46 (3): 317–35.

235 Apes don't develop hardened vessels or have heart attacks: K. Kawanishi et al. (2019). "Human species-specific loss of CMP-N-acetylneuraminic acid hydroxylase enhances atherosclerosis via intrinsic and extrinsic mechanisms." *PNAS* 116 (32): 16036–45. doi: 10.1073/pnas.1902902116.

237 men who can do more than ten pushups in one go: Justin Yang et al. (2019). "Association between push-up exercise capacity and future cardiovascular events among active adult men." *JAMA* Network Open 2 (2): e188341. doi: 10.1001/jamanetworkopen.2018.8341.

237 Older adults who can cover at least 1,200 feet: A. Yazdanyar et al. (2014) "Association between 6-minute walk test and all-cause mortality, coronary heart disease-specific mortality, and incident coronary heart disease." *Journal of Aging and Health* 26 (4): 583–99. doi: 10.1177/0898264314525665.

237 Vigorous activity, defined as anything demanding 6 METS: "Examples of Moderate and Vigorous Physical Activity," Harvard T. H. Chan School of Public Health, accessed March 20, 2020, https://www.hsph.harvard.edu/obesity -prevention-source/moderate-and-vigorous-physical-activity/.

237 triggering the release of nitric oxide: G. Schuler, V. Adams, and Y. Goto (2013). "Role of exercise in the prevention of cardiovascular disease: Results, mechanisms, and new perspectives." *Eur. Heart J.* 34: 1790–99.

238 slowing the rate of cognitive decline: G. Kennedy et al. (2017). "How does exercise reduce the rate of age-associated cognitive decline? A review of potential mechanisms." *J. Alzheimers Dis.* 55 (1): 1–18. doi: 10.3233/JAD-160665.

238 walking and running improve cognitive function: D. A. Raichlen and G. E. Alexander (2017). "Adaptive capacity: An evolutionary neuroscience model linking exercise, cognition, and brain health." *Trends Neurosci.* 40 (7): 408–21. doi: 10.1016/j.tins.2017.05.001.

238 Dan Lieberman details in his book *Exercised*: Daniel Lieberman, *Exercised: Why Something We Never Evolved to Do Is Healthy and Rewarding* (Pantheon, 2020).

238 exercising muscles release hundreds of molecules: M. Whitham et al. (2018). "Extracellular vesicles provide a means for tissue crosstalk during exercise." *Cell Metab.* 27 (1): 237–51.e4.

240 subjected adult male mice to different degrees of calorie restriction: S. E. Mitchell et al. (2015). "The effects of graded levels of calorie restriction: I. Impact of short term calorie and protein restriction on body composition in the C57BL/6 mouse." *Oncotarget* 6: 15902–30.

240 children fighting an infection increase the energy spent: S. S. Urlacher et al. (2018). "Tradeoffs between immune function and childhood growth among Amazonian forager-horticulturalists." *PNAS* 115 (17): E3914–21. doi: 10.1073 /pnas.1717522115.

240 When exercise starts to take up a large chunk: H. Pontzer (2018). "Energy constraint as a novel mechanism linking exercise and health." *Physiology* 33 (6): 384–93.

242 exercise is an effective way to lower chronic inflammation: M. Gleeson et al. (2011). "The anti-inflammatory effects of exercise: Mechanisms and implications for the prevention and treatment of disease." *Nat. Rev. Immunol.* 11: 607–15.

242 used public speaking to induce a stress response: U. Rimmele et al. (2007). "Trained men show lower cortisol, heart rate and psychological responses to psychosocial stress compared with untrained men." *Psychoneuroendocrinology* 32: 627–35.

243 a study of college-age women with moderate depression: C. Nabkasorn et al. (2006). "Effects of physical exercise on depression, neuroendocrine stress hormones and physiological fitness in adolescent females with depressive symptoms." *Eur. J. Publ. Health* 16: 179–84.

244 endurance runners to age-matched sedentary men: A. C. Hackney (2020). "Hypogonadism in exercising males: Dysfunction or adaptive-regulatory adjustment?" *Front. Endocrinol.* 11: 11. doi: 10.3389/fendo.2020.00011.

244 most effective ways to decrease the risk of cancers: J. C. Brown, K. Winters-Stone, A. Lee, and K. H. Schmitz (2012). "Cancer, physical activity, and exercise." *Compr Physiol.* 2: 2775–809.

245 doping was present at the birth of competitive cycling: Lorella Vittozzi, "Historical Evolution of the Doping Phenomenon," *Report on the I.O.A.'s Special Sessions and Seminars 1997,* International Olympic Academy, 1997, 68–70.

246 testosterone and its synthetic relatives accounted for 45 percent: R. I. Wood and S. J. Stanton (2012). "Testosterone and sport: Current perspectives." *Horm. Behav.* 61 (1): 147–55. doi: 10.1016/j.yhbeh.2011.09.010.

247 food supplements to thirty-on women endurance athletes: K. Lagowska, K. Kapczuk, Z. Friebe, and J. Bajerska (2014). "Effects of dietary intervention in young female athletes with menstrual disorders." *J. Int. Soc. Sports Nutr.* 11: 21.

249 Hadza men and women average around 16,000 steps: B. M. Wood et al. (2018). "Step counts from satellites: Methods for integrating accelerometer and GPS data for more accurate measures of pedestrian travel." *J. Meas. Phys. Behav.* 3 (1): 58–66.

250 rack up less than two hours of physical activity: Estimated amount of time to cover their customary 2 to 3 km per day walking and about 100 meters climbing: H. Pontzer. "Locomotor Ecology and Evolution in Chimpanzees and Humans." In Martin N. Muller, Richard W. Wrangham, and David R. Pilbeam, eds., *Chimpanzees in Human Evolution* (Harvard Univ. Press, 2017), 259–85.

250 They average around 5,000 steps per day: Chimpanzees cover roughly half a meter per step: H. Pontzer, D. A. Raichlen, and P. S. Rodman (2014). "Bipedal and quadrupedal locomotion in chimpanzees." *J. Hum. Evol.* 66: 64–82.

250 followed nearly 5,000 U.S. adults for five to eight years: P. F. Saint-Maurice et al. (2018). "Moderate-to-vigorous physical activity and all-cause mortality: Do bouts matter?" *J. Am. Heart Assoc.* 7(6): e007678. doi: 10.1161/JAHA.117.007678.

250 study of 150,000 Australian adults: E. Stamatakis et al. (2019). "Sitting time, physical activity, and risk of mortality in adults." *J. Am. Coll. Cardiol.* 73 (16): 2062–72. doi: 10.1016/j.jacc.2019.02.031.

250 the famed Copenhagen Heart Study: P. Schnohr et al. (2015). "Dose of jogging and long-term mortality: The Copenhagen City Heart Study." *J. Am. Coll. Cardiol.* 65 (5): 411–19. doi: 10.1016/j.jacc.2014.11.023.

251 a study of postal workers in Glasgow: W. Tigbe, M. Granat, N. Sattar, and M. Lean (2017). "Time spent in sedentary posture is associated with waist circumference and cardiovascular risk." *Int. J. Obes.* 41: 689–96. doi: 10.1038/ijo.2017.30.

251 one of the lowest life expectancies in Western Europe: "Scotland's public health priorities," Scottish Government, Population Health Directorate, 2018, accessed March 20, 2020, https://www.gov.scot/publications/scotlands-public-health-priorities/pages/2/.

251 traditional populations sleep about as much: G. Yetish et al. (2015) "Natural sleep and its seasonal variations in three pre-industrial societies." *Curr. Biol.* 25 (21): 2862–68. doi: 10.1016/j.cub.2015.09.046.

251 increase our risk of cardiometabolic disease: A. W. McHill et al. (2014) "Impact of circadian misalignment on energy metabolism during simulated nightshift work." *PNAS* 111 (48): 17302–07. doi: 10.1073/pnas.1412021111.

251 Hadza adults also accumulate the same amount of resting: D. A. Raichlen et al. (2020) "Sitting, squatting, and the evolutionary biology of human inactivity." *PNAS*, Epub ahead of print. doi: 10.1073/pnas.1911868117.

253 billionaire recluse who lives for months in the dark: Wikipedia, accessed March 20, 2020, https://en.wikipedia.org/wiki/Howard_Hughes.

253 teamed up with a dietician and medical officer: J. Mayer, P. Roy, and K. P. Mitra (1956). "Relation between caloric intake, body weight, and physical work: Studies in an industrial male population in West Bengal." *Am. J. Clin. Nutr.* 4 (2): 169–75.

253 followed nearly two thousand men and women: L. R. Dugas et al. (2017). "Accelerometer-measured physical activity is not associated with two-year weight change in African-origin adults from five diverse populations." *Peer J.* 5: e2902. doi: 10.7717/peerj.2902.

254 the brain regulates hunger and metabolism: A. Prentice and S. Jebb (2004). "Energy intake/physical activity interactions in the homeostasis of body weight regulation." *Nutr. Rev.* 62: S98–104.

255 attributable to sedentary lifestyles: I. Lee et al. (2012). "Effect of physical inactivity on major non-communicable diseases worldwide: An analysis of burden of disease and life expectancy." *Lancet* (London) 380 (9838): 219–29. doi: 10.1016/S0140-6736(12)61031-9.

255 a study of obese policemen in Boston: K. Pavlou, S. Krey, and W. P. Steffee (1989). "Exercise as an adjunct to weight loss and maintenance in moderately obese subjects." *Am. J. Clin. Nutr.* 49: 1115–23.

255 National Weight Control Registry: "The National Weight Control Registry," accessed March 20, 2020, http://www.nwcr.ws/.

257 Registry members spent nearly an hour more each day: D. M. Ostendorf et al. (2018). "Objectively measured physical activity and sedentary behavior in successful weight loss maintainers." *Obesity* 26 (1): 53–60. doi: 10.1002/oby.22052.

Chapter 8: Energetics at the Extreme: The Limits of Human Endurance

262 only eight had completed the crossing: Ocean Rowing, "Atlantic Ocean Crossings West–East from Canada," August 4, 2018, accessed March 21, 2020, http://www.oceanrowing.com/statistics/Atlantic_W-E__from_Canada.htm.

262 Bryce ate between 4,000 and 5,000 kilocalories: Christopher Mele, "Ohio teacher sets record for rowing alone across the Atlantic," *New York Times*, August

6, 2018, accessed March 21, 2020, https://www.nytimes.com/2018/08/06/world/bryce-carlson-rows-atlantic-ocean.html.

262 Tour de France cyclists burn 8,500 kilocalories: K. R. Westerterp, W. H. Saris, M. van Es, and F. ten Hoor (1986). "Use of the doubly labeled water technique in humans during heavy sustained exercise." *J. App. Physiol.* 61 (6): 2162–67.

262 Triathletes can burn that much energy: B. C. Ruby et al. (2015). "Extreme endurance and the metabolic range of sustained activity is uniquely available for every human not just the elite few." *Comp. Exer. Physiol.* 11(1): 1–7.

263 reportedly ate 12,000 kcal each day: Mun Keat Looi, "How Olympic swimmers can keep eating such insane quantities of food," Quartz, August 10, 2016, accessed March 21, 2020, https://qz.com/753956/how-olympic-swimmers-can-keep-eating-such-insane-quantities-of-food/.

263 Alex Hutchinson's excellent book, *Endure*: Alex Hutchinson, *Endure: Mind, Body, and the Curiously Elastic Limits of Human Performance* (William Morrow, 2018).

264 mental fatigue reduces endurance: See S. Marcora et al. (2018). "The effect of mental fatigue on critical power during cycling exercise." *Eur. J. App. Physiol.* 118 (1): 85–92. doi: 10.1007/s00421-017-3747-1.

266 type of fuel your body burns during exercise: J. A. Romijn et al. (1993). "Regulation of endogenous fat and carbohydrate metabolism in relation to exercise intensity and duration." *Am. J. Physiol.* 265: E380–91.

268 eating your dogs one by one: Mike Dash, "The most terrible polar exploration ever: Douglas Mawson's Antarctic journey," *Smithsonian,* January 27, 2012, accessed March 21, 2020, https://www.smithsonianmag.com/history/the-most-terrible-polar-exploration-ever-douglas-mawsons-antarctic-journey-82192685/.

271 averaging an incredible 6,200 kcal per day: C. Thurber et al. (2019). "Extreme events reveal an alimentary limit on sustained maximal human energy expenditure." *Science Advances* 5 (6): eaaw0341. doi: 10.1126/sciadv.aaw0341.

271 showing up in the AEE component: See, for example: H. Pontzer et al. (2016). "Constrained total energy expenditure and metabolic adaptation to physical activity in adult humans." *Curr. Biol.* 26 (3): 410–17. doi: 10.1016/j.cub.2015.12.046; S. S. Urlacher et al. (2019). "Constraint and trade-offs regulate energy expenditure during childhood." *Science Advances* 5 (12): eaax1065. doi: 10.1126/sciadv.aax1065.

272 non-exercise activity thermogenesis, or NEAT: J. A. Levine (2002). "Non-exercise activity thermogenesis (NEAT)." *Best Pract. Res. Clin. Endocrinol. Metab.* 16 (4): 679–702.

272 studies measuring the NEAT response to exercise: E. L. Melanson (2017). "The effect of exercise on non-exercise physical activity and sedentary behavior in adults." *Obes. Rev.* 18: 40–49. doi: 10.1111/obr.12507.

272 a daily roller-coaster trajectory: K.-M. Zitting et al. (2018). "Human resting energy expenditure varies with circadian phase." *Curr. Biol.* 28 (22): 3685–90.e3. doi: 10.1016/j.cub.2018.10.005.

275 he shaved mouse mothers with nursing pups: E. Król, M. Murphy, and J. R. Speakman (2007). "Limits to sustained energy intake. X. Effects of fur removal on reproductive performance in laboratory mice." *J. Exp. Biol.* 210 (23): 4233–43.

277 injecting intravenous doses of lipids and glucose: "The Dutch Doping Scandal—Part 3," Cycling News, November 29, 1977, accessed March 21, 2020, http://autobus.cyclingnews.com/results/archives/nov97/nov29a.html.

278 mom is being pushed to the brink: H. M. Dunsworth et al. (2012). "Metabolic hypothesis for human altriciality." *PNAS* 109 (38): 15212–16. doi: 10.1073/pnas.1205282109.

278 affecting this metabolic trigger: J. C. K. Wells, J. M. DeSilva, and J. T. Stock (2012). "The obstetric dilemma: an ancient game of Russian roulette, or a variable dilemma sensitive to ecology?" *Am. J. Phys. Anthropol.* 149 (55): 40–71. doi: 10.1002/ajpa.22160.

280 12,000 kcal per day figure floating around: Curtis Charles, "Michael Phelps reveals his 12,000-calorie diet was a myth, but he still ate so much food," *USA Today*, June 16, 2017, accessed March 21, 2020, https://ftw.usatoday.com/2017/06/michael-phelps-diet-12000-calories-myth-but-still-ate-8000-to-10000-quote.

281 Katie Ledecky, another star Olympic swimmer: Sabrina Marques, "Here's how many calories Olympic swimmer Katie Ledecky eats in a day. It's not your typical 19-year-old's diet," Spooniversity, accessed March 21, 2020, https://spoonuniversity.com/lifestyle/this-is-what-olympic-swimmer-katie-ledecky-s-diet-is-like.

281 Michael Phelps is a large guy, well above average: Ishan Daftardar, "Scientific analysis of Michael Phelps's body structure," Science ABC, July 2, 2015, March 21, 2020, https://www.scienceabc.com/sports/michael-phelps-height-arms-torso-arm-span-feet-swimming.html.

282 the earliest avian ancestors as insulation: M. J. Benton et al. (2019). "The early origin of feathers." *Trends in Ecology & Evolution* 34 (9): 856–69.

282 human ancestors began walking on two legs: Charles Darwin, *The Descent of Man: And Selection in Relation to Sex* (J. Murray, 1871).

283 the French Academy famously banned any discussion: S. Számadó and E. Szathmáry (2004). "Language evolution." *PLoS Biology* 2 (10): e346. doi: 10.1371/journal.pbio.0020346.

Chapter 9: The Past, Present, and Uncertain Future of *Homo energeticus*

285 for any trip longer than a mile: Y. Yang and A. V. Diez-Roux (2012). "Walking distance by trip purpose and population subgroups." *Am. J. Prev. Med.* 43 (1): 11–19. doi: 10.1016/j.amepre.2012.03.015.

287 over five million kilocalories worth of jet fuel: A Boeing 747 on an 8,800 mile flight burns 6,000 kilowatt hours per passenger: David J. C. MacKay, *Sustainable Energy: Without the Hot Air* (UIT Cambridge Ltd, 2009), https://www.withouthotair.com/c5/page_35.shtml.

288 existential crises: obesity and climate change: "Syndemics: Health in context." *Lancet* 389 (10072): 881.

290 discovery of fossil remains from an extinct hominin: L. S. B. Leakey, P. V. Tobias, and J. R. Napier (1964). "A new species of the genus *Homo* from Olduvai Gorge." *Nature* 202: 7–9.

290 Discoveries over the subsequent decades: Glenn C. Conroy and Herman Pontzer, *Reconstructing Human Origins: A Modern Synthesis*, 3rd ed. (W. W. Norton, 2012).

291 the force with which they pull the bowstring: H. Pontzer et al. (2017). "Mechanics of archery among Hadza hunter-gatherers." *J. Archaeol. Sci.* 16: 57–64. doi: 10.1016/j.jasrep.2017.09.025.

292 *Homo erectus*, over a million years ago: F. Berna et al. (2012). "Acheulean fire at Wonderwerk Cave." *PNAS* 109 (20): E1215–20. doi: 10.1073/pnas.1117620109.

292 puts the date at around 400,000 years ago: W. Roebroeks and P. Villa (2011). "On the earliest evidence for habitual use of fire in Europe." *PNAS* 108 (13): 5209–14. doi: 10.1073/pnas.1018116108.

293 his excellent book *Catching Fire*: Richard Wrangham, *Catching Fire: How Cooking Made Us Human* (Basic Books, 2010).

293 Wood fires release about 1,600 kcal per pound of fuel: Wikipedia, accessed March 22, 2020, https://en.wikipedia.org/wiki/Wood_fuel.

293 men and women following raw food diets: C. Koebnick, C. Strassner, I. Hoffmann, and C. Leitzmann (1999). "Consequences of a long-term raw food diet on body weight and menstruation: Results of a questionnaire survey." *Ann. Nutr. Metab.* 43: 69–79.

294 Fires could be used to change the landscape: D. W. Bird, R. Bliege Bird, and B. F. Codding (2016). "Pyrodiversity and the anthropocene: The role of fire in the broad spectrum revolution." *Evol. Anthropol.* 25: 105–16. doi: 10.1002/evan.21482; F. Scherjon, C. Bakels, K. MacDonald, and W. Roebroeks (2015). "Burning the land: An ethnographic study of off-site fire use by current and historically documented foragers and implications for the interpretation of past fire practices in the landscape." *Curr. Anthropol.* 56 (3): 299–326.

295 learned to use kilns to made bitumen: P. R. B. Kozowyk et al. (2017). "Experimental methods for the Palaeolithic dry distillation of birch bark: Implications for the origin and development of Neandertal adhesive technology." *Sci. Rep.* 7: 8033. doi: 10.1038/s41598-017-08106-7.

295 building fires hot enough to fire pottery: Cristian Violatti, "Pottery in Antiquity," Ancient History Encyclopedia, September 13, 2014, accessed March 22, 2020, https://www.ancient.eu/pottery/.

295 smelt ore to make copper and other metals: "Smelting," Wikipedia, accessed March 22, 2020, https://en.wikipedia.org/wiki/Smelting.

295 figured out how to make iron and glass: "History of Glass," Wikipedia, accessed March 22, 2020, https://en.wikipedia.org/wiki/History_of_glass.

295 converge on a game-changing insight: J. Diamond and P. Bellwood (2003). "Farmers and their languages: The first expansions." *Science* 300 (5619): 597–603.

297 a horse can comfortably produce around 640 kcal of work: R. D. Stevenson and R. J. Wassersug (1993). "Horsepower from a horse." *Nature* 364: 6434.

297 She could do the work of ten men: Eugene A. Avallone et al, *Marks' Standard Handbook for Mechanical Engineers*, 11th ed. (McGraw-Hill, 2007).

297 On horseback, a person could easily cover thirty miles in a day: Nicky Ellis, "How far can a horse travel in a day?" Horses & Foals, April 15, 2019, accessed March 22, 2020, https://horsesandfoals.com/how-far-can-a-horse-travel-in-a-day/.

298 fertility rates accelerated: J.-P. Bocquet-Appel (2011). "When the world's population took off: The springboard of the Neolithic demographic transition." *Science* 333 (6042): 560–61. doi: 10.1126/science.1208880.

298 A typical Hadza woman will have six children: N. G. Blurton Jones et al. (1992). "Demography of the Hadza, an increasing and high density population of savanna foragers." *Am. J. Phys. Anthropol.* 89 (2): 159–81.

298 a Tsimane woman, with the caloric benefits: M. Gurven et al. (2017). "The Tsimane Health and Life History Project: Integrating anthropology and biomedicine." *Evol. Anthropol.* 26 (2): 54–73. doi: 10.1002/evan.21515.

298 calls the collective brain: M. Muthukrishna and J. Henrich (2016). "Innovation in the collective brain." *Phil. Trans. R. Soc.* B 371: 20150192. doi: /10.1098/rstb.2015.0192.

298 how to harness the power of the wind to sail: Oldest evidence for sailing is from around 7,500 years ago in the Persian Gulf; see R. Carter (2006). "Boat remains and maritime trade in the Persian Gulf during the sixth and fifth millennia BC." *Antiquity* 80 (3071): 52–63. Also see "Ancient Maritime History," Wikipedia, accessed March 22, 2020, https://en.wikipedia.org/wiki/Ancient_maritime_history.

298 harness the energy of a flowing river: "Watermill," Wikipedia, accessed March 22, 2020, https://en.wikipedia.org/wiki/Watermill.

299 Windmills joined them a few centuries later: "Windmill," Wikipedia, accessed March 22, 2020, https://en.wikipedia.org/wiki/Windmill.

299 fossil fuels combine to provide over 35,000 kcal of energy: Energy data: "World Energy Balances 2019," International Energy Agency, accessed March 23, 2020, https://www.iea.org/data-and-statistics; **Population data:** "World Population Prospects 2017," United Nations, Department of Economic and Social Affairs, Population Division, 2017—Data Booklet (ST/ESA/SER.A/401), accessed April 28, 2020, https://population.un.org/wpp/Publications/Files/WPP2017_DataBooklet.pdf.

299 farmers made up 69 percent of the American workforce: U.S. Census Bureau, *Historical Statistics of the United States 1780–1945* (1949), 74, accessed March 23, 2020, https://www2.census.gov/prod2/statcomp/documents/HistoricalStatisticsoftheUnitedStates1789-1945.pdf.

299 farmers and ranchers make up only 1.3 percent: 2.6 million farmers in 2018: "Ag and Food Sectors and the Economy," USDA Economic Research Service, March 3, 2020, accessed March 23, 2020, https://www.ers.usda.gov/data-products/ag-and-food-statistics-charting-the-essentials/ag-and-food-sectors-and-the-economy/; **the U.S. population in 2018 was 327 million:** U.S. and World Population Clock, accessed March 23, 2020, https://www.census.gov/popclock/.

300 consumes roughly 500 trillion kilocalories each year: Randy Schnepf, *Energy Use in Agriculture: Background and Issues*, Congressional Research Service Report for Congress, November 19, 2004, accessed March 23, 2020, https://nationalaglawcenter.org/wp-content/uploads/assets/crs/RL32677.pdf.

300 Hadza adults acquire about 1,000 to 1,500 kcal per hour of foraging: Hadza and Tsimane rates of food energy acquisition (Figure 9.2) calculated from production and activity data: Frank W. Marlowe, *The Hadza: Hunter-Gatherers of Tanzania* (Univ. of California Press, 2010); M. Gurven et al. (2013) "Physical activity and modernization among Bolivian Amerindians." *PloS One* 8 (1): e55679. doi: 10.1371/journal.pone.0055679.

301 a manufacturing job could buy you more than 3,000 kcal: E. L. Chao, and K. P. Utgoff, *100 Years of U.S. Consumer Spending: Data for the Nation, New York City, and Boston*, U.S. Department of Labor, 2006, accessed March 23, 2020, https://www.bls.gov/opub/100-years-of-u-s-consumer-spending.pdf.

302 Sugar was a luxury item: Anup Shah, "Sugar," Global Issues, April 25, 2003, accessed March 23, 2020, https://www.globalissues.org/article/239/sugar.

302 the most calories per gram are also the cheapest: A. Drewnowski and S. E. Specter (2004). "Poverty and obesity: The role of energy density and energy costs." *Am. J. Clin. Nutr.* 79 (1): 6–16.

302 beet sugar and high-fructose corn syrup: S. A. Bowman et al., "Retail food commodity intakes: Mean amounts of retail commodities per individual, 2007–08," USDA, Agricultural Research Service, Beltsville, MD, and USDA, Economic Research Service, Washington, D.C., 2013.

302 The energy density of an industrialized diet: H. Pontzer, B. M. Wood, D. A. Raichlen (2018). "Hunter-gatherers as models in public health." *Obes. Rev.* 19 (Suppl 1):24–35.

303 median time between births: C. E. Copen, M. E. Thoma, and S. Kirmeyer (2015). "Interpregnancy intervals in the United States: Data from the birth certificate and the National Survey of Family Growth." *National Vital Statistics Reports* 64 (3).

303 half a year shorter than we see among the Tsimane: A. D. Blackwell et al. "Helminth infection, fecundity, and age of first pregnancy in women." *Science* 350 (6263): 970–72. doi: 10.1126/science.aac7902.

303 cultural and biological factors behind this change: O. Galor (2012). "The demographic transition: Causes and consequences." *Cliometrica* 6 (1): 1–28. doi: 10.1007/s11698-011-0062-7.

304 40 calories of food for every calorie they spend foraging: H. Pontzer (2012). "Relating ranging ecology, limb length, and locomotor economy in terrestrial animals." *Journal of Theoretical Biology* 296: 6–12. doi:10.1016 /j.jtbi.2011.11.018.

304 we burn 8 calories for every calorie of food we produce: "U.S. Food System Factsheet," Center for Sustainable Systems, University of Michigan, 2019. http:// css.umich.edu/sites/default/files/Food%20System_CSS01-06_e2019.pdf.

304 we consume a staggering 25 *quadrillion* kilocalories: "U.S. energy facts explained," U.S. Energy Information Administration, accessed March 23, 2020, https://www.eia.gov/energyexplained/us-energy-facts/.

304 In a few countries, per capita energy consumption: Data and Statistics, "Total primary energy supply (TPES) by source, World 1990–2017," International Energy Agency, 2019, accessed March 23, 2020, https://www.iea.org/data-and -statistics.

305 we've got around fifty years' worth of oil and natural gas: Hannah Ritchie and Max Roser, "Fossil Fuels," Our World in Data, 2020, https://ourworldindata .org/fossil-fuels.

305 the Earth 0.8°C (1.4°F) warmer than it was in the late 1800s: National Academy of Sciences, *Climate Change: Evidence and Causes* (National Academies Press, 2014). doi: 10.17226/18730.

305 an additional 8°C warming globally: R. Winkelmann et al. (2015). "Combustion of available fossil fuel resources sufficient to eliminate the Antarctic ice sheet." *Science Advances* 1 (8): e1500589. doi: 10.1126/sciadv.1500589; K. Tokarska et al. (2016). "The climate response to five trillion tonnes of carbon." *Nature Clim. Change* 6: 851–55. doi: 10.1038/nclimate3036.

305 during the Paleocene-Eocene Thermal Maximum: J. P. Kennett and L. D. Stott, "Terminal Paleocene Mass Extinction in the Deep Sea: Association with Global Warming," ch. 5 in National Research Council (US) Panel, *Effects of Past Global Change on Life* (National Academies Press, 1995). https://www.ncbi.nlm .nih.gov/books/NBK231944/.

305 at least 100 meters (328 feet) higher than today: B. U. Haq, J. Hardenbol, and P. R. Vail (1987). "Chronology of fluctuating sea levels since the Triassic." *Science* 235 (4793): 1156–67.

305 the largest cities, are less than ten meters above sea level: G. McGranahan, D. Balk, and B. Anderson (2007). "The rising tide: Assessing the risks of climate change and human settlements in low elevation coastal zones." *Environment and Urbanization* 19 (1): 17–37. doi: 10.1177/0956247807076960.

305 half of us live less than a hundred meters above sea level: J. E. Cohen and C. Small (1998). "Hypsographic demography: The distribution of human population by altitude." *PNAS* 95 (24): 14009–14. doi: 10.1073/pnas.95.24.14009.

306 steadily, if slowly, declining since the 1970s: Hannah Ritchie and Max Roser, "Energy," Our World in Data, 2020, accessed March 23, 2020, https:// ourworldindata.org/energy.

307 Work commutes in the United States and Europe: U.S.: Elizabeth Kneebone and Natalie Holmes, "The growing distance between people and jobs in metropolitan America," Brookings Institute, 2015, https://www.brookings.edu

/wp-content/uploads/2016/07/Srvy_JobsProximity.pdf; Europe: "More than 20% of Europeans Commute at Least 90 Minutes Daily," sdworx, September 20, 2018, accessed March 23, 2020, https://www.sdworx.com/en/press/2018/2018 -09-20-more-than-20percent-of-europeans-commute-at-least-90-minutes-daily.

307 we need to get to zero carbon emissions globally by 2050: R. Eisenberg, H. B. Gray, and G. W. Crabtree (2019). "Addressing the challenge of carbon-free energy." *PNAS* 201821674. doi: 10.1073/pnas.1821674116.

307 there are several plausible strategies: David Roberts, "Is 100% renewable energy realistic? Here's what we know," Vox, February 7, 2018, accessed March 23, 2020, https://www.vox.com/energy-and-environment/2017/4/7/15159034/100 -renewable-energy-studies.

307 fossil fuels kill thousands more people: A. Markandya and P. Wilkinson (2007). "Electricity generation and health." *Lancet* 370 (9591): 979–90.

309 processed foods lead to overeating and weight gain: K. D. Hall et al. (2019). "Ultra-processed diets cause excess calorie intake and weight gain: An inpatient randomized controlled trial of ad libitum food intake." *Cell Metabolism* 30(1): 67–77.e3. doi:10.1016/j.cmet.2019.05.008.

309 Double Chocolate Dunkin' Donut holds 350 kilocalories: Dunkin' Donuts, accessed March 23, 2020, https://www.dunkindonuts.com/.

309 Taxes on soda and other sugar-sweetened beverages: A. M. Teng et al. (2019). "Impact of sugar-sweetened beverage taxes on purchases and dietary intake: Systematic review and meta-analysis." *Obes. Rev.* 20 (9): 1187–1204. doi: 10.1111/obr.12868.

310 Americans with low incomes lived in food deserts: "Food Access Research Atlas," USDA Economic Research Service, accessed March 23, 2020, https://www .ers.usda.gov/data-products/food-access-research-atlas.

310 cheaper per kilocalorie than fresh fruit and vegetables: A. Drewnowski and S. E. Specter (2004). "Poverty and obesity: The role of energy density and energy costs." *Am. J. Clin. Nutr.* 79 (1): 6–16.

310 billions of dollars in subsidies each year: Kimberly Amadeo, "Government Subsidies (Farm, Oil, Export, Etc): What Are the Major Federal Government Subsidies?" The Balance, January 16, 2020, accessed March 23, 2020, https:// www.thebalance.com/government-subsidies-definition-farm-oil-export-etc -3305788.

310 As Stephan Guyenet and others have argued: Stephan Guyenet, *The Hungry Brain: Outsmarting the Instincts That Make Us Overeat* (Flatiron Books, 2017).

311 has tripled, from roughly 25 percent in 1910: I. D. Wyatt and D. E. Hecker (2006). "Occupational changes during the 20th century." *Monthly Labor Review* 129 (3): 35–57.

311 13 percent of all jobs in the U.S. are classified as "sedentary": "Physical strength required for jobs in different occupations in 2016 on the Internet," The Economics Daily, Bureau of Labor Statistics, U.S. Department of Labor, accessed March 23, 2020, https://www.bls.gov/opub/ted/2017/physical-strength-required -for-jobs-in-different-occupations-in-2016.htm.

311 increasing daily physical activity and reducing disease: D. Rojas-Rueda et al. (2016). "Health impacts of active transportation in Europe." *PloS One* 11 (3): e0149990. doi: 10.1371/journal.pone.0149990.

312 People living in poverty suffer from higher rates of obesity: O. Egen et al. (2017). "Health and social conditions of the poorest versus wealthiest counties in the United States." *Am. J. Public Health* 107 (1): 130–35. doi: 10.2105/AJPH.2016.303515.

312 marginalized communities have worse health: J. R. Speakman and S. Heidari-Bakavoli (2016). "Type 2 diabetes, but not obesity, prevalence is positively associated with ambient temperature." *Sci. Rep.* 6: 30409. doi: 10.1038/srep30409; J. Wassink et al. (2017) "Beyond race/ethnicity: Skin color and cardiometabolic health among blacks and Hispanics in the United States." *J. Immigrant Minority Health* 19 (5): 1018–26. doi: 10.1007/s10903-016-0495-y.

313 Loneliness has become so prevalent: N. Xia and H. Li (2018). "Loneliness, social isolation, and cardiovascular health." *Antioxidants & Redox Signaling* 28 (9): 837–51. doi: 10.1089/ars.2017.7312.

313 Time outside can relieve stress: K. M. M. Beyer et al. (2018). "Time spent outdoors, activity levels, and chronic disease among American adults." *J. Behav. Med.* 41 (4): 494–503. doi: 10.1007/s10865-018-9911-1.

313 typical American spends 87 percent of his life in buildings: N. E. Klepeis et al. (2001). "The National Human Activity Pattern Survey (NHAPS): A resource for assessing exposure to environmental pollutants." *J. Expo. Anal. Environ. Epidemiol.* 11 (3): 231–52. https://www.nature.com/articles/7500165.pdf?origin=ppub

INDEX

oxidative stress, 98–99
oxygen, 57–61, 98–99, 105, 106
    consumption of, 67–69, 74–75
    discovery of, 66–67
oxygen-18, 107
oxygenic photosynthesis, 57–59
Oz, Memhet, 208, 209

pace of life, 11–12
palatability, 221–24, 226–27
paleoanthropologists, 120, 142
paleoanthropology, 125–26
Paleocene-Eocene Thermal
    Maximum, 305
Paleo diet, 54, 193–94, 196, 201, 202–4,
    203, 205, 206, 210–11
Paleolithic era, 197, 230
PAL ratio, 163
pancreas, 41, 45, 211
pandas, 165
Paranthropus, 126
parasites, 90
Pasteur, Louis, 36
pastoralism, 202, 203, 204
pastoralists, 313
Patara Dmanisi, 116, 118–19
peak aerobic power, 139
Pearl, Raymond, 98
Pennington Biomedical Research
    Center, 172–73, 176, 180
pepsin, 47
pepsinogen, 47
Perlmutter, David, 201
Phelps, Michael, 262–63, 280–82
Phinney, Stephen, 202–3, 205–6, 218
phlogiston, 66
photosynthesis, 57–59
physical activity, 230, 313. *See also*
    exercise
    activity energy expenditure (AEE)
        and, 271–72
    apes and, 250–51
    chimpanzees and, 250–51
    daily energy expenditure and, 161–64
    effects of speed, training, and
        technique on, 78–81

evolution and, 180
Hadza and, 154–57, 158, 162,
    165, 251
ideal amount of, 249–52
importance of, 259, 311
increases in, 136–37
metabolic compensation and, 170
metabolic expenditure and,
    239, *241*
metabolic response and, 180–81
moderate, 237–38, 249, 257
overeating and, 253–54
Tsimane and, 162
vigorous, 237, 249, 251, 257
weight and, 253–55
physical activity ratio (PAR), basal
    metabolic rates (BMR) and, 102–3
physical stress, 227
Pinasaouri River, 114, 118–20
placebo effect, 207
placental mammals, 95
    energy expenditure of, 19, 21–22
    longevity and, 100
Plains cultures, 202
plant-based diets, 227. *See also*
    herbivores
plants
    domestication of, 296–98, 300
    photosynthesis and, 57–59
polysaccharides, 40, 41
population growth, slowing of, 303
positive feedback, 135–44
potato diet, 217
poverty, obesity and, 312
pregnancy, 92, 93
    constraints on energy absorption and,
        278–79
    daily energy expenditure and,
        273–75
    sedentary lifestyle, consequences of
        and, 279
    as ultimate ultramarathon, 274, *274*
Prentice, Andrew, 107
Priestley, Joseph, 66–67
primage energetics, evolution of,
    21–22
primate energetics project, 13–22,
    25–26